Medieval Islamic medicine

Medieval Islamic medicine

PETER E. PORMANN
EMILIE SAVAGE-SMITH

GEORGETOWN UNIVERSITY PRESS
WASHINGTON, D.C.

As of January 1, 2007, 13-digit ISBN numbers have replaced the 10-digit system.

13-digit		10-digit	
Paperback:	978-1-58901-161-8	Paperback:	1-58901-161-9
Cloth:	978-1-58901-160-1	Cloth:	1-58901-160-0

Cover illustration: A physician with two patients, illustrating the Arabic translation of Dioscorides's treatise on medicinal substances. Washington, D.C., Arthur M. Sackler Gallery, Smithsonian Institution; Purchase-Smithsonian Unrestricted Trust Funds, Smithsonian Collections Acquisition Program, and Dr. Arthur M. Sackler, SI986.97a (copied in Baghdad, 1224). Reproduced with permission from the Sackler Gallery, Smithsonian Institution.

First published in the United Kingdom by Edinburgh University Press.

Georgetown University Press, Washington, D.C.

Pormann, Peter E.
Medieval Islamic medicine / Peter E. Pormann, Emilie Savage-Smith.
p. ; cm.
Includes bibliographical references and index.
ISBN-13: 978-1-58901-160-1 (hardcover : alk. paper)
ISBN-10: 1-58901-160-0 (hardcover : alk. paper)
ISBN-13: 978-1-58901-161-8 (pbk. : alk. paper)
ISBN-10: 1-58901-161-9 (pbk. : alk. paper)
1. Medicine, Arab. 2. Medicine, Medieval. 3. Medicine–Religious aspects–Islam. I. Savage-Smith, Emilie. II. Title.
[DNLM: 1. History, Medieval. 2. Medicine, Arabic–history. 3. Islam–history. WZ 54 P836m 2007]
R128.3.M4344 2007
610–dc22

2006031180

♾ This book is printed on acid-free paper meeting the requirements of the American National Standard for Permanence in Paper for Printed Library Materials.

14 13 12 11 10 09 08 07   9 8 7 6 5 4 3 2
First printing

Printed in the United Kingdom

Contents

To Manfred Ullmann

... nos esse quasi nanos gigantum umeris insidentes, ut possimus plura eis et remotiora uidere, non utique proprii uisus acumine, aut eminentia corporis, sed quia in altum subuehimur et extollimur magnitudine gigantea.

... we are like dwarfs perched on the shoulders of giants, so that we can see more, and things farther away, than they, not because of the sharpness of our own eyesight or the height of our body, but because we are lifted up high and elevated by their gigantic size.

– Bernard of Chartres (d. c. 1130), quoted by John of Salisbury (d. c. 1180), *Metalogicon*, bk 3, ch. 4.

Acknowledgements

In the course of writing this book, we have accumulated many debts of gratitude. We wish to thank first and foremost those who read an earlier draft of the entire manuscript with great care and made numerous suggestions, namely Anna A. Akasoy, Cristina Álvarez-Millán, Monica Green, Peregrine Horden, Yossef Rapoport, and Simon Swain. We are particularly grateful to Cristina Álvarez-Millán for making available to us her draft edition of al-Rāzī's *Book of Experiences*, as well as a preliminary version of the *Book of Moderation* by Ibn Zuhr, edited and translated into Spanish by the late Rosa Kuhne Brabant, which she is currently preparing for publication. Apart from the scholars already mentioned, others have lent their assistance and council in individual matters, or provided us with references to primary and secondary sources of which we would not otherwise have been aware; they include Charles Burnett, Bill Granara, Remke Kruk, Karine van 't Land, Vivienne Lo, Fergus Millar, Chase Robinson, P. Oktor Skjærvø, Natalia Smelova, Ronit Yoeli Tlalim, Manfred Ullmann, and Fritz W. Zimmermann. The comments and suggestions of all these colleagues proved invaluable, though of course the infelicities and inaccuracies that remain are entirely our responsibility.

We were fortunate in being able to include in this book a number of attractive illustrations, and we wish to thank the various museums, libraries, and individuals for permitting their reproduction in this volume. We would particularly like to single out the director of the St Petersburg Branch of the Institute of Oriental Studies (Russian Academy of Sciences), Dr Irina F. Popova, for her kind cooperation, as well as Nigel N. James, of the Map Room of the Bodleian Library, who generated the outline map from digital data.

We are also most grateful to Carole Hillenbrand, the editor of the New Edinburgh Islamic Surveys series, who encouraged the undertaking of this volume. Finally our thanks are due to the staff of Edinburgh University Press – in particular Senior Commissioning Editor Nicola Ramsey and Eddie Clark of the desk-editing department – for their patience and assistance in the production of the book.

The Khalili Research Centre for the Art and Material Culture of the

Middle East, at the University of Oxford, has provided, for one of the authors, many reams of paper, cartridges for the printer, and a lovely office, along with the services of an IT expert, Dan Burt, who assisted with the mechanics of producing the map and diagrams. The Warburg Institute elected the other author to a Frances A. Yates Long-Term Fellowship which permitted him to work on this project. The Warburgian atmosphere of fierce intellectual rigour coupled with great generosity of spirit and a library which is second to none proved the ideal environment to write this book. Moreover, Corpus Christi College and St Cross College, both at Oxford, catered not only for our spiritual but also our culinary needs, and many a discussion about the book took place in their Common Rooms.

London, August 2006 Peter E. Pormann
Oxford, August 2006 Emilie Savage-Smith

Notes on general format, dates, and transliteration

The world of medieval Islam is both foreign and familiar to the Western reader: foreign, in that most of its literature, whether prose or poetry, remains untranslated and often even unedited; yet familiar, because of the shared history which has tied the fates of the Islamic and the Christian worlds closely together for centuries. In the arrangement of this book, we have endeavoured to find ways to bring this foreign world to the reader of English as much as possible. For this reason, we have translated virtually everything: not only the quotations from various sources in a whole host of languages such as Arabic, Persian, Syriac, and Hebrew, but also the titles of the many essays, epistles, and encyclopedias discussed here. Similarly, the bibliography favours recent English literature, although we also thought it desirable to provide some references to works of scholarship and sources in other European languages. Since our essay is often based on material inaccessible to the general reader, and since we advance some new theses and interpretations, we thought it desirable to provide the necessary documentation, especially to sources hitherto unpublished.

In order to reconcile these two exigencies, readability and scholarly rigour, we have opted for the following system. Before the note section to each chapter, there is a short bibliographical essay providing suggestions for further general reading on the topics covered in that chapter. A separate full bibliography lists all the literature in English and other European languages cited in the endnotes. The Index of names and works enumerates the authors and their treatises that we discuss; in addition, it also contains the names of all historical personalities to which we refer. Because there are no standard English designations for most of our primary sources, we give, in the Index, both the English titles which we have adopted and the Arabic originals. Since such Arabic titles often rhyme, some of their beauty may even be appreciated in transliteration. Moreover, in the Index the reader can also find references to translations as well as editions, when such have been published.

For the purpose of not cluttering the volume, the references to Arabic editions in the Index are, where possible, abbreviated according to the scholarly conventions laid down by Manfred Ullmann in his monumental Dictionary of Classical Arabic (*Wörterbuch der Klassischen Arabischen Sprache*). Where there are no standard abbreviations, we provide the necessary information after the Arabic title. Specialists should have no trouble locating the primary sources which we cite, while those coming to the subject for the first time will find the translations to be a useful guide.

For convenience, all dates given in the body of the text are those of the Christian calendar, unless otherwise specified. The designation AD is used only when there is need to distinguish a date from an earlier BC date. General references to a century rather than a specific year refer to centuries of the Christian era. For example, ninth century refers to years AD 800–99 (which in the Muslim calendar would be 184–287). The Muslim calendar is designated by H; it is a lunar one of 354 days beginning from the day of the Emigration (*Hijrah*) of the Prophet Muḥammad from Mecca to Medina, which occurred on 16 July 622 of the Christian calendar. Consequently, Muslim dates do not correspond directly to those of the Christian era (AD) commonly used today in Europe and the Americas (and sometimes called Common Era).

We have transliterated Arabic according to a system which readers of English should find relatively easy. A dot under the letters *ḍ*, *ṣ*, *ṭ*, and *ẓ* means that they are pronounced in an 'emphatic' way, that is to say a bit deeper and more sombre. An *ḥ* with a dot is articulated as a heavily aspirated h, whilst *th* and *dh* are respectively an unvoiced ('think') and voiced ('there') 'th' in English; the combination *kh* is pronounced like gh in Scotland as for instance in the name 'Naughtie'. A macron above the vowels *ā*, *ī*, and *ū* means that they are long and often stressed.

Figures acknowledgements

0.1 (p. xiv) Map of the medieval world, c. 600–1400.
Outline map created from digital map data © Collins Bartholomew Ltd [5/01/06]. Reproduced by Kind Permission of HarperCollins Publishers

1.1 (p. 11) Aristotle giving instruction to Alexander the Great.
London, British Library, APAC, MS Or. 2784, fol. 96a (undated, Baghdad, 13th cent.?). Reproduced with permission of The British Library

1.2 (p. 14) Branch diagrams from the *Summary (Jawāmiʿ) of the Treatise by Galen on Simple Drugs*, with explanatory translation alongside.
Oxford, Bodleian Library, Oriental Collections, MS Hunt. 600, fol. 15b (undated, 12-13th cent.?). Reproduced with permission of The Bodleian Library

1.3 (p. 34) The *Abridgment* (*Talkhīṣ*) by Ibn Maymūn (Maimonides, d. 1204) of Galen's *Method of Healing*.
Paris, BnF, MS heb. 1203, folio 45b (12th cent.). Reproduced by permission of the Bibliothèque nationale de France

2.1 (p. 42) Arabic translation of Galen's *On [Medical] Sects for Beginners*, with important owners' signatures.
Paris, BnF, MS arabe 2859, fol. 1a (early 11th cent.). Reproduced by permission of the Bibliothèque nationale de France

2.2 (p. 43) The four elements, humours, primary qualities, and temperaments as they relate to the seasons, the ages of man, the months, and the zodiacal constellations.
© E. Savage-Smith

2.3 (p. 46) The movement of blood according to the Galenic model and according to Ibn al-Nafīs.
© E. Savage-Smith

2.4 (p. 52) The illustration of 'horsetail', a variety of *Equisetum sylvaticum* L., from a copy of the Greek treatise by Dioscorides on medicinal substances.
Vienna, Österreichische Nationalbibliothek, Cod. med. grec. 1, folio 144v (copied c. 510). Reproduced with permission of the Austrian National Library, picture archives

2.5 (p. 66) The muscles of the eye, from Ḥunayn ibn Isḥāq's *Ten Treatises on the Eye*.
Cairo, Dār al-Kutub, MS Ṭibb Taymūr 100 (copied in Syria, 1197), page 316. Reproduced with permission from Dār al-Kutub al-Miṣrīyah, Cairo

2.6 (p. 69) A Karshuni copy of *The Almanac of Bodily Parts for the Treatment of People* by Ibn Jazlah.
Glasgow, University Library, Spec. Coll., MS Hunter 40, fols. 15b–16a (undated, c. 15th cent.). Reproduced with permission of The University Library, Glasgow

3.1 (p. 97) Cupping, as depicted in a thirteenth-century copy of the *Assemblies* (*Maqāmāt*) by al-Ḥarīrī.
St Petersburg, Institute of Oriental Studies, MS C23, fol. 165a. Reproduced courtesy of the St Petersburg Branch of the Institute of Oriental Studies, Russian Academy of Sciences

3.2 (p. 99) The Manṣūrī hospital complex, from Pascal Xavier Coste, *Architecture arabe ou monuments du Kaire* (Paris: Firmin-Didot, 1839), Plate XV. The labels have been added on the basis of identifications given by Coste. Reproduced with permission of the Bodleian Library, shelfmark Mason Y 60

3.3 (p. 106) The hour of birth in a copy of the *Assemblies* (*Maqāmāt*) by al-Ḥarīrī.
Paris, BnF, MS arabe 5847, fol. 122b (painted in 1237, probably in Baghdad). Reproduced by permission of the Bibliothèque nationale de France

4.1 (p. 123) A physician with two patients, illustrating the Arabic translation of Dioscorides' treatise on medicinal substances.
Washington, D.C., Arthur M. Sackler Gallery, Smithsonian Institution; Purchase-Smithsonian Unrestricted Trust Funds, Smithsonian Collections Acquisition Program, and Dr Arthur M. Sackler, SI986.97a (copied in Baghdad, 1224). Reproduced with permission from the Sackler Gallery, Smithsonian Institution

4.2 (p. 126) The instruments illustrated in *The Sufficient Book on Ophthalmology*, by Khalīfah ibn Abī al-Maḥāsin al-Ḥalabī.
Paris, BnF, MS arabe 1043, fols. 42b–43a (copied in Syria, c. 1256–75). Reproduced by permission of the Bibliothèque nationale de France

4.3 (p. 137) A scene in a steam bath (*ḥammām*), illustrating a copy of the *Khamsah* ('Quintette') by Nizāmī.
Dublin, Chester Beatty Library, Persian MS 195, fol. 33a (painted in 1529). © The Trustees of the Chester Beatty Library, Dublin

5.1 (p. 147) The *budūḥ* magic square.
© E. Savage-Smith

5.2 (p. 149) A design for a gemstone from *The Book of the Oblique* by al-Būnī.
London, The Nasser D. Khalili Collection of Islamic Art, MS 300, fol. 71a (copied in 1425). Reproduced by permission of the Nasser D. Khalili Collection of Islamic Art

5.3 (p. 152) A magic-medicinal bowl made in 1169–70 for Nūr al-Dīn Maḥmūd ibn Zangī.
London, The Nasser D. Khalili Collection of Islamic Art, MTW 1443. Reproduced by permission of the Nasser D. Khalili Collection of Islamic Art

6.1 (p. 163) A 'portrait' of al-Rāzī in a copy made in 1443 of the ninth book of the Latin translation of *The Book for al-Manṣūr* by al-Rāzī.
Oxford, Bodleian Library, Dept. of Western Manuscripts, MS Canon. Misc. 566, fol. 1r (copied in 1443). Reproduced with permission of The Bodleian Library

6.2 (p. 174) A traditional Unani doctor (*ḥakīm*) surrounded by pouches of medicines, with a servant seated alongside.
London, British Library, APAC, MS Add. Or. 1585, fol. 2r (drawn in c. 1856). Reproduced with permission of The British Library

6.3 (p. 176) A vendor of traditional remedies in the city of Ta'iz in Southern Yemen.
Photo taken in July 1993 by Prof. L. P. H. M. Buskens. © L. P. H. M. Buskens, reproduced here with his kind permission

The publisher is grateful to the various libraries, institutions, and individuals for permission to reproduce the illustrations.

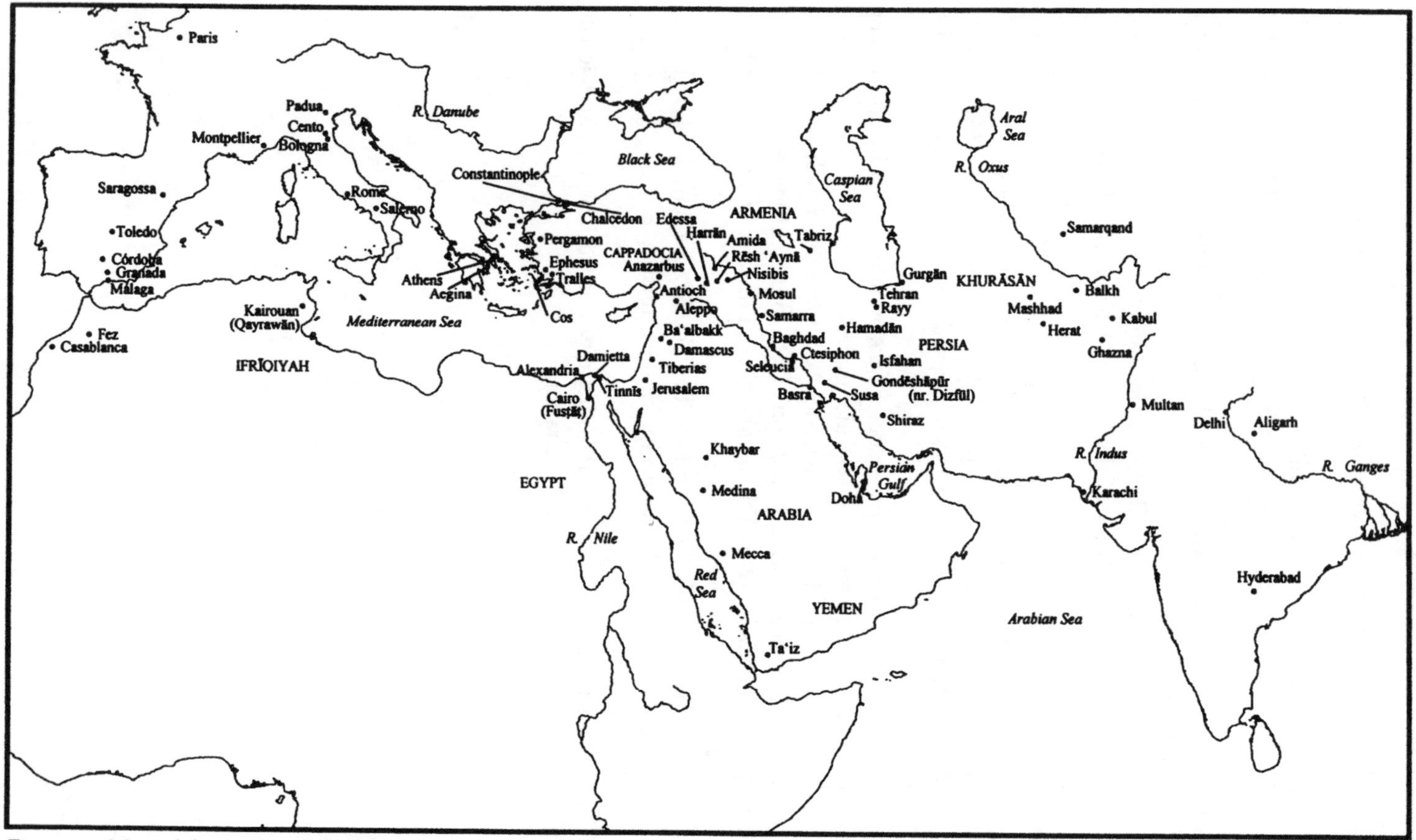

Figure 0.1 Map of the medieval world, c. 600–1400. Localities indicated are those mentioned in this volume.

Introduction

The medical tradition that developed in the lands of Islam during the medieval period has, like few others, influenced the fates and fortunes of countless human beings. It is the story of contact and cultural exchange across countries and creeds, affecting caliphs, kings, courtiers, courtesans, and the common crowd. In addition to being fascinating in its own right, medieval Islamic medicine is also important because of its influence on Europe where it formed the roots from which modern Western medicine arose. To be sure, the earlier Graeco-Roman scholarly medical literature was the stem from which much Islamic medicine grew, just as, several centuries later, Islamic medicine was to be at the core of late medieval and early modern European medical education. As will be seen in the following chapters, however, medieval Islamic medicine was not simply a conduit for Greek ideas, which is the stereotypical picture, but it was a venue for innovation and change.

The geographical contours of the medieval Islamic world extended from Spain and North Africa in the west to Central Asia and India in the east, with the central lands of Egypt, Syria, Iraq and Persia playing a pivotal role (see the map in Figure 0.1). In temporal terms it covered a period of roughly nine centuries – from the middle of the seventh to the end of the fifteenth century, by which time it had broken up into three distinct empires, the Ottoman, the Safavid, and the Mughal. For the purposes of this study, our consideration of medieval Islamic medicine will not extend past the emergence of the Safavid empire in Persia (modern Iran) and the Mughal empire in India, both of which coincided with the golden age of the Ottoman empire, centred in Turkey. The Ottoman dynasty in fact arose at the end of the thirteenth century, but the theoretical and practical approaches to medicine in the areas under its domain during the first two centuries of its existence firmly belonged to the medieval Islamic medical tradition. In the sixteenth century, however, the courts of the three empires came into contact with the courts of Europe. With new commercial and military undertakings and increased travel between Europe and the Middle East, medical education and practice began to change subtly. This 'transitional' medicine between the medieval and the early modern will only be lightly touched upon in our final chapter.

The medical needs and practices of the medieval Islamic world over such a vast area and time-span of nine centuries were of course neither uniform nor unchanging. The everyday medical practices and the general health of the Islamic community were influenced by many factors: the dietary and fasting laws as well as the general rules for hygiene and burying the dead of the various religious communities of Muslims, Jews, Christians, Zoroastrians, and others; the climatic conditions of the desert, marsh, mountain, and littoral communities; the different living conditions of nomadic, rural, and urban populations; local economic conditions and agricultural successes or failures; the amount of travel undertaken for commerce, for attendance at courts, or as a pilgrimage; the maintenance of a slave class and slave trade; the injuries and diseases attendant upon army camps and battles; and the incidence of plague and other epidemics as well as the occurrence of endemic conditions such as dysenteries and certain eye diseases.

The institutions and policies responsible for dispensing medical care were subject to political and social fluctuations. Moreover, the medical practices of the society varied not only according to time and place, but also according to class. The economic and social level of the patient determined to a large extent the type of care sought, just as it does today, and the expectations of the patients varied along with the approaches of the practitioners. Throughout medieval Islamic society a medical pluralism existed that may be viewed as a continuum running from the scholarly theories and practices of learned medicine to those of local custom and magic. Woefully little evidence is available as to the patient's perspective in all of this, but we have tried in this volume to tease out a few pertinent testimonies.

The medieval Islamic community comprised Muslims and non-Muslims speaking many languages: Arabic, Persian, Syriac, Hebrew, Turkish, and various local dialects. Islam became the dominant faith, and Arabic (the language of the Qur'ān) served as the *lingua franca*, a common language for all educated and official discourse, much as Latin did in Europe for several centuries. Use of the Arabic language enabled a mix of diverse peoples speaking different languages to communicate with one another. Thus, whether the authors were Persian or Arab, Jewish or Christian, and whether they spoke Greek, Syriac, or Turkish, for the most part they wrote in Arabic. The resulting medical literature and medical practice involved a rich and diverse mixture of religions and cultures to be seen in both the physicians and the patients. For this reason, the term 'Islamic culture' or 'Islamic medicine', in this context, is not to be interpreted as applying only to the religion of Islam.

The aim of this book is not to compress the entire history of medieval Islamic medicine into a single small volume. Rather, it presents an overview, highlighted with particular examples. The volume also incorporates a considerable amount of hitherto unpublished material (details of which are given in the endnotes), which in many instances has allowed us to expand our perceptions of the medical care at that time. Because so many topics have yet to receive proper scholarly attention, we are still in no position to undertake a comprehensive history of medicine in the Muslim World, even when limiting it to the medieval Islamic period. Nonetheless, we did wish to address some aspects of the social history of medicine, such as female patients and practitioners, hospitals, public health care, rural and urban provisions, medical ethics and education, and so on. Moreover, we wanted to tackle the problem of how patients were actually treated, rather than simply confining ourselves to a description of the medical theory and a chronology of famous physicians.

We have organised the essay around five major topics, reflected by the titles of the first five chapters: (1) the emergence of medieval Islamic medicine and its intense cross-pollination with other cultures, notably by way of translation, but also by trade and travel; (2) the theoretical medical framework and extensive literature that guided learned doctors in their work; (3) how physicians from various backgrounds functioned within the larger society; (4) what case histories tell us about the application of medical practices to specific patients and what remedies they really resorted to; and (5) the role of magical therapies, folkloric traditions and devout religious invocations in scholarly as well as everyday medicine. The sixth, and final, chapter is on the 'afterlife' of medieval Islamic medicine – that is, how it came to form the basis of the European medical tradition and how medieval Islamic medicine still continues to be practised today. It should be noted that treatments for animals – horses, camels, falcons, domestic animals of various sorts – are not included amongst the subjects of this book, though medieval Arabic and Persian treatises exist on many such topics. Here, we are concerned only with humans and their attempts to understand and regulate their health and well-being.

The medical tradition which we describe in this book is intimately linked to the European one. It had its origins primarily in parts of the Greek-speaking world located in modern Turkey and Egypt, and it subsequently greatly contributed to late medieval and Renaissance medicine in Europe. This constant movement of ideas between the different shores of the Mediterranean belies the dichotomy of 'East' and 'West'.

Late medieval and early Renaissance European medical education owed much to the medieval Islamic medical tradition. In fact the debt was so great that the history of medieval Islamic medicine is in essence the history of the origins of early modern Western medicine. Of course it must be stressed that, following the absorption in Europe of Arabic medical writings (and the Greek medicine that they also contained), medical theory as well as anatomical and pathological knowledge changed radically, particularly in the nineteenth and twentieth centuries. Yet the origins of the approaches and methodology of modern Western medicine can be traced in large part to medieval Islamic medicine (in its Latin garb), while the institutionalisation of both teaching and the provision of medical care was foreshadowed by Islamic institutions.

While some elements of medieval Islamic medicine can be viewed as forerunners of modern practices, other features may seem strange, or quaint, or even irrelevant to the modern world. Magical procedures, folkloric practices of local custom, and devout religious measures formed as much a part of the society's reaction to pain and illness as did those elements we now consider more 'rational'. A modern reader should not approach medieval Islamic medicine with an attitude of amused indulgence or contempt, nor should one hunt the present in the past.

In the last part of this introduction, it is necessary to place the present project in the context of previous scholarship. In 1968 Manfred Ullmann finished the manuscript of his monumental *Die Medizin im Islam*, which set the agenda for all subsequent research into the topic. In it, he deliberately chose not to write a history of medicine, but rather to survey the evidence available in manuscripts, printed sources, and secondary literature. In his much shorter and more discursive *Islamic Medicine* completed in 1976, he specifically excluded a number of topics from his discussion, because of the 'state of contemporary research'. These included 'surgery and hospital institutions', and 'the doctor's social standing, the doctor-patient relationship, [and] medical teaching'.[1] Some thirty years later, we are in a slightly better position to deal with these subjects, for scholars such as the late and lamented Michael W. Dols, as well as Cristina Álvarez-Millán, Lawrence I. Conrad, and Avner Gil'adi, have tackled different social and practical aspects of the history of medicine in the medieval Islamic world. We are, nonetheless, profoundly indebted to Manfred Ullmann, whose earlier volume of *Islamic Medicine* was published in the *Islamic Surveys* by the Edinburgh University Press. The volume we have written is intended not to replace it, but to succeed and supplement it, focusing upon issues and topics that at the time of the first volume were not sufficiently studied by scholars to permit even a preliminary survey.

In the course of the following six chapters, we hope to reveal complexities and contradictions, encourage comparisons, raise – and perhaps to offer a few answers to – questions such as: How did Islamic medical writers arrive at such a high standard of medical knowledge and such successful treatments? What was the position of the physician in medieval Islamic society and how did one become a physician? How do the many theoretical treatises relate to the actual practice of medicine? What role did the Islamic hospitals play in the provision of medical care and in the education of physicians?

The diversity of medieval Islamic society is so great that it cannot be painted but with a broad brush. We hope that our picture of medical theory and practice in medieval Islam, given the limited sources presently at hand, is sound and not too far off the mark.

Suggested reading

For general surveys of Islamic medicine, see our predecessor volume Ullmann, *Islamic Medicine*; Conrad, 'The Arab-Islamic Medical Tradition'; E. Savage-Smith, '*Ṭibb*', *EI*² x. 452–60; Savage-Smith, 'Medicine'; Haskell, 'Arabic Medical Literature'; Strohmaier, 'Reception and Tradition'; and the long introduction to Dols, *Medieval Islamic Medicine*. For medicine in Muslim Spain, the volume edited by Maribel Fierro and Julio Samsó is a good starting point (Fierro and Samsó, *The Formation of al-Andalus, Part 2*). Still useful, but to be used with some caution, are Plessner, 'Natural Sciences and Medicine'; and Browne, *Arabian Medicine*.

For individual figures, as well as topics, see the comprehensive bibliography by Ullmann, *Medizin im Islam*, as well as that by Sezgin, *Medizin-Pharmazie*. For major figures and topics, the corresponding entries in the *Encyclopaedia of Islam*, both the printed second edition and its more recent on-line version, are invaluable, as are the articles in the *Encyclopedia Iranica*, which is still in the course of publication. The website '*Islamic Medical Manuscripts at the National Library of Medicine*' (in Bethesda, Maryland, USA, www.nlm.nih.gov/hmd/arabic) also provides useful biographies of authors and short essays on types of medical writings.

Note

1 Ullmann, *Islamic Medicine*, p. xiii.

I

The emergence of Islamic medicine

> It is a remarkable fact that, with few exceptions, most Muslim scholars both in the religious and in the intellectual sciences have been non-Arabs (*'ajam*) ...
>
> We have mentioned before that sedentary people cultivated the crafts and that, of all peoples, the Bedouins are least familiar with them. Thus, the sciences came to belong to sedentary culture, whilst the Arabs were not familiar with them or with their cultivation.
>
> – Ibn Khaldūn (d. 1406), *Introduction* [*to World History*][1]

Health and disease preoccupied man from the earliest days of his existence, and all cultures, however rudimentary, have developed means to preserve health and to restore it when absent. This universal concern for physical and mental well-being led different civilisations to develop a whole host of diverse strategies to cope with illness. The bedouin Arab population, like other peoples, were exposed to bodily harm and disease, and they, too, used different techniques for treatment. By the tenth century, Arabs in the major urban centres had developed a highly sophisticated framework of medical theory and practice, admired by friend and foe. Ideas about maintaining health and avoiding or curing disease that existed in the deserts of pre-Islamic Arabia, however, varied greatly from those of the urban elite in the capital of the 'Abbāsid empire, Baghdad. The story of how Islamic medicine arose from a diverse background of earlier medical traditions will be told in this chapter.

To begin, it is important to note that Islam as a religious and cultural venture was not born in a vacuum. Looking at the affinities between the Qur'ān on the one hand, and the Hebrew Bible, the Greek New Testament, and the Talmud on the other, scholars have argued that early Islam was heavily influenced by Christian and Jewish ideas; some went even so far as to state that Islam was initially little more than another Jewish sect. Be that as it may, it is clear that the Muslim holy writ appeared in a context where Arabic was the predominant language, and the poetry of the Bedouins, transmitted orally, represented the most revered form of literary expression. On the other hand, certain aspects of Greek culture pervaded even into the deserts of pre-Islamic Arabia. In the realm of medicine, a creative tension between intrinsic Arabic developments and foreign influence was keenly felt. The emergence of Islamic medicine can only be appreciated against the background of these two trends – namely, the indigenous Arab tradition and the foreign influence. Consequently, we investigate them in turn in order to understand how Islamic civilisation was eventually able to develop such an impressive system of healthcare.[2]

Bedouin medicine

> Many a wailing woman have I sent away, when the star Belletrix rose,
> who wailed, whilst examining the wound so that her palm and wrist disappeared [in the wound],
> [the wound] of a man, whose head is bent and whose wounds exhaled blood,
> [a woman] who separated his joints with a probe as the comb separates the hair hanging down.
> – al-Burayq ibn ʿIyād (*fl.* c. 600–30)[3]

> Civilized Bedouins have a kind of medicine which is mainly based upon individual experience [*tajribah qaṣīrah*]. They inherit its use from the old men and women of the tribe. Some of it may occasionally be correct, yet it is neither based upon any natural law [*qānūn ṭabīʿī*] nor is it consistent with the temperament [*mizāj*]. Much of this sort of medicine existed among the Arabs [Bedouins].
> – Ibn Khaldūn (d. 1406), *Introduction* [*to World History*][4]

In this second extract, Ibn Khaldūn – the greatest Arab historian, who created a philosophy of history foreshadowing modern sociology and political theory – contrasts Bedouin medicine based on individual experience with the learned medical tradition, in which 'natural law' and the 'temperament' were of the utmost importance. In his day, the two existed side by side in a certain creative tension, as we will see later. Yet, this was not always the case on the Arabian peninsula, and in the present section, the medical ideas and provisions of pre-Islamic and early Islamic times will be explored, since they formed the central background against which the Islamic medical tradition emerged.

There are five main sources for our knowledge of how the Arabs lived in pre-Islamic times: archaeological remains, inscriptions, Islamic religious texts such as the Qur'ān and *ḥadīths* (sayings attributed to the Prophet and collected by later authors), historical accounts, and Arabic poetry. All these sources have their limitations. Such archaeological remains as have been uncovered tell us little about attitudes towards health and disease, and the inscriptions are equally silent. The Qur'ān says nothing about medical practice. The *ḥadīths* do contain information about how Muḥammad (d. 632) treated certain illnesses and what he advised. They later gave rise to a medical genre, the so-called 'Medicine of the Prophet (*ṭibb al-nabī*)' or 'Prophetic Medicine (*al-ṭibb al-nabawī*)'. *Ḥadīths*, however, pose a major problem in source criticism. Medieval Muslim scholars such as al-Bukhārī (d. 860) distinguished between genuine traditions, called 'sound' (*ṣaḥīḥ*), and others. The traditions collected in the books of Prophetic Medicine were not all considered genuine by medieval religious scholars. But even when they were, some 'sound' *ḥadīths* were later shown to be of highly questionable origin, with many being thought not to go back to the Prophet.[5]

Arabic-language histories and chronicles for this period date from the eighth century onwards, but they also have come under the scrutiny of historical source criticism and been found wanting. Scholars have therefore supplemented their resources by turning to historical writings of Byzantine Greek, Syriac or Armenian authors, although they, too, do not necessarily convey an accurate picture of pre-Islamic Arabia. What is more, none of these historiographic works contains an account of medical practices for this time period.[6]

Because of these methodological difficulties, poetry remains the major avenue through which we can learn about the Arabs' attitudes to body and soul in pre-Islamic and early Islamic times, and observe what means they had at their disposal to treat illness and injury. The passage from the ode quoted above by the poet al-Burayq, who lived in the early seventh century, has two salient features. Firstly, in the scene painted by the poet, it is a woman who treats the wounded warrior, even if her actions are portrayed as the ultimate act of desperation in the face of horrendous wounds. There are many instances where women appear as carers in early Arabic poetry, so that this depiction blends in well with the general image of women being responsible for curing. In other pre-Islamic odes, female practitioners are referred to as physicians (*ṭabā'ib*, singular *ṭabībah*; *awāsin/āsiyah*), soothsayers (*kawāhin/kāhinah*), and sick-nurses (*'awā'id/'ā'idah*).[7]

Secondly, the fourth line of the poem highlights the Greek influence present even in the desert of Arabia. For the probe used to straighten the injured limbs is called *mīl*, a loan-word derived from Greek *mēlē*, also meaning 'probe'. That Greek words and concepts are found in Arabic poetry is not all that surprising, for, over many centuries, the Byzantine empire and the Arabs shared borders, and were, at various times, in both hostile and friendly contact with each other. Some Arabs, such as the Ghassānids, a Christian tribe, even joined forces with Byzantium in their struggle against the Sasanians (about whom more shortly). As a result, there is much evidence for intense cultural exchange even at this early stage.[8]

The war wounds described in this poem were not the only medical problems with which the desert-dwelling Arabs were faced. A great number of terms found in early Arabic poetry signify a variety of illnesses. Some were later used in the medical literature to denote specific diseases such as *zukām* (a cold), *su'āl* (cough), *khunāq* (constriction of throat and inability to breathe) and *kalab* (rabies). Others were rather vague and undefined, never making it into the technical vocabulary of later physicians; the latter include *qudād* (grumbling stomach) and *'araj* (lameness). Other frequently mentioned complaints included ophthalmia (eye inflammation, *ramad*) and fevers (*ḥummá*). The latter were often interpreted in terms of supernatural causation as is apparent from a learned explanation, a so-called scholion, to a verse by the poet al-Akhnas Shihāb al-Taghlibī. According to this scholion, people in the oasis of Khaybar brayed liked donkeys ten times before entering the area infested by a violent fever. They did this in order to deceive the *jinn*, who they believed inflicted the fever only upon humans: as donkeys, they could escape the scourge. In addition to such apotropaic measures, cupping, cautery, and simple remedies such as camel urine reduced through boiling were employed. Many of these folk remedies reoccur in the later manuals of Prophetic Medicine.[9]

Greek medicine

Ibn Khaldūn contrasted these rather basic procedures of the Bedouins with a medicine guided by 'natural law' (or 'the law of nature') and in accordance with 'temperament'. These two terms refer to concepts which the Greeks had developed and which were later adopted by both the European and the Islamic medical traditions. One cannot appreciate the development of medical theory and practice in the Islamic medieval period without understanding its Greek antecedents.

When mentioning the 'temperament', Ibn Khaldūn alluded to the idea that the human body is made up of four humours (or 'juices') which are in a state of relative balance, resulting in health, or imbalance, resulting in illness. This idea – known in modern scholarship as 'humoral pathology' and to be described in greater detail in the next chapter – was first developed in the Hippocratic treatise *On the Nature of Man*. This text is part of the so-called *Hippocratic Corpus*, a collection of writings attributed to Hippocrates of Cos (mid-fifth century BC), the 'father of medicine' in the view of both Europe and the medieval Islamic world. In Hippocrates' time as well as in the centuries to follow, there was a great plurality of approaches to medicine. This is especially apparent from the writings of the most important Greek physician, Galen of Pergamon (d. c. 216), who was born in 129 in Asia Minor, modern Turkey. He argued against different rivalling medical 'sects' or schools such as the rationalists, favouring the use of reason and analogy (Greek *logos*, Arabic *qiyās*); the empiricists, advocating that experience (*empeiria, tajribah*) ought to take centre stage in medical investigations; and the methodists, followers of a specific method (*methodos, ḥīlah*) (not to be confused with the modern protestant movement founded by John Wesley in the eighteenth century).

Galen's own approach was characterised by a strong eclecticism. He did not believe that any of these sects held the key to correct medical practice. On the other hand, Galen was responsible for establishing Hippocrates as *the* medical authority. He did so by writing a number of commentaries to different treatises in the *Hippocratic Corpus*. He reshaped Hippocrates, so to speak, in his own image. Those treatises which he could reconcile or interpret in accordance with his own medical ideas he declared to be genuine, whilst dismissing others which were in conflict with his thought. Galen also succeeded in establishing himself as the 'new Hippocrates', as the model physician whose doctrine was to dominate the medical discourse, not only in Europe but also in the Islamic world, for a least the next millennium and a half. The resulting medical system has been aptly called 'Galenism' by Oswei Temkin. It silenced most dissenting voices by developing and further refining the all-encompassing system of humoral pathology to take into account new material and ideas. This system linked the four humours (blood, phlegm, yellow bile, and black bile) to the four primary qualities (wet or dry, and cold or warm), the four elements (fire, water, earth, and air), and the four major organs. The latter were only three in Galen's system (heart, brain and liver), but a fourth (spleen) was added to make up the numbers.[10]

One important vehicle for this theoretical outlook was the medical encyclopedia, that is to say the comprehensive handbook on a wide-ranging variety of medical topics organised in ways that makes it easy to find the required information. Oribasius of Pergamon (d. after 395), the physician to the Byzantine emperor Julian the Apostate, was the first prominent proponent of this genre. Others such as Alexander of Tralles (d. after 500), Aëtius of Amida (*fl.* c. 500–50), or Paul of Aegina followed in his footsteps. The last one, a seventh-century physician who lived and worked in Alexandria 'at the first time of Islam', and witnessed its conquest at the hands of the Arabs in 642, is especially important, since he symbolises both the end of the Greek and the beginning of the Arabic encyclopedic tradition. These encyclopedic authors drew mostly on the writings of Galen, thus representing the Galenism of Late Antiquity. They did include, however, material from other authors who predate Galen, the three most prominent being: Rufus of Ephesus (*fl.* c. 100), who wrote on melancholy, amongst other things; Soranus of Ephesus (*fl.* c. 100), a methodist physician well-known for his gynaecological writings; and Dioscorides of Anazarbus (d. c. 90), author of the celebrated *On Medicinal Substances*. Since Galen had already accepted them as competent physicians, they were more easily incorporated into these late antique encyclopedias.

Ibn Khaldūn mentioned 'natural law' as lacking in Bedouin medicine. This is an allusion to the principle, important already in Greek medical thought, that there are certain laws of nature which rule the universe and which, when properly understood, allow one to diagnose diseases and treat maladies correctly. These questions of causation and causality – strictly speaking philosophical quandaries – occupied the minds of many physicians. They also raise the question of the relationship between medicine and philosophy, which was

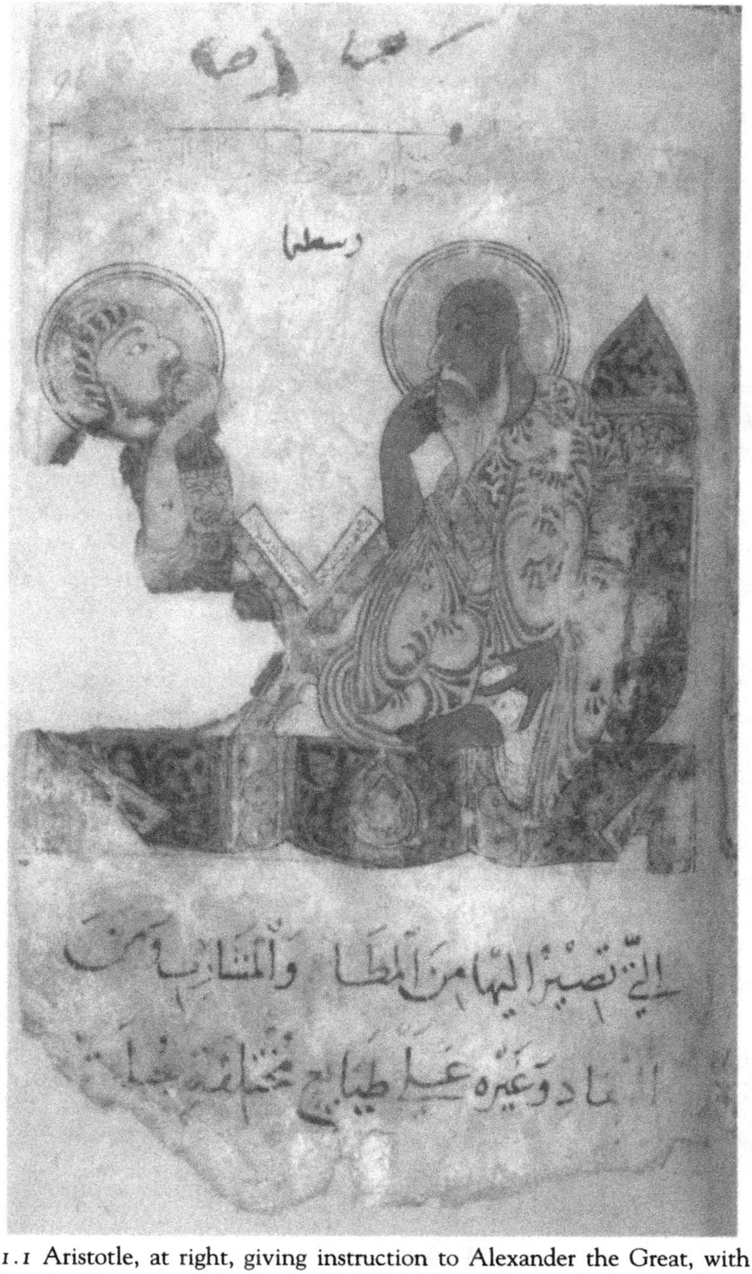

Figure 1.1 Aristotle, at right, giving instruction to Alexander the Great, with a text open on a stand between them. From *The Description and Uses of Animals*, an anonymous compilation made from the works of Aristotle and 'Ubayd Allāh ibn Bukhtīshū' (d. after 1058). The undated copy was probably made in Baghdad in the first half of the thirteenth century.

often intimate but not always unproblematic. The theory of humoral pathology as set out in the Hippocratic treatise *On the Nature of Man* originated against the background of speculations about the first cause (Greek *archē*), a dominant concern in pre-Socratic philosophy. On the other hand, in another Hippocratic treatise, *On Ancient Medicine*, the author attacked philosophy and conceived the art of medicine as a discipline in which one should stick to empirical facts rather than indulge in vain and futile philosophical speculations. This rejection of philosophy within the *Hippocratic Corpus* could have posed a potential problem to Galen, who wrote a treatise with the programmatic title *That the Best Physician is Also a Philosopher*. He solved it, however, by declaring that *On Ancient Medicine* was not written by Hippocrates, but falsely attributed to him. This represents one of the instances in which Galen shaped Hippocratic doctrine in the light of his own understanding and requirements.

By establishing a firm link between medicine and philosophy, Galen strove to provide medicine with the veneer of respectability which philosophy generally enjoyed at the time. This connection was further enhanced in Late Antiquity. At that time, philosophers often endeavoured to reconcile the views of Plato (427–347 BC), as elaborated in the neo-Platonic tradition by such luminaries as Plotinus (d. AD 270) and Porphyry (d. c. AD 304), with those of Aristotle (384–322 BC).

One famous area of difference between Plato and Aristotle regards the problem of the seat of the intellect. The latter had argued that reason is located in the heart, whilst the former thought it to be in the brain. Galen had already proven by experiment that Plato's opinion was correct. Yet, many Aristotelian ideas, such as the theory of the four causes (formal, material, effective, and final), were employed to explain the origin of diseases and bodily functions. Late antique philosophers continued the efforts to reconcile the two great philosophers in terms of medical thought, and this syncretic medical philosophy became immensely popular in subsequent centuries. Aristotle's fame in later Islamic centuries is visible also in many manuscript illuminations. Figure 1.1 shows him giving instruction to his pupil, Alexander the Great (d. 323 BC), the eponymous founder of Alexandria.

Alexandria in late antiquity

Although both Hippocrates and Galen were the undisputed masters and models for the subsequent medical traditions, it was late antique Alexandria that to a large extent shaped medieval Islamic medicine. Soon after its establishment in 332 BC, the city rose to prominence in the medical field through the works of Herophilus and Erasistratus, two eminent anatomists active in the early third century BC. With the presence of the acclaimed Library of Alexandria and under the enlightened and tolerant rule of the Ptolemies, it continued to grow in fame for its literary and scientific achievements. Under Roman and Byzantine administration, it went through some difficult times: the Library and its successor institutions were burnt down on different occasions. With the rise of Christianity, Greek philosophy came under ever-increasing pressure and was pejoratively labelled 'pagan'. After the closure of the Academy in Athens in 529 at the behest of Justinian I, many a philosopher came to Alexandria, and the creative tension between Christians and pagans increased. In the field of medicine, Alexandria in Late Antiquity could draw on the legacy of nearly a thousand years, and it attracted promising students and proficient masters of the medical art. The Library of Alexandria no longer existed, but there were numerous *akadēmias* ('academies') and *museions* (literally 'museums'), medico-philosophical schools-cum-libraries where both medicine and philosophy were taught side by side.[11]

It is not surprising that in such a congenial environment, some of the most eminent philosophers wrote also on medicine. A good example is the renowned Christian philosopher John Philoponus (the 'lover of toil', as his name suggests; d. c. 570s), who composed a commentary on Galen's *On Usefulness of the Parts*. Authors such as John of Alexandria (*fl.* early seventh century; different from John Philoponus) and Stephen of Alexandria (*fl.* c. 570–80s) wrote commentaries on Galenic works, which used philosophical concepts to illustrate how the body functioned and reacted to environmental influences and disease. In addition to these commentaries, Alexandria also produced abridgements and paraphrases of Galenic and Hippocratic works, presumably to fulfil educational needs.[12]

The Alexandrian medical curriculum had an important impact on how the subject was taught in early Islamic times. Its core comprised the *Sixteen Books of Galen*, a selection of treatises which Galen himself had written 'for beginners'. Galen's *On the [Medical] Sects for Beginners* was the starting point, and Figure 2.1 on p. 42, shows a copy of this treatise once owned by Ibn Sīnā. Other Galenic texts followed in varying orders, including: *On the Art of Medicine (Small Art)*; *On the Pulse for Beginners (to Teuthros)*; and *Therapeutics to Glauco*. Similarly, Hippocratic treatises were read and commented upon, though not to the same extent as Galenic ones.[13]

Moreover, for teaching purposes, the material in these *Sixteen Books*, as well as in other Galenic treatises, was abridged into the so-called *Alexandrian Summaries (Jawāmiʿ al-Iskandaranīyīn)*. Although originally written in Greek, they only survive in Arabic, Hebrew, and Latin translations. Despite their common appellation, they did not just represent shorter versions of the Galenic original, but mixed commentary and paraphrase, often interpreting Galen in light of the syncretic philosophy of Late Antiquity. They enjoyed great popularity, for they

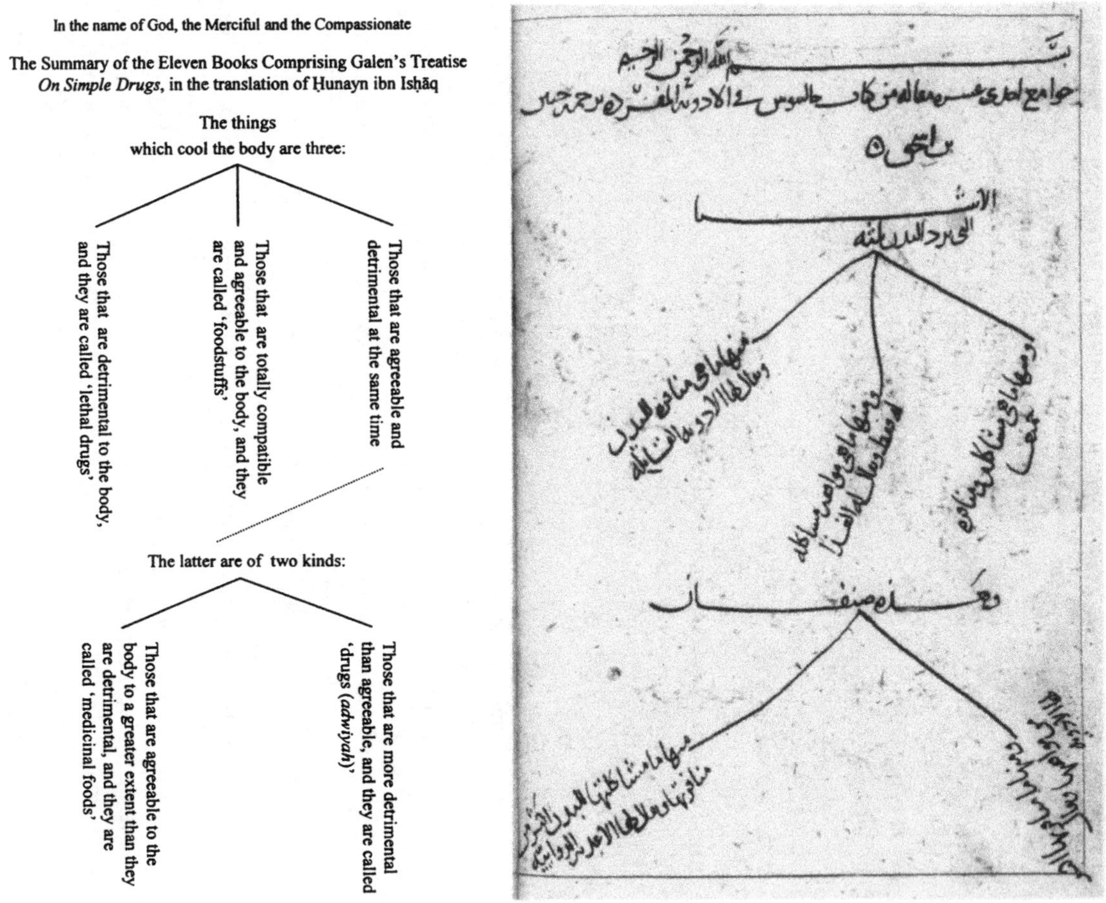

بسم الله الرحمن الرحيم
In the name of God, the Merciful and the Compassionate
The Summary of the Eleven Books Comprising Galen's Treatise On Simple Drugs, in the translation of Ḥunayn ibn Isḥāq
The things which cool the body are three:
Those that are agreeable and detrimental at the same time
Those that are totally compatible and agreeable to the body, and they are called 'foodstuffs'
Those that are detrimental to the body, and they are called 'lethal drugs'
The latter are of two kinds:
Those that are more detrimental than agreeable, and they are called 'drugs (adwiyah)'
Those that are agreeable to the body to a greater extent than they are detrimental, and they are called 'medicinal foods'

Figure 1.2 Branch diagrams opening the *Summary (Jawāmiʿ)* of *the Treatise by Galen on Simple Drugs*, with explanatory translation alongside.

provided effective didactic and mnemonic devices. One method for teaching medicine employed in them was that of division (*dihairesis*): the subject matter was divided, sub-divided, and sub-sub-divided so as to be easily digestible. For instance, medicine was divided into theory and practice; theory into physiology, aetiology, and semiotics; and practice into prophylactics and therapeutics. Physiology could be further sub-divided into elements, temperaments, parts of the body, and so on. These classifications presented in the *Alexandrian Summaries* were also sometimes arranged in the form of branch diagrams. A visualised text could be more easily remembered. Figure 1.2, for instance, shows material from one such summary in a diagrammatic format.[14]

The two genres of the encyclopedia and the commentary (the latter closely linked to paraphrase and abridgement) achieved great popularity in the medical circles of late antique Alexandria. The theoretical outlook was Galenic – that is to say, the medical authors of Alexandria adopted humoral pathology as championed by Galen and adapted it to their specific educational and practical needs. The Galenism as digested in these Alexandrian compositions was to have immense influence on the Arabic medical tradition. This happened both directly and indirectly. Directly, in the sense that the medical literature composed and studied in late antique Alexandria was made available in Arabic through a vast translation movement. Indirectly, in that the medical teachings and techniques which pervaded Alexandria also percolated into other neighbouring cultures. Two other important medical traditions, the Persian and the Syriac, influenced developments in the Islamic world, and they also had come under the spell of Greek culture.

Medicine in the Sasanian empire

Persia was ruled, from the third century to the middle of the seventh, by the Sasanian dynasty. Its founder Ardashir I (r. 224–41) defeated the Parthians and created an enormous empire. Under his successor Shāpūr I (r. 241–71), it reached its largest extension, roughly encompassing modern Iraq, Iran, Afghanistan, and Pakistan as well as the eastern parts of Saudi Arabia and Oman along the Persian Gulf. The Sasanians, like their predecessors the Achaemenids and Parthians, were Zoroastrians, professing the ancient Iranian religion of the Avesta, their holy book. This religion is commonly referred to either as Zoroastrianism, after Zoroaster, the Greek form of Zarathustra, its mythical prophet, or as Mazdaism, after the name of the supreme god, Ahura Mazdā. The Avesta is a collection of mostly ritual texts that had been composed and transmitted orally for millennia before they were written down, probably sometime in the sixth century. It was composed in the ancient 'Avestan' language, which in the sixth century was no longer a living language; for this reason the religious texts (including translations of the Avesta) were therefore in Middle Persian, or Pahlavi, the then current language.

The Sasanian empire was in unremitting conflict with Byzantium, and this near constant war of attrition led to the former's demise in 652, when, tired and exhausted, it was conquered by Muslim armies in a matter of months. Paradoxically, although hostile to Christian Byzantium, the Sasanian empire had become a safe haven for certain Christian refugees from Byzantium who were considered to hold heretical views and hence were persecuted. The Nestorians, for example, were expelled from the church after the Council of Chalcedon in 451 because of Christological quarrels. They fled to various localities within the Sasanian empire, including Nisibis (now Nusaybin in south-eastern Turkey) and the twin cities of Seleucia and Ctesiphon (30km south-east of modern Baghdad), where they established monasteries, schools, and hospices.

An even earlier influence in Sasanian lands came from a different quarter. When Alexander the Great (d. 323 BC) conquered the territory of the future Sasanian empire, he pursued a deliberate programme of Hellenisation, continued by his successors, so that Greek culture exerted a considerable influence there for centuries to come. The earliest Sasanians even had their inscriptions composed in Greek, as well as Parthian and Pahlavi.[15]

In order to appreciate medical theory and practice in the politically and militarily powerful realm of the Sasanian empire, it is necessary to look at the three influences just mentioned. In the religious texts of Zoroastrianism, concepts of health and disease played a role, and certain therapeutic methods were advocated. Then, there are the translations of Greek medical writings into Pahlavi, some of which were later rendered into Arabic. Finally, Nestorian Christians living under Sasanian rule created their own medical tradition by drawing heavily on Greek models.

The Pahlavi (Middle Persian) texts are preserved in manuscripts the earliest of which date from the thirteenth century, though most are much later. They are generally anonymous compilations whose individual items cannot be dated, but some have authors known to have lived in the ninth century. This poses the problem as to whether the picture emerging from these later sources accurately reflects medical ideas of the earlier Sasanian period. Nonetheless, they constitute our best evidence for concepts of health and disease in pre-Islamic Persia, and ought therefore to be exploited. The two most prominent treatises are the ninth-century *Dēnkard* (literally 'Acts of Religion') and the *Wizīdagīhā ī Zādsparam* ('Selections of Zādsparam'). The *Dēnkard* is a compilation of traditional Zoroastrian religion and culture, of which most of books three to nine have been preserved. One section in the third book deals specifically with medicine. It is by far the longest portion of the book and probably circulated as an independent text prior to being incorporated into the *Dēnkard*;

it serves as the basis for the following discussion.

A key feature of Zoroastrianism is a strong belief that the universe is made up of a tangible 'material' world (called 'the world of living beings' or 'the world with bones') and an intangible 'spiritual' world (called 'the world of thought'). In keeping with being a religious text, the *Dēnkard* divides the medical art into two corresponding constituents: the spiritual and the material (or bodily). The high-priests (*dastwars*, today called *dasturs*) are the physicians of the soul, while 'healers of this world' are the physicians of the body. Diseases of the soul are best avoided or dispelled through observance of the 'good religion (*dēn*)'. Diseases of the body are brought about through an imbalance of heat and cold, and moisture and dryness, with blood (*xōn*), the primary bodily fluid, being directly affected. These four qualities are linked to the four elements of fire, water, air, and earth, which also need to be balanced, and food should be administered with regard to the specific qualities of the elements present in it. Surgery is mentioned as a means to restore health in the case of wounds and fractures; it had already been an important part of medical care in the Avesta.[16]

The *Wizīdagīhā ī Zādspaoram* is a Pahlavi compilation written by the ninth-century priest-physician Zādsparam. The third part, entitled 'On the Constitution of Man', explains in a systematic and detailed fashion how the author conceived of the body and its different parts. Man is made up of body (*tan*), life-giving fire (*gyānīg-ātaxsh*) and soul (*ruwān*), with the body containing four different humours (*ābs*), namely, blood (*xōn*), phlegm (*drēm*), red bile (*wish ī suxr*) and black bile (*wish ī syā*). Each of these four humours was assigned two primary qualities: blood is hot and moist; phlegm cold and moist; red bile hot and dry; and black bile cold and dry. The three main organs are the heart (*dil*), the lungs (*sush*) and the brain (or 'marrow', *mazg*). Other important parts of the body were associated with the celestial planets: hair with Saturn; skin with Jupiter; blood vessels with Mars; nerves with the Sun; flesh with Venus; bones with Mercury; and marrow with the Moon.[17]

The parallels with Greek humoral pathology are immediately evident. The concept of humours, primary qualities, and balance is important both in Pahlavi medical texts and in the Greek medical tradition. These similarities go beyond mere coincidence. In fact, the notional complex of four humours and associated attributes arose in Greece and reached Persia via two channels: translations of Greek medical texts into Pahlavi, and the presence of a Syriac medical tradition within the Sasanian empire.

The Syriac tradition

The Council of Chalcedon in 451 adopted the Nicene creed and declared that Christ combined in himself two natures (divine and human) and two persons (divine and human). It explicitly banned the doctrine of Nestorius (d. c. 451) who claimed that Christ's divine and human natures existed in separate persons and were only loosely united. And it rejected Monophysitism, the belief that Christ had only one (divine) nature. These Christological decisions led to some momentous divisions within Christendom that were to have significant repercussions for the history of medicine. As a result of this council, the Byzantine authorities persecuted two communities, the Nestorians and the Jacobites, both of whom later emerged as the transmitters of Greek medicine to the Persians and the Arabs. The followers of Nestorius fled to the Sasanian empire to set up the Nestorian church (more properly called the Syrian Church of the East). The inhabitants of Antioch expelled their bishops, who accepted Chalcedon, and openly declared themselves Monophysites in defiance of orthodoxy. Their church was later organised by Jacob Baradaeus (d. 578), and hence became known as Jacobite, although it is more correctly called Syrian Orthodox, or Western Syrian.

Both these Christian confessions share a common language and literature. Their language is Syriac, a Christian Aramaic dialect, and their literature is largely religious in content. The most important text is the Syriac translation of the Bible, but many homilies and hagiographical Greek works were also rendered into Syriac. As a result of this process, and through other contacts with Greek culture, the Syriac language was thoroughly Hellenised, with many Greek words and concepts being absorbed into it. The Syriac literature also continues discussions originating in Greek theological, philosophical, medical, and scientific literature. Against this cultural and linguistic backdrop, the Syriac Christians played a major role in the transmission of Greek science and medicine in both the Pahlavi and the Arabic traditions. They also developed their own medical literature, of which, unfortunately, little is extant. Syriac Christian scholars continued, however, to prepare versions of Arabic texts for their own communities, as is illustrated in Figure 2.6 on p. 69. It shows a popular Arabic therapeutic treatise written in the Syriac alphabet during the fifteenth century.

The most important translator of Greek medical texts into Syriac was Sergius of Rēsh ʿAynā (d. 536). He exemplifies well the medical trends in the Syriac-speaking world, being a Jacobite priest who studied medicine and philosophy in Alexandria. His three main interests were theology, philosophy, and medicine. In all of these subject areas, the Alexandrian tradition set the agenda for his activity as a writer and translator, and it is evident from his compositions that he could assume on the part of his readership a certain familiarity with general Hellenistic culture. In philosophy his favoured authors for translation were Aristotle and the Aristotelian commentators such as Alexander of Aphrodisias (*fl.* 200); in theology, Pseudo-Dionysius (the author of a number of works attributed to Dionysius the Areopagite, the first Bishop of Athens converted by the Apostle Paul); and in medicine, Galen and, to a lesser extent, Hippocrates. Sergius translated all of the so-called *Sixteen Books of Galen*, a selection of Galenic writings which constituted, as we have seen, the core of the medical curriculum at Alexandria. Some of his work was commissioned by Theodorus, Bishop of Karkh Juddān (in modern Samarrā', north of Baghdad), as is apparent from the dedications.[18]

Since Sergius' translations of Greek medical texts into Syriac were popular with the larger educated public of his day, his medical outlook must have been in tune with the trends of the time. The Syriac medical milieu as represented by Sergius was heavily influenced by the Alexandrian tradition. Philosophy, by then often related to Christian theology, was closely linked to medicine in the curriculum, and the latter was largely based on Galen. Galen's medical philosophy, however, had been transformed and harmonised in Late Antiquity, and it was in such an adjusted form that it was present not only in Alexandria, but also in the Syriac centres of learning such as Edessa and Nisibis.

Despite Sergius' popularity and influence on the subsequent Syriac tradition, most of his writings have not come down to us. The reason for this was simple: another translator, Ḥunayn ibn Isḥāq (d. 873 or 877) acquired even greater fame and favour, and his translations superseded those by Sergius. In an anecdote about Ḥunayn's life preserved in a thirteenth-century Syriac source, Jibrīl ibn Bukhtīshū' (d. 827) is reported to have said about Ḥunayn: 'If this man lives, then there shall be no memory (*'ūhdānā*) of Sergius of Rēsh 'Aynā left in the world.'[19] And indeed, Ḥunayn's success meant that, from the ninth century onwards, Sergius ceased to be used and copied.

Before turning the page, so to speak, and taking the story into Islamic times, it is necessary to discuss briefly the most important and well-known Syriac medical text still extant, the so-called *Syriac Book of Medicines*, first edited and translated in 1913. Much mystery surrounds it: different scholars have speculated when it might have been written, with suggestions ranging from the sixth to the thirteenth centuries. Whatever the moment of the final compilation, it is evident that this text contains much material dating back to the sixth and seventh centuries. It is composed of three parts that differ significantly in character from each other. Part One is based for the most part on Galen, in particular his *On the Affected Parts* and *On the Composition of Drugs according to Places in the Body*. The second part describes the relationship of the planets and the signs of the zodiac with human health and disease: certain alignments of stars are more propitious than others. Numerology also plays an important role; for instance, the numerical value of the letters in the patient's name is used in calculations to ascertain the best therapy. Finally, the recipes in Part Three contain many folk remedies: some are based on the natural properties of certain medicinal substances, while others rely on their magical powers, such as the advice to 'hang a dog's tooth around you[r neck]' to avoid being bitten by a rabid dog. The *Syriac Book of Medicines* highlights important pursuits in Late Antiquity apart from Galenism – namely astrology, numerology, and magic. All three were part not only of popular culture but also of the world of ideas of the Greek-speaking elite. These evidently filtered down into the Syriac medical tradition, eventually to become important in the Islamic world as well.[20]

The myth of Gondēshāpūr and the origin of the hospital

Since Islam developed a highly innovative and sophisticated system of hospital provision, one ought to understand its antecedents. Until fairly recently the conventional account of the origin of hospitals in Islam would begin with a version of what scholars now refer to as 'the myth of Gondēshāpūr'. The story goes something like this: The city of Gondēshāpūr (known in Arabic as Jundaysābūr), now a ruined site to the southeast of Dizfūl in southwest Iran, had become an outpost of Hellenism, with many Greek and Syriac-speaking scholars resident there. As early as the fourth century, so the story continues, Nestorian Christians had founded a medical academy or school which supported the translation of Greek and possibly Sanskrit texts into Middle Persian (Pahlavi) and Syriac, and associated with this academy was a large hospital which then served as a model for subsequent Islamic hospitals.[21]

This claim, however, has been challenged and found to be without substance. There seems to be no evidence that there was a hospital in Gondēshāpūr nor a formal medical school. There may have been a modest infirmary where Galenic medicine was practised and a forum where texts could be read, as was the case in other towns such as Susa nearby to the west. The 'myth' was based mostly on an account given by the thirteenth-century medical historian al-Qifṭī (d. 1248). One of the main arguments against it is the following: If such a large institution had existed, we would not hear of it for the first time only in such a late source, and a source, moreover, containing many anecdotes of little historical value, told more to entertain than to inform.[22]

Then how did the story arise? The myth can best be explained in terms of a retrospective historiography. For eight generations, from the mid-eighth century well into the second half of the eleventh century, twelve members of the Bukhtīshū' family of Nestorian Christian physicians served the caliphs in Baghdad as physicians and advisors. Hailing originally from Gondēshāpūr, the family rose to great prominence in Baghdad and were involved in hospital medicine during 'Abbāsid times (750s onwards). It would seem that they or their entourage forged a narrative which would provide them with a mythical and glorious past to give more weight and depth to their position at the court. In other words, if the Bukhtīshū' family could claim the hospital as their idea which they had brought with them from Gondēshāpūr, then their prestige and medical authority would be greatly enhanced.[23]

If, however, the hospital of Gondēshāpūr did not serve as the model for the subsequent Muslim tradition, and did not constitute the 'first hospital', then where are we to find the antecedents to later Islamic institutions? The most obvious candidate is the hospices attached to monastic foundations which developed in the eastern part of the Greek-speaking world from the fourth century onwards. Moved by the ideal of Christian charity, but also by a desire to promote their own image, a variety of church dignitaries set up shelters for the relief of the poor and the infirm. Some of these hospices had monks of some medical training attached to them, although the details of how they cared for or cured patients remain elusive.[24]

Similarly, the Syriac-speaking Christians developed a system of hospices and overnight shelters for the pilgrims and the sick. It was inspired by Greek models, and would prove crucial to the formation of the Islamic hospital. A letter by the Nestorian patriarch Timothy I (d. 823) illustrates the continuity between the Greek, the Syriac, and the later Islamic tradition. In it, Timothy I says:

> We built a *xenodocheion*, that is, a *bīmāristān*, in the catholic city [the see of the Catholicos, Seleucia/Ctesiphon, southeast of Baghdad], and spent on its building more or less 20,000 *zuzē* [a considerable sum of money].[25]

The institution is called both *xenodocheion* from the Greek meaning 'a place where one received guests or strangers', and *bīmāristān*, from the Persian meaning 'place of the sick'. The latter term became the standard word in Arabic to refer to hospitals. Little is known about the *xenodocheion*, how it operated, or who took shelter there, but it illustrates the importance of Nestorian Christians in the transmission of late Greek ideas regarding poor relief.

Indian and Chinese medicine

Two great medical traditions – those of India and China – also influenced the Islamic one, though only marginally. Through trade and travel, the Arabs came into direct contact with these two civilisations, and they imported many medicinal substances which were previously unknown in the Islamic heartlands or to Graeco-Roman physicians. Moreover, through intermediary Persian translations of Indian, and, to a lesser extent, Chinese medical texts, the medical theory of these two cultures became known.

Traditional Indian medicine, also called Ayurvedic, literally meaning 'science (*veda*) of life/longevity (*āyus*)', is based on the idea of three humours rather than four – wind (*vāta*), bile (*pitta*), and phlegm (*kapha*) – which interact with seven body tissues and the waste products. Disease occurs when these different constituents of the body are misaligned, misplaced, or imbalanced.

The two most ancient and important texts expounding Indian medical theory are Caraka's *Compendium* and Suśruta's *Compendium*. Both are composite works, containing elements from different periods; however, since they are mentioned in a sixth-century manuscript, the so-called Bower manuscript, they must have been compiled before that time. Their earliest parts may well date back to the third or second century BC. Both are multi-faceted and multi-layered compilations which, although important achievements in their own right, lack a coherent structure. A third (and last) book to be mentioned here, Vāgbhaṭa's *Heart of Medicine* (*Aṣṭaṇgahṛdaya*) written around 600, systematised and organised the medical knowledge contained in these earlier two compendia. It enjoyed great popularity in all of India, and beyond, so not surprisingly it was translated into Persian and from Persian into Arabic, together with the other two classics of Indian medicine. Yet, even if a basic outline of the Indian medical system was available in Arabic from the mid-ninth century onwards, it is evident that this system did not have much impact on the Islamic tradition. The greatest contribution of India to Islamic medicine was certainly the many new drugs imported from that part of the world.[26]

From roughly the third century BC, a Chinese medical theory developed which endeavoured to explain bodily functions and diseases in terms of natural causation, rather than demonic domination as often happened earlier in China. The medical ideas of the time were set out, for instance, in the *Inner Canon of the Yellow Thearch*, sometimes translated as the *Inner Canon of the Yellow Emperor* (*Huáng Dì Nèi Jīng*). There are three fundamental concepts: *yīn* and *yang*, the five evolutive phases, and *qì*. *Yīn* and *yáng* are complementary opposites which require each other to form a unity. *Yīn* is associated with female, earth, night, moon and water, whilst *yáng* is linked to male, heaven, day, sun, and fire. The five evolutive phases are wood, earth, water, fire, and metal, which conquer and generate each other in a circular fashion (for example, wood conquering earth; earth conquering water and so forth). *Qì* is the fundamental vitality in nature that powers transformations in the world and in the human body.[27]

Indian and Chinese medicine share certain features with the Greek and Persian medical traditions, without there being a generic link between them. All four strive to explain disease in terms of certain natural or bodily functions. They do this by referring to principles, elements or fundamental forces which animate life. The idea of outer (environmental) conditions influencing the inner workings of the body is also apparent in all these traditions, with various ideas about the interaction between the microcosm and the macrocosm. Often a misalignment or imbalance of these will lead to disease, whilst therapy is based on restoring the balance, or rearranging the constituent parts which are out of place. Scholars have pointed out the parallels between the Indian theory of three humours and Greek humoral pathology employing four humours; between the Chinese idea of *qì* and Greek *pneuma* (spirit); or between the Persian idea of a fire of life and Greek 'innate heat' (*emphuton thermon*), an energy source powering the vital functions of the body. It is important, however, to resist the temptation to explain the other medical systems in terms of Greek theory.[28]

Other earlier medical traditions which had flourished in the territories later to be conquered by Islam are the Egyptian, Mesopotamian, and Ancient Iranian ones. Because certain concepts or drugs filtered through to the Islamic world, often via numerous intermediaries, it might seem that they deserve fuller discussion here. Their impact in the realm of medicine, however, was very limited, and this may partially be explained by the fact that they placed emphasis on surgery and medication, whilst the Greek tradition favoured diet and regimen.

The immediate environment into which Islam erupted is the world of Late Antiquity where Greek thought pervaded not only Alexandria and other traditional strongholds of Hellenism, but also the Persian- and Syriac-speaking lands. When conquering peoples of different cultures and creeds, Islam adopted and adapted the scientific and medical heritage of those who came under its sway. Moreover, the structural parallels of humours and balances between the Greek medical tradition and those of India and China facilitated the process of integrating some of their drug lore into the system of humoral pathology. A translation movement of unprecedented scale, which put the Islamic medical tradition firmly on the map, largely fuelled this process of transferring medical knowledge.

Transformation through translation

> The Works of the Indians are rendered [into Arabic], the wisdom of the Greeks is translated, and the literature of the Persians has been transferred [to us Arabs]. As a result, some works have increased in beauty, while others have remained virtually unchanged. If one were to transpose the wisdom of the Arabs [into another tongue], however, then the wonderful splendour of the metre would be lost, and those attempting to do so would not comprehend the meaning. For this reason, non-Arabs do not mention it [Arabic poetry] in their works, which they [the non-Arabs] composed for their livelihood, intelligence and wisdom. These [foreign] books were transmitted from nation to nation, from century to century, and from language to language, until they ended up in our possession. We are the last to inherit and study them. It is true that these books are more successful in recording the achievements [of past generations] than monuments and poetry.
> – al-Jāḥiẓ, *The Book of Animals*[29]

Translation was fundamental to the formation of the Islamic medical tradition, and, more generally, has played a pivotal role in the fate of many a nation throughout history from the earliest times until today. For instance, when the Assyrians defeated the Sumerians, the former translated the works of the latter to forge their own literary tradition, which, in turn, had an impact on the nascent Greek literature. The story of Gilgamesh first told in Sumerian texts and then rendered into Akkadian, indirectly inspired Homer's *Odyssey*. Not only was the literature of Ancient Greece influenced by 'eastern' models, but the Greek medical tradition was as well. Recent research has shown that Hippocratic concepts of epilepsy have their precursors in Babylonian medical texts. Greek medical theory and practice were later also adopted and adapted by the Romans from the late third century BC onwards, even if some proud inhabitants of the eternal city such as Cato the Elder (d. 149 BC) deplored what they perceived as foreign and pernicious influence. He called Greek doctors 'butchers' and advised his fellow countrymen to stick to Roman virtues such as exercise and frugality, rather than the complicated medical tradition of these 'charlatans'. Greek medical ideas were again transmitted by translation to others, such as speakers of Persian and Syriac, who, in their turn, transformed and altered them according to their own needs. The importance of these translations, however, pales in comparison with what happened in ninth-century Baghdad, where virtually all the Greek medical texts then available were rendered into Arabic.[30]

The Graeco-Arabic translation movement

Islamic medicine is largely a continuation and further development of the Greek medical tradition. So great was the influence of Greek medicine that it had an impact not only on the learned medicine found in works by such famous authors as al-Rāzī (Rasis, d. 925) and Ibn Sīnā (Avicenna, d. 1037), but also, to a lesser extent, on treatises about Prophetic Medicine. For this reason, the formative period of Islamic medicine is the time of translation, when the medical concepts which were to govern Islamic medical thought were first expressed in Arabic.

There are some legendary reports about translations from Greek into Arabic being produced in Damascus during the reign of the first Islamic dynasty, the Umayyads (661–750). It was said, for example, that prince Khālid ibn al-Yazīd (d. 704) commissioned the translation of Greek medical and alchemical works, but, for the most part, such accounts lack any historical foundation. In general we know precious little about medical literary activity – let alone medical practice – during the Umayyad period.[31]

The first powerful patron systematically to have sponsored Graeco-Arabic translations appears to have been al-Manṣūr (r. 754–75), the second 'Abbāsid caliph. This occurred after the 'Abbāsid dynasty had moved the centre of power from Damascus (a thoroughly Hellenised city) to newly established Baghdad. Reportedly, al-Manṣūr asked Jurjīs ibn Jibrīl ibn Bukhtīsū' (d. 768) and al-Biṭrīq, both Nestorian Christians, to translate a number of medical works. While no translation which can securely be attributed to the former has come down to us, we are in the fortunate position to possess some Arabic versions by the latter. They represent the earliest stage of Graeco-Arabic translation activity. This translation movement received its major impetus, however, during the reigns of renowned caliphs such as Hārūn al-Rashīd (r. 786–809), al-Amīn (r. 809–813), and al-Ma'mūn (r. 813–33). They and their heirs extended patronage to physicians able to translate Greek medical works, the most illustrious examples being Yuḥannā ibn Māsawayh (d. c. 857) and his precocious pupil Ḥunayn ibn Isḥāq (d. c. 873). The latter ultimately surpassed his master both as translator and as a medical author in his own right.

We are extremely well informed about Ḥunayn Ibn Isḥāq's activity as a translator. He wrote an epistle (*risālah*) in which he gave a detailed report of all the Galenic works (some 129 in total) which he and his collaborators translated into Syriac and Arabic. Among the latter, we find his son Isḥāq ibn Ḥunayn (d. 910) and his nephew Ḥubaysh ibn al-Aʿsam (*fl.* c. 860). Ḥunayn described the practicalities of translation in a number of entries, the one about the *Method of Healing* lending itself particularly well to illustrating a number of points:

> Galen's *Book on the Method of Healing* [*Therapeutikē methodos*, consisting of 15 books]: … [1] The first six books of this work were translated into Syriac by Sergius [of Rēsh ʿAynā] when he was still a very weak translator. After he had acquired experience as a translator, he translated the remaining eight books and produced a better translation than that of the earlier books …
>
> [2] A few years later I translated the work from the beginning for Bukhtīshūʿ ibn Jibrīl. [3] For the last eight books, a number of Greek manuscripts were at my disposal. These I collated and produced a single correct copy from them, which I then translated with the utmost accuracy (*istiqṣā'*) and in the best style (*balāghah*) I was able to master. [4] For the first six books only a single manuscript, and moreover a very faulty one, was at my disposal at the time. I was therefore unable to produce these books in the manner required. [5] Later I came across another manuscript and collated the text with it and corrected it as much as possible. It would be better if I could collate a third manuscript with it, if only I were fortunate enough to find one. [6] For Greek manuscripts of this work are rare, since it does not belong to the works that were read in the school (*kuttāb*) of Alexandria.
>
> [7] From the Syriac manuscripts of my translation Ḥubaysh ibn al-Ḥasan translated this work for Muḥammad ibn Mūsá. [8] Then, after he had translated the work, he asked me to go through the last eight books critically for him and correct possible mistakes, and I did this for him successfully.[32]

This short account shows a number of salient features of Ḥunayn's activity: he often translated into Syriac first, not into Arabic directly, although he sometimes also did the latter. He consulted previous translations, insofar as they existed [1]. In this instance, there is one by Sergius of Rēsh ʿAynā, whom we have encountered earlier. Ḥunayn's work was commissioned by prominent patrons: he prepared the Syriac version for a member of the Bukhtīshūʿ family originally from Gondēshāpūr [2]. Bukhtīshū' ibn Jibrīl (d. 870), referred to here, was the personal physician of three caliphs: al-Ma'mūn and his successors al-Wāthiq (r. 842–7) and al-Mutawakkil (r. 847–61). The Arabic translation, on the other hand, was ordered by one of the Banū Mūsá, three sons of the infamous highwayman turned plutocrat Mūsá ibn Shākir [3]. Their father Mūsá, who had close connections to the caliph al-Ma'mūn, gave his sons an impeccable education, so that they became proficient in subjects such as medicine, mathematics, mechanics and astronomy. The most famous of the three sons was Muḥammad, mentioned here, some of whose works on scientific subjects are still extant today. Both Bukhtīshū' ibn Jibrīl and Muḥammad ibn Mūsá were intimately linked to the caliphal palace, which eagerly sponsored Graeco-Arabic translation activity.[33]

The question arises, however, why the 'Abbāsid elite would want to fund Nestorian Christians to translate Greek texts into Arabic, or, to put it differently, what their political agenda was in doing so. The causes for this phenomenon, as for most momentous historical events, are multiple. Unlike the Umayyads in Damascus, the 'Abbāsids were a dynasty which did not hail from Arab stock, but came from the Persian East. As such, they had an interest in promoting a cultural policy which went beyond the restricted remit of pure Arab heritage to forge a more cosmopolitan identity. Another factor was their wish to portray themselves in some way as successors to the Sasanians, whose medical system, as we have seen, was already influenced by Greek ideas. Moreover, the Nestorian milieu in Mesopotamia – especially in the newly founded capital of Baghdad, the 'City of Peace (*Madīnat al-Salām*)', as it was then called – was itself heavily Hellenised, and this also helped increase the interest in Greek learning. The Greek medical system in the form of humoral pathology had already penetrated and influenced many other cultures. Finally, there was the attraction for elite scholars of the day to Greek thought in its own right. For all these various reasons, it is not surprising that the 'Abbāsids came under its spell as well.

Apart from the importance of patronage, the extract from Ḥunayn's epistle makes manifest two significant features of his translation method: philological acumen and stylistic accuracy [3]–[5]. Ḥunayn states that for part of the work he had only one Greek manuscript at his disposal, which rendered his task more difficult. When he later got hold of a second one, he collated it with the first in order to emend the text – that is to say, he compared the two in order to arrive at the correct reading. He even remarks that he would have preferred to have a third one, in order to improve it further. This technique of collation and emendation is essentially the same used by scholars today, and Ḥunayn had already adopted it over a millennium ago.

Ḥunayn was, however, not only concerned with questions of textual criticism and philological accuracy, but also with style. As he himself states at the end of [3], he prepared the Syriac translation 'in the best style I was able to master'. Likewise, when working on Arabic versions, he strove to be idiomatic rather than following his source too closely. In an oft-quoted passage, the fourteenth-century historian al-Ṣafadī (d. 1363) put his appreciation of Ḥunayn's translation technique thus:

> The translators use two methods of translation. One of them is that of Yuḥannā ibn al-Biṭrīq, Ibn al-Nā'imah al-Ḥimṣī and others. According to this method, the translator studies each individual Greek word and its meaning, chooses an Arabic word of corresponding meaning and uses it. Then he turns to the next word and proceeds in the same manner until in the end he has rendered into Arabic the text he wishes to translate. This method is bad [...]
>
> The second method is that of Ḥunayn ibn Isḥāq, al-Jawharī and others. Here the translator considers a whole sentence, ascertains its full meaning and then expresses it in Arabic with a sentence identical in meaning, without concern for the correspondence of individual words. This method is superior, and hence there is no need to improve the works of Ḥunayn ibn Isḥāq.[34]

These two methods are sometimes also called *verbum de verbo* (word for word) and *sensum de sensu* (meaning for meaning) after a well-known expression by Cicero, the famous Roman statesman, orator, and philosopher (d. 43 BC). Although this characterisation is not entirely true, as can be seen from the extant Arabic versions by these translators, yet it is still the case that Ḥunayn surpasses his colleagues and competitors not only in philological accuracy but also in style.[35]

To return to Ḥunayn's account of the translation of Galen's *Method of Healing*, it is Ḥubaysh ibn al-Ḥasan called al-A'sam ('having withered limbs'), the nephew and pupil of Ḥunayn, who translates the text from Syriac into Arabic in the first place [7]. Ḥunayn later corrects and improves this Arabic, presumably by comparing it to the Greek source [8]. In general, the picture which emerges from the entry on the *Method of Healing* in Ḥunayn's epistle is confirmed by the other entries and can be summarised as follows. Quite a number of people participated in the translation of Galen's compostions into Syriac and Arabic. Patrons of these translations were part of the Christian and Muslim elite of the time and belonged to, or had ties with, the 'Abbāsid ruling class. They paid handsomely for the privilege to be able to read the works in question. Most of the translators working with Ḥunayn ibn Isḥāq were Nestorian Christians, and although they sometimes drew on previous work, they generally produced new Syriac and Arabic translations.

Common misconceptions about the translation movement

Three misconceptions regarding the translation movement have arisen in scholarly and popular literature. The first concerns the factors which motivated the translation process. Raymond Le Coz has claimed that, in essence, Nestorian physicians such as Ḥunayn ibn Isḥāq instigated the translation movement and taught the Greek sciences, and especially medicine, to the Arabs. Dimitri Gutas, on the other hand, has amply demonstrated that the translation movement was the result of intense patronage by 'Abbāsid rulers who became increasingly interested in Greek science, medicine, philosophy, and astronomy for reasons discussed above. Although some Syriac-speaking Christians in pre-Islamic times, such as Sergius of Rēsh 'Aynā, had translated certain Greek medical texts into Syriac, the vast majority of Graeco-Syriac translation activity took place under the aegis of the 'Abbāsids. Surely, Nestorian Christians played a crucial role in the transmission of medical knowledge from the Greeks to the Arabs. To call them 'masters of the Arabs', however, as Le Coz does, overlooks the historical and intellectual forces at work in ninth-century Baghdad, where the ruling elite and their entourage set not only the political, but also the cultural and scientific, agenda.[36]

The second misconception regards the selection of texts to be translated, allegedly made primarily for reasons of taste, interest, or inclination. Bernard Lewis has claimed that they were deliberately chosen for their usefulness, and that Muslims had no interest in Greek literature, poetry or drama, saying:

> This was clearly a cultural rejection: you take what is useful from the infidel; but you don't need to look at his absurd ideas or to try and understand his inferior literature, or to study his meaningless history.[37]

The reality was quite different. As Ḥunayn himself stated, the availability of Greek manuscripts (and hence Greek texts) depended on whether or not they were read in the 'School of Alexandria' (see [6] in the previous section). It is true that some Muslim authors such as al-Jāḥiẓ, quoted above on p. 23, believed that it is impossible or extremely difficult to translate poetry, because metre and diction cannot be transferred adequately. This did not, however, stop many Muslim authors, including al-Jāḥiẓ, from taking a keen interest in Greek history and legend, or even Greek poetry.[38]

The availability of Greek poetry in Arabic translation depended heavily on the fads and fashions of Late Antiquity. A good example is Greek drama. By the time of the Arab conquest in the mid-seventh century, the classics of tragedy and comedy were no longer performed. Instead, the more popular genre of the pantomime, in which a sole actor entertained the audience through dance, song, and monologue, found favour with the audience. No wonder, then, that the Arabs turned to Sophocles (d. c. 406 BC) and Aristophanes (d. c. 386 BC) only during their modern Renaissance (c. 1870–1950), and did not translate them in ninth-century Baghdad. Likewise, the most prominent exponent of the New Comedy, Menander (342–291 BC), had long ceased to be put on stage. Certain memorable one-liners (*monostichoi*) from his plays, however, enjoyed the favour of the public and were copied, as the papyrus record shows, and these *monostichoi* circulated in different Arabic collections.[39]

Another extremely well-liked text in Late Antiquity was the so-called *Alexander Romance*, an account of the great conqueror's exploits, in which fact and fiction were intimately intertwined. Its reception in the Arabic world ranges from the Qur'ān (18:82–98) to longwinded narratives. Moreover, there is much Arabic historical writing which explores the ancient Greek past as well as contemporaneous Byzantium. There can therefore be no doubt that most members of the Muslim intelligentsia would not consider Greek ideas absurd or Greek history meaningless, as Lewis polemically put it. Rather, to cite Franz Rosenthal, 'the fundamental importance of the ancient Greeks and their intellectual achievements for the formation of Islamic civilisation was fully realised among Muslims'. The choice of what to translate was determined by the availability of texts as well as the taste and tendencies in Late Antiquity, and not by some innate philistinism.[40]

The third and most prevalent misconception or 'myth' about the translation movement is that it took place in a famous House of Wisdom (*Bayt al-Ḥikmah*). This 'House of Wisdom', it is said, was a translation academy with a library, founded by Hārūn al-Rashīd's successor, al-Ma'mūn, where Ḥunayn and his colleagues carried out their tasks. Reliable evidence for this legend, however, is virtually non-existent. Dimitri Gutas, who has recently reviewed the available sources, concludes that if such a 'House of Wisdom' ever existed, it is best explained as a library where translations from Persian into Arabic were stored. In any case, it was completely unrelated to the Graeco-Arabic translation movement of the ninth century.[41]

Graeco-Arabic translation techniques

Ever since Max Simon in 1905 published those parts of the Arabic translation of Galen's *Anatomical Procedures* which were lost in Greek, academics have endeavoured to describe by what means and through what mechanisms Greek words, expressions and phrases were rendered into Arabic. Generally speaking, with time, scholars have grown less and less confident that they have found specific linguistic criteria which would allow them to identify individual translators. There is, however, a notable exception, afforded to us in a recent study by Manfred Ullmann. Because of a curious quirk of fate, two different Arabic versions of book six of Galen's *On the Powers of Simple Drugs* have come down to us: the older by al-Biṭrīq or his son Ibn al-Biṭrīq (version **A**), and the younger produced by Ḥunayn towards the end of his life, in the 870s (version **B**). These two versions represent respectively the initial and the mature stage of Graeco-Arabic translations, since al-Biṭrīq was one of the first to render Greek medical texts into Arabic, whilst Ḥunayn brought this activity to an impressive level of sophistication. Is it then true that al-Biṭrīq's version is exceedingly literal, as al-Ṣafadī claimed?[42]

There are some differences between these two versions, the most striking of which are the following. Version **A** often both transliterates and translates Greek medicinal terms, where **B** only translates them; for instance, the Greek heading '*Peri iou* ('On violet [*ion*]') is rendered in Arabic as '*Al-qawlu fī yyw*', *wa-huwa l-banafsaju* (The discussion on *ion*, that is, violet [*banafsaj*])' in **A**, while **B** merely says: '*Al-qawlu fī l-banafsaji* (The discussion on violet [*banafsaj*]). One might interpret this as greater precision in **A**, but such an assessment would be unjustified. By omitting transliterated terms, Ḥunayn strove to produce an idiomatic and jargon-free translation, as can be seen when looking at how the two translators handled other challenges. There are many cases where **A** paraphrases the original, whilst **B** endeavours to bring out all the subtle nuances contained in the source. For example, we can look at how the following Greek phrase, referring to different varieties of the resin bdellium, is translated. The original Greek reads:

> *chrōntai de autois tines ... epi te bronchokēlōn kai hudrokēlōn, asitōi ptuelōi deuontes, hōs emplastrōdē sustasin echein*
> Some use them [different kinds of bdellium] for goitres and hydroceles, moistening them with 'fasting [*asitos*]' saliva [i.e., saliva produced during fasting], so that they get a plaster-like consistency.

In **A** it is rendered in a paraphrastic way:

> *Wa-mina l-nāsi man yasta'milu hādhā l-dawā'a mina l-adwiyati wa-yudhībuhū bi-rīqihī wa-yaṣna'uhū mithla l-laṣūqi*
> Some people use this drug; they dissolve it in their saliva and make it into something like a sticking plaster.

B, on the other hand, follows the Greek much more closely:

> *Wa-mina l-nāsi qawmun yasta'milūna l-muqla ... fī mudāwāti l-warami l-ḥādithi fī l-ḥanjarati wa-fī qīlati l-mā'i wa-idhā arādū sti'mālahū layyanūhu bi-rīqi insānin lam ya'kul shay'an wa-lā yaẓālūna ya'jinūnahū bihī ḥattá yaṣīra ka-l-marhami*
> Some people use bdellium ... in order to treat a swelling occurring in the throat and hydrocele. When they want to use it, they soften it with the saliva of a man who has not eaten anything, kneading it constantly so that it becomes like cream.[43]

There are a number of points which **A** omits, whilst **B** renders them faithfully and idiomatically. First, there are the two diseases, goitre and a hydrocele, which **A** fails to mention. Nor does **A** render the Greek *asitos* ('fasting'), whilst **B** understands it accurately as 'of a man who has not eaten anything'. The process of preparing the remedy is described in **B** in greater detail than in the original; the translator uses his knowledge to clarify the source. Therefore, in one sense, al-Ṣafadī is right in saying that Ḥunayn 'considers a whole sentence, ascertains its full meaning and then expresses it in Arabic with a sentence identical in meaning, without concern for the correspondence of individual words'. Yet al-Ṣafadī is wrong in qualifying al-Biṭrīq's approach as a literal one. On the contrary, he is less literal than Ḥunayn, paraphrasing and summarising rather than translating the original. Ḥunayn's version is superior not only in the greater precision displayed in it, but also from a stylistic point of view. It uses more complex syntactical structures, often reflecting those of the source, where **A** merely employs parataxis, that is to say, main clauses linked by conjunctions such as 'and'. **B** is generally more idiomatic, using, for instance, the generic article such as in *al-insān*, 'man', where **A** omits it. Although these few examples can only illustrate certain trends in Graeco-Arabic versions, it is clear that translation technique had come a long way in the seventy years between 800, when **A** was produced, and Ḥunayn's own heyday.

Creating a medical terminology

The language of pre-Islamic Arabia did contain a number of names for a variety of common ailments such as coughs, diarrhoea, and fevers, as we have seen at the beginning of this chapter. It lacked, however, a precise technical terminology to describe and classify symptoms and diseases, or to detail medicaments and therapies. The Graeco-Arabic translation movement forged an extensive medical vocabulary, such that, by the mid-ninth century, the Arabic language no longer lagged behind its Greek counterpart in this area.

Let us consider what strategies were employed to create technical terms for scientific medical discourse. When faced with the problem of rendering Greek medical terminology, one can basically adopt three different approaches: (1) to transliterate; (2) to resort to a loan translation (also called 'calque' in linguistic parlance); or (3) to employ a genuine term from the target language. In English, for instance, the first method is often used.

These three approaches are illustrated by the contrasting translations of two Greek medical terms into Arabic and English. The word 'alopecia', a technical term for baldness in English, is directly taken from the Greek *alōpekia*. The Greek term refers to a trichological condition in which the hair falls out 'like in a fox', since it comes from *alōpēx* (fox). Likewise the word 'spasm', referring to a 'sudden and uncontrollable tightening of the muscles', derives from the Greek *spasmos* (convulsion), which itself is a noun going back to *spaō* (to draw). In Arabic, however, neither of these two terms is merely transliterated. The first, *alōpekia*, is rendered as *dā' al-tha'lab*, literally meaning 'the disease of the fox'. In other words, a loan translation (a translation following the pattern of the source language) is used. The second, *spasmos*, is translated as *tashannuj* (convulsion), a purely Arabic form. Therefore, instead of simply transliterating, the Arabic coins its own words or expressions.

We can perceive a historical development in the Arabic medical terminology. There is a move from transliteration to translation, visible in a variety of areas. We have already encountered the case of Greek *ion* (violet) being both transliterated and translated at the early stage of the translation movement, whilst Ḥunayn only used a translation, *banafsaj*. Something similar happened with a variety of highly technical terms for disease such as 'erysipelas', denoting a red inflammation of the skin in both Greek and English. In Arabic, it is mostly transliterated at first, but is then replaced by the Arabic word '*ḥumrah* (redness)', which became a technical term in a medical context.[44]

Another instance where transliteration and translation exist side by side is the term for inflammation of the brain, called phrenitis in both Greek and English. It is sometimes transliterated as *farānīṭis* in Arabic, but also called *sirsām*. The latter term comes from the Persian *sarsām*, literally 'inflammation (*sām*) of the head (*sar*)'. Moreover, this example highlights two additional features of Arabic medical language: the problematic nature of transliteration, and the strong influence of Persian. Compared with translation, transliteration had some clear disadvantages. Greek words in their Arabic garb were prone to being misread, and hence misunderstood, because the Arabic language requires diacritics to distinguish between some letters. In the case of *farānīṭis*, the first letter was misread as *qāf* (two dots) rather than *fā'* (one dot), and hence the disease occasionally appears as *qarānīṭis*. Other letters easily confused are *nūn* (one dot above the letter), *tā'* (two dots above), *thā'* (three dots above), *bā'* (one dot below), and *yā'* (two dots below). This potential ambiguity led to some acute problems of identification, especially in the area of medicinal substances, where transliterations proliferated. The second feature is the presence of Persian in the Arabic medical vocabulary. Both *sirsām* and *banafsaj* are Persian words in an Arabised form. The influence of Syriac and, to a lesser extent, also Sanskrit is visible as well, particularly in the pharmacological nomenclature.

Cultural specifications

When rendering Greek texts into Arabic, whether or not a Syriac intermediary was present, the translators sometimes were faced with specific cultural sensitivities which they felt they had to take into consideration. A well-known example is the frequent references to the Greek pantheon and other polytheistic ideas which occur in Galen and other medical authors. To be sure, the Muslim audience knew that the ancient Greeks worshipped a variety of gods such as Zeus and Apollo. In a medical context, however, such references were not infrequently altered so as to be more acceptable to the monotheistic reader. For instance, Galen writes in his treatise *That the Powers of the Soul Follow the*

Mixtures of the Body: 'Here he [Plato in his *Timaeus*] says that *the gods* (*hoi theoi*) created man (*entha phēsi tous theous dēmiourgēsai ton anthrōpon*)'. The translator, probably Ḥunayn ibn Isḥāq, rendered this in the following manner: 'He said [...] that God (*Allāh*) – great and exalted is He – when he created man [...] (*Qāla inna llāha jalla wa-'azza ḥīna khalaqa l-insāna*)'. In this way, the Greek term for 'the gods (*hoi theoi*)' is translated as 'God (*Allāh*)', and, for good measure, the eulogy 'great and exalted is He' added. The polytheistic elements of the source are thus removed.[45]

Another well-known instance of this process occurs in the Arabic translation of the *Hippocratic Oath*. In the Greek original, it begins with an invocation to different deities: 'I swear by Apollo, the physician, and Asclepius, and Health (*Hugeia*) and Panaceia, and all male and female gods ... (*Omnumi Apollōna iētron kai Asklēpion kai Hugeian kai Panakeian kai theous pantas te kai pasas* ...)'. In the anonymous Arabic translation, however, Apollo, Health and Panaceia are brushed out, the 'male and female gods' become 'male and female "friends" of God (*awliyā' Allāh*)', and only Asclepius makes it through this process of transformation by translation: 'I swear by God (*Allāh*), lord of life and death, giver of health, creator of healing and all cure; I swear by Asclepius; and I swear by all male and female "friends" of God, taking them as my witness that ... (*Innī uqsimu bi-llāhi rabbi l-ḥayāti wa-l-mawti wa-wāhibi l-ṣiḥḥati wa-khāliqi l-shifā'i wa-kulli 'ilājin wa-uqsimu bi-Asqalībīyūsa wa-uqsimu bi-awliyā'i llāhi mina l-rijāli wa-l-nisā'i jamī'an wa-ushhiduhum 'alá anna* ...)'.[46]

Not only did the Greek gods pose a potential problem for a monotheistic audience; other features, too, could shock and were therefore expunged. To give just one final example: in a passage from his *Anatomical Procedures* where Galen talks about dissecting children who died after having been exposed, Ḥunayn changes the meaning by replacing 'the corpses of exposed children (*paidia* ... *tōn ektithemenōn nekra*)' with 'aborted infants (*aṭfāl asqāṭ*)'. This suggests that he and his audience felt a deep reluctance and repugnance to exposing children; there are, after all, strong injunctions in the Qur'ān against such practices (6:151; 17:31).[47]

Translating Greek medical texts therefore meant to transpose them into a different culture and, by doing so, also to transform them.

Arabic as the scientific lingua franca

As the major tongue of Islam, in which the Qur'ān was written, boasting a literary and poetic tradition of great refinement, Arabic was in pole position, so to speak, to dominate the race for linguistic hegemony. Moreover, through the efforts of translators such as Ḥunayn, Arabic developed into a powerful linguistic tool, able to express the most subtle and complicated philosophical, medical, and scientific

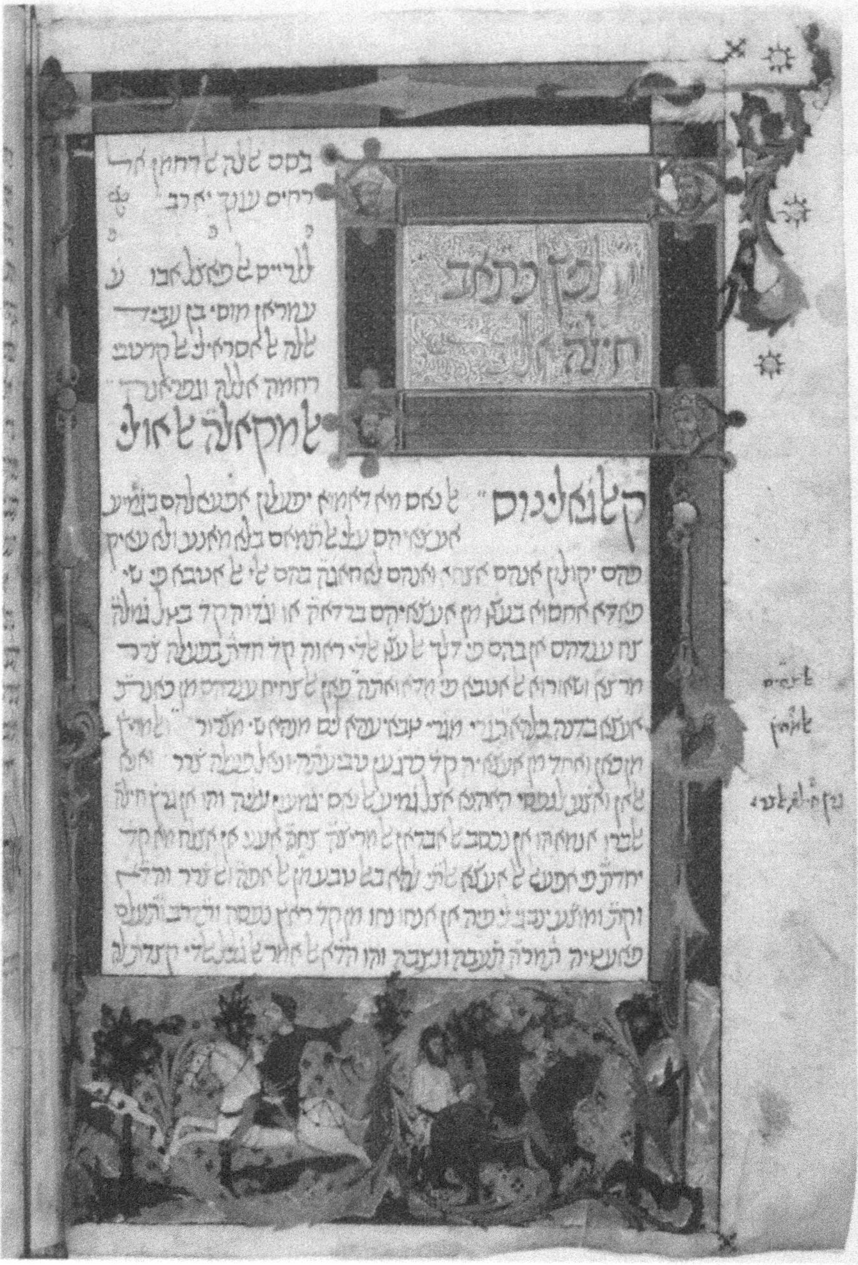

Figure 1.3 The *Abridgement* (*Talkhīṣ*) by Ibn Maymūn (Maimonides, d. 1204) of Galen's *On the Method of Healing*, in a twelfth-century manuscript written in Judeo-Arabic. It was possibly illuminated in the workshop of Ferrer and Arnau Bassa in Barcelona.

ideas. For centuries, the scientific discourse in the Muslim world – whether on the shores of the Guadalquevir or the Ganges – took place in Arabic. To be sure, with the reawakening of Persian nationalism in the tenth century, some people began to write also in Persian on medical topics. Yet, one had to wait until the late eleventh century to see any significant medical treatises being composed in this tongue, which later was used as the language of culture not only in Persia, but also on much of the Indian subcontinent. Likewise, it is useful to point out that Jewish authors living under Muslim governance drafted most of their works in Arabic, except for books on purely Jewish subjects. For instance, Ibn Maymūn (Maimonides, d. 1204), the most famous Jewish scholar of the Middle Ages, wrote most of his œuvre, including many letters and responsa (religious legal advice), in Arabic, with the notable exception of his great compendium of Jewish law called *Mishne Torah* ('Repetition of the Law', also known as *Yad Ḥazakah*, 'Strong Hand'). Figure 1.3 shows his *Abridgement* (*Talkhīṣ*) of Galen's *Method of Healing*, written in Judaeo-Arabic, that is to say Arabic in Hebrew letters.

The omnipresence of Arabic as the *lingua franca* of science in large parts of the medieval Muslim world might also explain why so few medical works in Syriac survive today. One could even say that Ḥunayn himself created the conditions for the loss of his own Syriac versions. The vast corpus of Greek medical texts in Arabic translations proved so popular and influential that interest in Syriac works waned. Ḥunayn operated in a world in which Greek medical and philosophical thought dominated; the interest of the age, however, was not limited to Greek ideas, but also extended to other cultural traditions.

Translations from other languages

Although Greek medical theory constituted the framework in which Islamic medicine was to evolve, other traditions also contributed to its development. For the earlier period until the end of the tenth century, Arabic versions of Syriac and Pahlavi medical texts were the most important. Apart from those already discussed above, one Syriac author deserves special mention, namely Ibn Sarābiyūn. He lived in the second half of the ninth century and wrote two medical encyclopedias, one consisting of seven, and another of the twelve books, circulating under the titles *Small* and *Large Compendium*, respectively. The former, also known as the 'famous (*shahīr*)', was translated no fewer than three times into Arabic. It continued the tradition of medical handbooks, containing a digest of the most important information arranged in a logical order.

As Syriac was often an intermediary in the transmission of Greek texts into Arabic, so was Persian for Indian and later also Chinese medical works. Some of the most famous Indian compendia were translated into Arabic via Persian.

We have already seen that Caraka's *Compendium*, Suśruta's *Compendium*, and Vāgbhaṭa's *Heart of Medicine* became available in Arabic. Ibn al-Nadīm, a tenth-century Baghdad bookseller and bibliographer, informs us in his *Catalogue* (*Fihrist*) that Caraka's *Compendium* was first translated into Persian, and then from Persian into Arabic by a certain 'Abd Allāh ibn 'Alī. This translation served as an important source of information for 'Alī ibn Rabban al-Ṭabarī (*fl.* 850), who drew on it, as well as the other two medical works, when describing the Indian medical system in his *Paradise of Wisdom*. Similarly, al-Rāzī, writing fifty years later, quoted all three profusely in his *Comprehensive Book* (*al-Kitāb al-Ḥāwī*).[48]

Translations of Chinese medical texts appeared at a much later stage, and had even less influence on the Islamic medical tradition than the Indian ones. The first to have come down to us was prepared at the behest of the Rashīd al-Dīn Faḍl Allāh (d. 1318), also known as Rashīd al-Dīn Ṭabīb ('the physician') because in his youth he had studied medicine. Born into a Jewish family in the Persian city of Hamadān, he converted to Islam at around the age of 30 and eventually became a high-ranking official in the service of the Īlkhānids, the Mongol successors to Genghis Khan (d. 1227) in Iran. He not only had a general interest in universal history, but also, and more to the point in our context, in Chinese medicine. For this reason he ordered a student of his to go to China and bring back books on medicine. From Persian translations of these, Rashīd al-Dīn himself compiled a collection of the most relevant material in an illustrated treatise under the title *Book of Precious* [*Information*].[49]

Acculturation

> The inhabitants of the middle zones [3rd–5th climes] are temperate in their physique and character and in their ways of life. They have all the natural conditions necessary for a civilized life, such as ways of making a living, dwellings, crafts, sciences, political leadership, and royal authority. They thus have had prophecy, religious groups, dynasties, religious laws, sciences, countries, cities, buildings, horticulture, splendid crafts, and everything else that is temperate. Now, among the inhabitants of these zones about whom we have historical information are, for instance, the Arabs, the Byzantines, the Persians, the Israelites, the Greeks, the Indians and the Chinese.
> – Ibn Khaldūn, *Introduction*[50]

By the mid-ninth century, numerous Greek medical texts were available in Arabic. The Islamic medical tradition built on these translations: both medical theory and practice were overwhelmingly a continuation of the Greek one. It was, however, not merely a watered-down and corrupt version of glorious Greek medical achievements, as scholars from the Renaissance onwards have often claimed. It incorporated other elements such as Syriac, Persian and Indian medical concepts into the general framework of humoral pathology, and we shall shortly investigate how health care in the medieval Islamic world, although largely inspired by Greek ideas, introduced innovation on the theoretical, social, and practical levels.

The quotation by Ibn Khaldūn, as well as that by al-Jāḥiẓ given earlier (p. 23), illustrate two important points: that Muslims in general were aware that they inherited 'the sciences' from non-Arabs and non-Muslims, and that they made them their own. Ibn Khaldūn insisted that 'the Byzantines, the Persians, the Israelites, the Greeks, the Indians and the Chinese' all belong to climes adjacent to that of the Arabs, and therefore share in the benefits of civilisation. Similarly, the 'Abbāsids promoted legendary accounts of the Greeks having plundered the storehouses of Persian wisdom, thereby saying that Greek science, medicine, and philosophy are, in essence, Persian – that is to say, from their own background. In both cases, the aim was to acclimatise or assimilate the foreign elements by forging bonds of intellectual kinship. This is the ultimate result of the translation movement: Greek medicine as well as some elements of other medical traditions were transformed and not merely given permanent right of abode as aliens; rather, they were assimilated, adapted, and finally adopted in the truest sense of the word into Islamic society.

Suggested reading

For Greek medicine in general, see, Nutton, *Ancient Medicine*; for the problem of medicine and philosophy in the Greek world, see Eijk, *Medicine and Philosophy*.

On the different Persian empires in general, see Brosius, *Persians*; more specifically on medical ideas, see Gignoux, *Man and Cosmos* and Hampel, *Medizin der Zoroastrier*. On Syriac Medicine, see Bhayro, 'Syriac Medical Terminology'.

On translation as a general means to transfer scientific knowledge, see Montgomery, *Science in Translation*. On the Greek-Arabic translation movement, see Gutas, *Greek Thought*; and Rosenthal, *Classical Heritage*. For a specific example of Greek-Syriac-Arabic translation, see Pormann, *Oriental Tradition*.

Notes

1 tr. [modified] Rosenthal, *Muqaddimah*, iii. 311, 312–13; Arabic text iii. 270, 10–12; 272, 1–4.
2 See Humphreys, *Islamic History*, 84–5 for foreign influences on the early Muslim community with further literature.
3 Wellhausen, *Skizzen und Vorarbeiten*, German translation 128; Arabic text 22–3; see Ullmann, *WKAS*, ii. 1313b12–21.
4 tr. Rosenthal, *Muqaddimah*, iii. 150, Arabic text iii. 118, ult.–119, 4.
5 See Humphreys, *Islamic History*, ch. 3; Motzki, *Ḥadith*.
6 See Robinson, *Islamic Historiography*; Hoyland, *Arabia*.

7 For example, Goldz., *Abh.*, ii. 16, 9; Qais b. -Ḫ., no. 1, 9; Muf. no. 15, 15 [quoted according to Ullmann, *WKAS*].

8 See Shahîd, *Byzantium and the Arabs in the Sixth Century*.

9 For the scholion see Lyall (ed.), *Mufaḍḍalīyāt*, i. 411, 10.

10 Temkin, *Galenism*.

11 For early Alexandria, see Von Staden, *Herophilus*; for the history of the Alexandrian Library, see El-Abbadi, *The Life and Fate*; for medicine and medical teaching in late antique Alexandria, see Scarborough (ed.), *Symposium on Byzantine Medicine*; Roueché, 'Did medical students'.

12 Pormann, 'Jean le Grammairien'.

13 Iskandar, 'Attempted Reconstruction'.

14 See Pormann, 'Alexandrian Summary'; and Savage-Smith, 'Galen's Lost Ophthalmology'. The English word 'dieresis' is derived from Greek *dehairesis* (division), but is generally employed in a more restricted sense.

15 For these trilingual inscriptions, see Rubin, '*Res Gestae Divi Saporis*'.

16 See Sigerist, *History of Medicine*, ii. 203–4, for a discussion of the Avestan material.

17 See Ph. Gignoux, art. 'Health, i. Pre-Islamic Period', *Enc. Ir.* xii. 102a–4a for further literature. Section 157 of the third book of the *Ḍēnkard* is available in an unreliable English translation by Sanjana, *Ḍinkarḍ*, iv. 220–41; for a more scholarly rendering see Menasce, *Troisième livre*, 158–68.

18 For Sergius, see Hugonnard-Roche, 'Note sur Sergius'. It has previously been thought that Sergius also translated Porphyry's *Introduction* [*to Philosophy*] and Aristotle's *Categories*, the first of his logical works known as the *Organon* ('Tool'); Hugonnard-Roche has shown this to be erroneous. See also Bhayro, 'Syriac Medical Terminology'.

19 Budge, *Chronography*, i. 148 (tr.) and ii. fol. 53b18–19 (txt); cf. Bhayro, 'Syriac Medical Terminology', 154.

20 Budge, *Syriac Book of Medicines*; the quotation is found i. 577, last two lines (text), ii. 687 (tr.).

21 For this earlier conventional view about Gondēshāpūr, see M. W. Dols, *Medieval Islamic Medicine*, 5–6, with further literature. For the location of Gondēshāpūr, whose ruins are today called Shāhābād, see Barthold, *Historical Geography of Iran*, 180, 187–8.

22 See particularly the challenges made by Michael Dols and Peregrine Horden: Horden, 'Byzantine Welfare State'; Dols, 'Origins of the Islamic Hospital'.

23 See L. Richter-Bernburg, art. 'Bok̲tīšū'', *Enc. Ir.* iv. 333a–6a.

24 For a recent survey of the question, see Horden, 'Earliest Hospitals', with further literature (we disagree, however, with his interpretation of the Islamic evidence); Horden, 'How Medicalized were Byzantine Hospitals?'; and, for the monastic developments, Crislip, *From Monastery to Hospital* (to be used with caution).

25 Birmingham, Mingana Collections, MS 587, fol. 342a18–20 (we are grateful to N. Smelova for inspecting this manuscript for us, and copying the relevant passage); see also Pormann, 'Islamic Hospitals'.

26 This outline of Indian medicine is based for the most part on Wujastyk, *Roots*.

27 This sketch of early Chinese medical ideas is based on Unschuld, *Chinese Medicine*, ch. 2; the definition of *qì* – in slightly modified form – has been provided by Vivienne Lo.

28 See specifically Wujastyk, *Roots*, xviii, xxix, and Sigerist, *History of Medicine*, ii. 326;

and more generally Lloyd and Sivin, *The Way and the Word*; and Kuriyama, *Expressiveness of the Body*.

29 Arabic text i. 75, 9.

30 For eastern influence on early Greek culture, see West, *The Eastern Face*; more specifically in the realm of medicine and magic, Horstmanshoff and Stol, *Magic and Rationality*; for Greek influence on Roman medicine, Cruse, *Roman Medicine*.

31 For Khālid ibn al-Yazīd, see M. Ullmann, 'Ḫālid ibn al-Yazīd'; another 'myth' will come under scrutiny below p. 129.

32 Translation with slight modifications by Rosenthal, *Classical Heritage*, 20; Arabic text, Bergsträsser, *Ḥunain ibn Isḥāq*, 17, 15–18; 18, 6–18. The numbers in square brackets have been added here for discussion's sake.

33 See D. Pingree, art. 'Banū Mūsā', *Enc. Ir.* iii. 716b–17b.

34 Quoted according to Rosenthal, *Classical Heritage*, 17.

35 For a discussion of these translation approaches, see Brock, 'Aspects of Translation Technique', 69.

36 Le Coz, *Les médecins nestoriens*; the programmatic title of his book, *Les médecins nestoriens au Moyen Âge: Les maîtres des Arabes* (Nestorian Physicians in the Middle Ages: The Masters of the Arabs), reflects his approach to the subject matter. Dimitri Gutas, *Greek Thought*, gives a very different version.

37 Lewis, *What Went Wrong*, 139.

38 Paul Kunitzsch, 'Über das Frühstadium', 269–70, had already made the point in 1975 that Alexandria determined the agenda.

39 Giuseppe Serra has recently investigated the impact of the Arabic translation of Aristotle's *Poetics* on ideas about Greek comedy and tragedy, and emphasised that not only the Arabic, but also the Greek and Syriac traditions of Late Antiquity, had no first-hand experience of their performance; see Serra, *Da 'tragedia'*, esp. 59; and also Heinrichs, *Arabische Dichtung*. For the *monostichoi*, see Ullmann, *Arabische Überlieferung*; for the papyrus fragments of Menander, see Easterling, 'Menander'. For reception of poetry and drama in the modern Arabic world, see Pormann, 'The Arab "Cultural Awakening (*Nahḍa*)"'.

40 Franz Rosenthal's quotation is found in art. 'Yūnān (Greece)', *EI*² xi. 343b–345a, on 344a; for the reception of the Alexander Romance, see Doufikar-Aerts, *Alexander Magnus Arabicus*; for the Arab view of Byzantium, El Cheikh, *Byzantium*.

41 Gutas, *Greek Thought*, 53–60, esp. 58–9.

42 See Ullmann, *WGAÜ*; and Pormann, *Oriental Tradition*, 127–32.

43 Quoted according to Ullmann, *WGAÜ*, entry *hydrokēlē*.

44 For a terminological study of ophthalmology, see Pormann, *Oriental Tradition*, 135–205; for 'erysipelas', see Ullmann, *WGAÜ*, entry *erysipelas*.

45 The example is taken from Endress and Gutas, *Greek–Arabic Lexicon*, entry *'lh*; Galen iv. 780 Kühn, Biesterfeldt, *Galens Traktat*, 43, 13.

46 Littré, *Œuvres complètes d'Hippocrate*, iv. 628; Ibn Abī Uṣaybi'ah, *Sources of Information*, i. 25, 18–19; this example is already mentioned in Ullmann, *Islamic Medicine*, 30–31; see Ullmann, *WGAÜ*, entry *Asklēpios*.

47 The quotation occurs in Galen, *Anatomical Procedures*, ii. 386, 5 (Kühn); i. 178, 15 (Garofalo). The passage was also translated and discussed by Savage-Smith, 'Attitudes toward Dissection', 89. For the general attitude of Islam towards children, see Gil'adi, *Children of Islam*.

48 For Ṭabarī, see Siggel, *Die Indischen Bücher*.
49 F. Klein-Franke, art. '*Ṭibb* 2', *EI*[2] x. 460a–61a; Klein-Franke and Zhu, 'Rashīd ad-Dīn as a Transmitter'; Klein-Franke and Zhu, 'Rashīd ad-Dīn and the *Tansuqnamah*'.
50 tr. [modified] Rosenthal, *Muqaddimah*, i. 61.

2

Medical theory

> Medicine is a science from which one learns the states of the human body with respect to what is healthy and what is not, in order to preserve good health when it exists and restore it when it is lacking.
> – Ibn Sīnā (d. 1037)[1]

> The physician, even though he has his doubts, must always make the patient believe that he will recover, for the state of the body is linked to the state of the mind.
> – attributed to al-Rāzī (d. 925)[2]

> Whoever has been occupied with the science of anatomy has increased his belief in God.
> – attributed to Ibn Rushd (Averroes, d. 1198)[3]

The definition of medicine with which Ibn Sīnā (later known to Europeans as Avicenna) opened his famous *Canon of Medicine* – and which begins this chapter as well – illustrates the continuation of the Graeco-Roman medical tradition, for it was derived from Galen's treatise *On [Medical] Sects for Beginners*. Remarkably, we have preserved today a copy of the Arabic translation of Galen's treatise that in the year 1016 was in the possession of Ibn Sīnā himself, some two decades before he died. The title page with the dated note in his handwriting is illustrated in Figure 2.1.

The laudable aim of restoring and preserving good health assumes the ability to recognise disease and its causes. Defining disease at this time, however, was problematic, and averting or curing it very difficult indeed. Symptoms in the modern sense were often classified as diseases. Fevers, for example, were considered medical conditions in their own right. These were difficult issues at a time when there was no way to observe the internal functioning of the human body and almost no methods of quantifying data. It must be remembered that physicians did not have x-rays or imaging techniques at their disposal, not even stethoscopes with which to listen to the working of the body, nor microscopes with which to observe bacteria or minute structures.

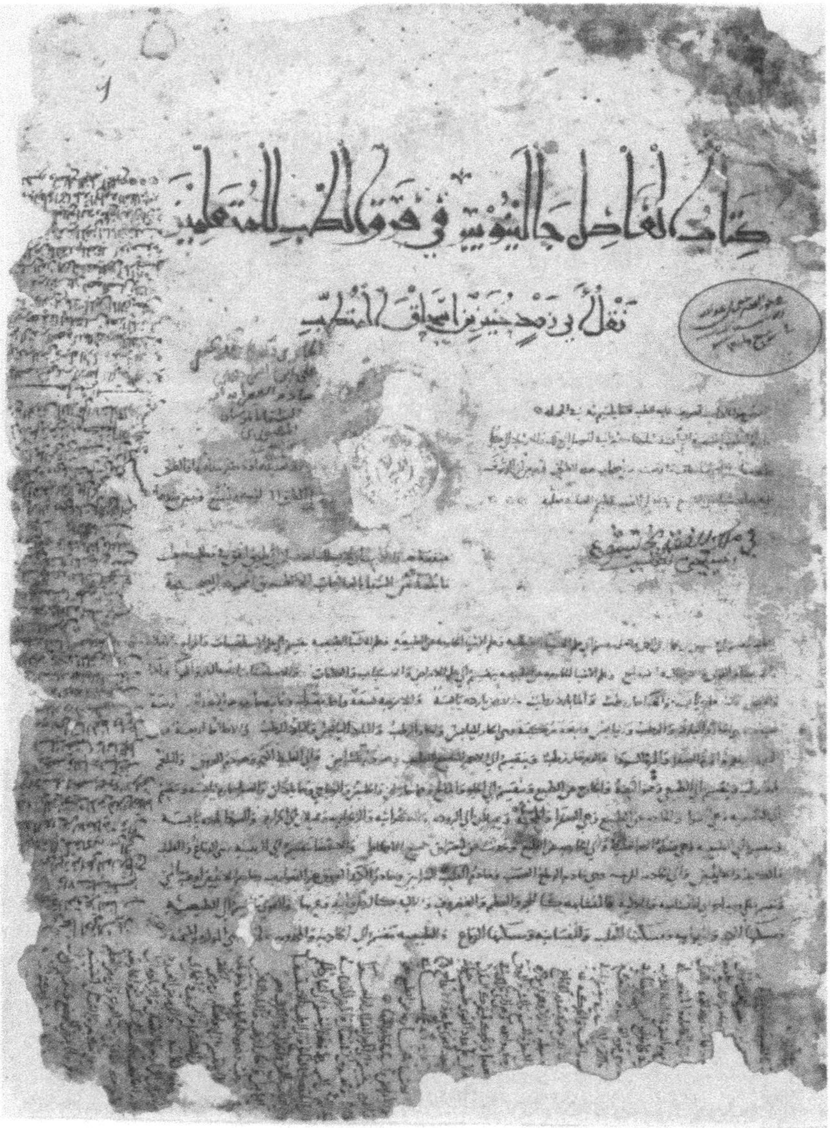

Figure 2.1 A copy of the Arabic translation of Galen's *On* [*Medical*] *Sects for Beginners*, with important owners' signatures. Circled, to the right beneath the title, is the *ex libris* of Ibn Sīnā, dated 1016 (407 H); it reads: 'In the possession of (*fī ḥawz al-faqīr*) Ḥusayn ibn 'Abd Allāh Ibn Sīnā, the physician (*mutaṭabbib*)'. At the middle right of the page another *ex libris* occurs for a member of the Bukhtīshū' family: 'Property (*fī mulk*) of the humble Bukhtīshū', the Christian physician (*mutaṭabbib*)'. In the left-hand margin, written upside down, is a note by one 'Alī ibn Ibrāhīm who signs himself a physician at the Manṣūrī hospital in Cairo.

Man, the Cosmos, and Humoral Pathology

The single most pervasive explanatory medical principle was that of humoral pathology inherited from the Greeks. In this theory, the body was thought to be made up of four humours (*akhlāṭ*, plural of *khilṭ*): blood, phlegm, yellow bile, and black bile. Each humour was associated with two of the four primary qualities (hot or cold, and dry or moist), one of the four seasons, and a 'temperament' (sanguine, phlegmatic, choleric, and melancholic). Finally, the four ages of man, the months, and the apparent rotation of the zodiacal signs were linked to this system. Thus the function of the human body (the microcosm) was related to and reflected the movements of the heavens (macrocosm); see Figure 2.2.

Though no person had a perfect balance, an excess of one of the humours (such as blood) was considered harmful and therefore needed to be counter-balanced through diet or removed through such measures as blood letting or purging. Two practices often advocated in medieval medicine – venesection (also called phlebotomy) and cupping – are to be understood in the context of this humoral pathology: a surplus of blood was removed either by opening a vein

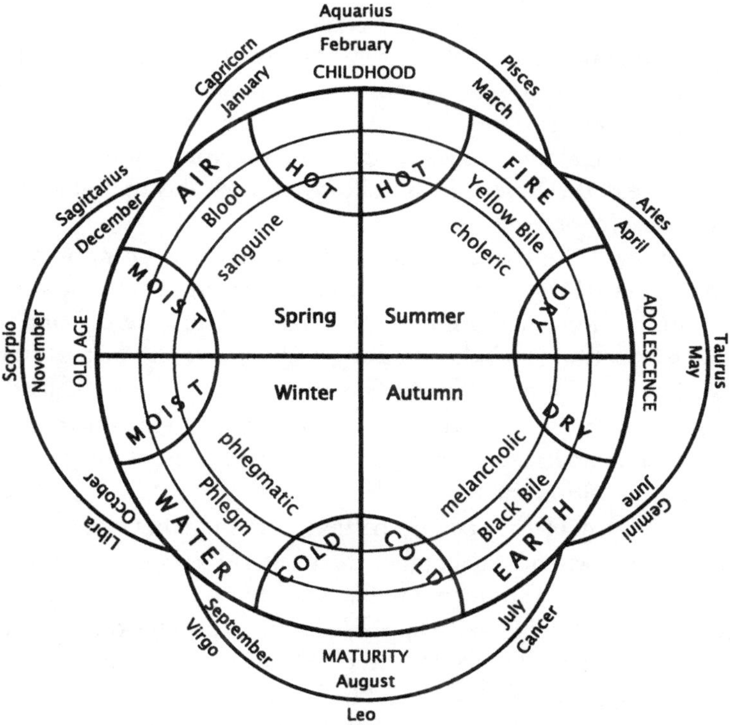

Figure 2.2 The four elements, humours, primary qualities, and temperaments as they relate to the seasons, the ages of man, the months, and the zodiacal constellations.

or by putting a heated cupping glass onto skin that had been lightly scarified. As proof that excess of blood was harmful, writers often cited the fact that women, by loosing blood during their menstrual cycle, suffer less than men from gout, arthritis, epilepsy, and apoplexy. Phlegm (*balgham* in Arabic, derived from the Greek word *phlegma*) was a viscous moisture or mucus readily evident in various discharges of the body. Yellow bile (*mirrah ṣafrā'*), often said to be red in colour despite its name, was generally considered a foam or scum produced during the formation of blood. After its production in the liver, half the yellow bile flowed with the venous blood while the other half was said to go to the gallbladder; several subcategories of yellow bile were enumerated. Black bile (*mirrah sawdā'*), the final in the sequence, was usually interpreted as a sedimentary dark material also produced during blood formation; half of it remained in the blood with the other half going to the spleen. Thus the fluid carried by the veins was considered a mixture of the pure humour blood plus yellow and black bile. Both the third and fourth humours were highly hypothetical, and speculations were rife and varied as to their natures. That portion of the yellow bile that was siphoned off to the gallbladder can be compared to what we know today as bile – a golden-brown to greenish-yellow and bitter fluid secreted by the liver and poured into the small intestines via the bile ducts, and concentrated in the gallbladder. The other portion of the yellow bile that was said to flow with the venous blood has no clear counterpart in today's physiology. Similarly, black bile has no obvious equivalent in modern terms, though the darkest part of coagulated blood is black, and dark material is occasionally found in vomit, urine, and excrement. The existence of these two biles was, however, necessary to postulate in order to complete the symmetry of the system.

Health could often be regained by adjustment of the 'six non-naturals' – that is, factors external to the body over which a person could have some control: surrounding air, food, and drink, sleeping and waking, exercise and rest, retention and evacuation (including bathing and coitus), and mental states (anger, sadness, joy, love, and so forth). The term 'non-natural' was used for those circumstances which a person could in part control, while 'natural' referred to the system of humours, elements, qualities, and other properties and forces (such as age) at work within the body itself.

That the first of the six non-naturals, air (together with other environmental aspects), was fundamental to the health of a population was made clear by Ibn Riḍwān (d. c. 1068), an irascible and argumentative Egyptian physician, in his treatise *On the Prevention of Bodily Ills in Egypt*. This tract was intended to refute the work of the North African physician Ibn al-Jazzār (d. 980), who had argued that Egypt was a very unhealthy place. Ibn Riḍwān in fact agreed with the conclusion of Ibn al-Jazzār, but felt that he was right for the wrong reasons, not having properly understood the cause of disease in Egypt. The Hippocratic treatise *Airs, Waters, and Places* was widely read by the general literate public as well as by physicians. Its assertion that the quality of the soil, the condition of the water, and the nature of wind and weather were constantly influencing the human body was crucial in shaping notions of a meteorological medicine and a geographical pathology. Its influence can be seen in the following comments by Ibn Riḍwān on the poor sanitary conditions of Old Cairo (Fusṭāṭ):

> Hippocrates has shown that low-lying places are hotter than elevated ones and that the air in the former is worse because of the accumulation of vapours. The higher districts surrounding them hinder the penetration of the wind. The alleys and streets of Fusṭāṭ are narrow, and their buildings are high ... The people of Fusṭāṭ are in the habit of throwing cats, dogs, and other domestic animals that die in their homes out into the streets and alleys where they decay, and their corruption mixes with the air. In addition, they customarily throw animal droppings and carrion into the Nile, from which they drink. The sewers from the latrines also empty into the Nile. Sometimes, when the flow of water is cut off, the people drink this corruption mingled with the water. In Fusṭāṭ there are large hearths for the baths, from which excessive smoke rises into the air. Moreover, there is a great deal of dust because the soil is fine, so that in the summertime the air appears dingy. It affects breathing, and clean clothes become dirty in one day ... Of all the inhabitants of Egypt, those of Fusṭāṭ are the ones who most quickly succumb to illnesses.[4]

Thus humoral theory, combined with the 'six non-naturals', provided the explanatory basis for the cause and nature of illness as well as the theoretical framework within which it was to be treated.

Structure and function of the body

The Greek concept of *pneuma* (literally, 'wind' or 'breath') formed an important part of the explanation of bodily functions, as did what were called 'faculties'. There were three pneumas: natural pneuma (*rūḥ ṭabīʿī*, in Arabic) that originated in the liver and was distributed throughout the body by way of the veins; animal or vital pneuma (*rūḥ ḥayawānī*) produced in the heart and distributed via the arteries; and psychic pneuma (*rūḥ nafsānī*) formed in the ventricles of the brain and dispersed through the nerves. Similarly, there were three faculties: the natural faculty (*quwá ṭabīʿīyah*), seated in the liver and responsible for maintaining growth and reproduction; the animal or vital faculty (*quwá ḥayawānīyah*), located in the heart and responsible for respiration and emotions; and the psychic faculty (*quwá nafsānīyah*), based in the brain and responsible for sensory perception and thought processes.

Food was digested or 'cooked' in the stomach, passed through the pylorus into the duodenum and then into the small intestine. From there the veins absorbed the nutritious constituents and transported them through the portal vein into the liver where they were converted into blood. The venous blood

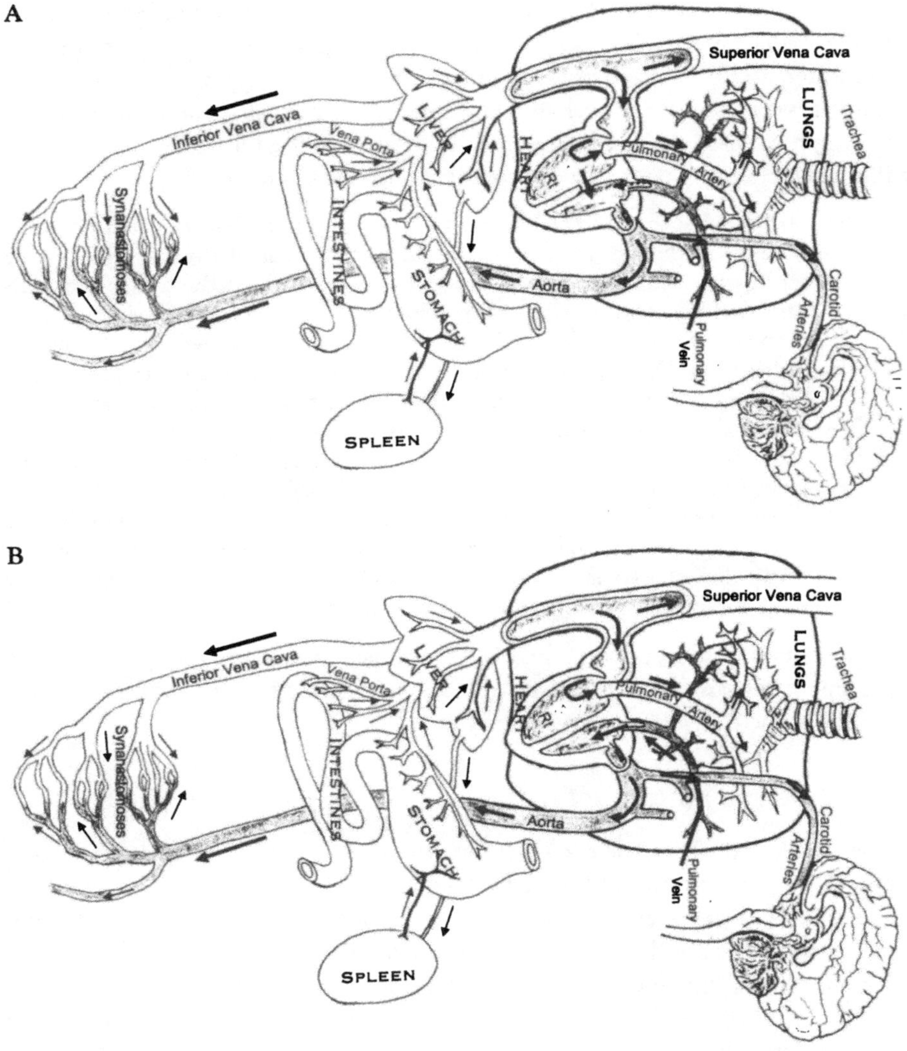

Figure 2.3 **A**: The movement of blood according to the Galenic model, followed by most Islamic physicians. **B**: The movement of blood according to Ibn al-Nafīs.

then moves through the vena cava to the other organs and parts of the body (see Figure 2.3A). Via the vena cava it also reaches the right ventricle of the heart, where a valve formed of three small membranes prevents the return of the blood back into the vena cava. From the right ventricle, the pulmonary artery (called the 'arterial vein', a vein with the structure of an artery) takes blood to the lungs. In the left ventricle, air from the lungs moves down the pulmonary vein (the 'venous artery', an artery with the structure of a vein) and mixes with blood, forming arterial blood, which is visibly different from venous blood. A movement in the opposite direction through the pulmonary vein allows the passage of this necessary arterial blood into the lungs. So, the question became: how did blood get into the left ventricle of the heart?

Galen had suggested that there were minute connections in the lungs between the branches of the pulmonary artery and pulmonary vein, but he also asserted that the majority of the blood was shunted from the right to left ventricle through small, essentially invisible, passages in the thick wall separating the left from the right side of the heart (see Figure 2.3A). Most Islamic physicians followed Galen in his explanation of pulmonary bloodflow, though reducing the number of tiny passages in the interventricular septum to one.

This interpretation was, however, challenged by the thirteenth-century Syrian physician Ibn al-Nafīs (d. 1288), who spent much of his working life in Cairo. Not only had he prepared a highly successful epitome of the *Canon of Medicine* by Ibn Sīnā (d. 1037), but he also composed a commentary on it. In his commentary on the anatomy in the *Canon*, preserved today in a copy completed 46 years before his death, Ibn al-Nafīs asserted, correctly, that the blood in the right ventricle of the heart must reach the left ventricle by way of the lungs alone and not through a passage connecting the ventricles, as Galen had maintained. This formulation of the pulmonary transit was an important challenge to the Galenic anatomy then universally accepted, though Ibn al-Nafīs' revision received little subsequent attention in the Islamic world, except for two fourteenth-century Arabic physicians who knew of it. The pulmonary transit is sometimes erroneously termed the pulmonary circulation or 'lesser' circulation. There is, however, no notion of a circular return of blood from the second chamber (the left ventricle) back to the first chamber (the right ventricle). The transit or circuit of blood through the lungs, from the first chamber of the heart to the second, implies connections between the arterial and venous systems in the lungs, but the direction of blood flow was essentially unidirectional.[5]

This 'discovery' of the pulmonary transit is of course not equivalent, as some modern writers have suggested, to the demonstration of the continuous circular motion of blood throughout the body published by William Harvey in 1628. According to the medieval (and earlier Greek) conception of the functioning of the system, nutritive blood produced by the liver was distributed through the veins to all the organs and peripheral parts of the body, while blood enhanced with vital pneuma flowed through the arteries to all parts of the body. Both the blood in the veins and that in the arteries was totally expended as it flowed outward to the peripheral organs, for all organs absorb and consume blood as part of their functioning and what we would call today metabolic processes.

Galen had allowed, however, that there must be at least some invisible end-to-end junctions ('synanastomoses') between peripheral blood vessels, since cutting an artery can drain the body of venous as well as arterial blood. Harvey, on the other hand, demonstrated conclusively that there had to be a direct connection between the venous and arterial systems throughout the body, and not just in the lungs. Most importantly, he argued that the beat of the heart produced a continuous circulation of blood through minute connections at the extremities of the body. This is a conceptual leap that was quite different from Ibn al-Nafīs' refinement of the anatomy and bloodflow in the heart and lungs.[6]

Mind and body

The importance of the patient's state of mind when treating an illness is a constant theme throughout the literature, exemplified by the aphorism attributed to the Baghdad clinician al-Rāzī (d. 925), known to Europeans as Rhazes or Rasis, quoted at the beginning of the present chapter. The relationship between mind and body had occupied Greek physicians and continued to be a subject of speculation amongst Islamic medical writers. The issue was of particular importance when defining and explaining mental illness, but also had a more general application. As we have just seen, one of the six non-naturals is the mental state of the patients, and, as such, it affects their health directly. Sadness and anxiety are to be avoided, and music, as well as pleasant company, and a quiet environment can contribute to the convalescence.[7]

In this context, moral philosophy also had ramifications for medicine. One aspect of moral philosophy concerned the achievement of happiness, which was thought to be conducive to good health. Consequently, physicians occasionally wrote works dealing with the topic. An early tenth-century example is al-Rāzī's treatise *On Spiritual Medicine*, in which he made a case for the pursuit of pure knowledge and the avoidance of 'afflictions of the soul' (*'awāriḍ al-nafs*). By the latter term he meant mental states – desire, regret, and fear – caused by a variety of human inclinations such as greed, lust, anger, envy, or fear of death. The reasons for avoiding the afflictions of the soul were philosophical arguments, as, for instance, that the 'man of intellect' should not resemble brute beasts. As a medical man, al-Rāzī used his knowledge of physiology to make his points more efficiently. To take a specific example: among the things to be avoided, al-Rāzī mentioned sexual intercourse (*jimā'*), 'because it weakens the eyesight, wrecks and exhausts the body, speeds up aging, senility, and withering, damages the brain and the nerves, and renders the [bodily] strength weak and feeble, in addition to many other conditions which would take too long to mention'. A sober life is a better and healthier life. Moral philosophy is thus applied as a means of avoiding afflictions of the soul that ultimately lead to ailments of the body. Al-Rāzī's general advice to avoid sex did not prevent him from writing a book entitled *On Sexual Intercourse, its Harmful and Beneficial Effects, and Treatment*. Injunctions to have sex with slave girls, in order to improve one's mood in the case of certain mental disorders such as melancholy, also occur in the medical as well as the specialist literature on sexual hygiene.[8]

A century after al-Rāzī, Ibn Sīnā composed a work titled *The Book of the Cure* (*Kitāb al-Shifā'*). It became a particularly famous treatise employing philosophy as a means of curing the soul. Its title could suggest that it is a medical work, but this is not the case; it actually is a philosophical encyclopedia with 'Cure' used in the title in the sense of curing the soul of ignorance. Yet, in choosing this title, Ibn Sīnā was perhaps motivated by the same idea that philosophy could provide spiritual health that in turn could influence bodily well-being.

Regimen and diet

Regimen and diet dominated the therapeutic arsenal, with non-interventionist techniques being preferred to more invasive practices. In other words, much of the medicine involved what today we would call a 'holistic' approach.

A great deal of common sense was employed in determining diet and regimen. When ill, for example, the diet was often restricted to broths, especially barley-water (ptisane), and honey mixed in water (hydromel) or honey mixed with water and vinegar (oxymel). The Egyptian Jewish doctor Ya'qūb ibn Isḥāq (d. c. 1208) showed particular concern about improper medical care during a visit to Damascus around the year 1202. In his *Treatise on the Errors of the Damascene Physicians*, he gave the following instructions:

> The physician must pay attention to the patient's strength, the matter of the disease, and its duration; for if the strength is weak, but the disease-matter plentiful and the duration long, then the patient should be offered from the very beginning something which sustains the strength while not increasing the disease-matter – and there is nothing more appropriate for that than the right amount of chicken broth. Moreover, the physician must consider what exactly to give the patient, for if the strength is good, and both disease-matter and duration are average, then barley-water on its own is normally sufficient. Yet, the physician may have to resort to something more nutritious than that. In general, there is no set time in the course of a disease at which to employ chicken broth and other such nutriment – which is to say that it is permissible to give it on the third, fourth, fifth, actually on any given day of the disease, as soon as it becomes apparent that the physical strength has weakened, particularly if accompanied by a symptom indicating a lengthy illness.[9]

A similar need for observation and intuition had been called for by Ibn Sīnā when assessing the causes and alleviation of pain in his *Canon of Medicine*, the most influential of all medieval Islamic medical encyclopedias:

> One can frequently make a mistake regarding pains, for their causes may be external, such as heat or cold, or an incorrect arrangement of the pillow, or a poor bed, or a fall during drunkenness, and other such things. For then one is wrong to seek in the body for the cause of the pain ... Frequently there is no need for strong measures such as evacuation and the like, since bathing and sound sleep are often sufficient ... By necessity there is a limit to the strength of the patient, and so the physician must determine which period of time will be the longer, that of strength or that of the pain, and also which is more harmful, the pain or the inherent danger of the pain-killer. For sometimes continuous pain can cause death by its intensity, and sometimes insensibility to pain can kill or be harmful in another way ... Water in an animal bladder may be applied as a compress, being safe and mild, but burns can occur if care is not taken ... Among the means of lessening pain is gentle, long walking, because of the relaxation in it. Similarly, methods of alleviating pain include [massage using] the well-known light fats and oils already mentioned, sweet music especially when accompanied by sleep, and being occupied with something very enjoyable.[10]

Such practical changes in diet and routine were presented both in chapters on general regimen in medical compendia, such as that by Ibn Sīnā, and in monographs on the topic. The most popular of all such monographs was the *Almanac of Health* by a Christian physician of Baghdad, Ibn Buṭlān (d. 1066), in which he set out the regimen of the 'six non-naturals'. In the course of 40 synoptic tables, he presented 210 plants and animals and 70 other items and procedures useful for maintaining good health, including the use of music, the regulation of sleep and exercise, bathing, fumigations, the alteration of air quality, and seasonal changes. He accompanied all 280 topics by recommendations from various authorities whose names were represented by abbreviations. Above and below each table he set out forty canons (*qānūns*), expounding the principles of dietetics and regimen. This imaginatively structured manual enjoyed wide currency not only in the Arabic-speaking world but also in medieval and Renaissance Europe where elaborate illustrations were introduced to enhance the visual structure.[11]

Medical compendia routinely had sections devoted to regimens for infants and for the elderly, both groups requiring special adjustments in diet and other routines. Occasionally regimen for travellers would be treated in a separate section. Another subtopic that attracted particular attention was that of sexual hygiene, with a considerable number of monographs devoted to the topic. The treatises often provided cosmetic procedures for making a person more attractive, such as removing unwanted hair, and they usually included procedures useful for enhancing the pleasure of sexual intercourse as well as recipes for aphrodisiacs, for ensuring the production of offspring, and occasionally for contraception. A typical example of a recipe for countering impotency is given in the influential treatise *Provisions for the Traveller and Nourishment for the Sedentary*, written in Kairouan by the physician Ibn al-Jazzār (d. 980):

> A recipe for a pastille which I have composed that will increase sexual desire, refresh the soul, warm the body, expel gas from the stomach, put an end to coldness of the kidneys and bladder, and increase memory: Taken in the winter, it will warm the limbs. Its uses are many, and it is one of the 'royal electuaries', and I have named it 'reliable against calamities' (*mā'mūn al-ghawā'il*). Take seven *mithqāls* each of Chinese cinnamon, sweet cost, Indian spikenard, saffron, fennel seeds, ginger, dried mint leaves, wild mountain thyme, mountain mint, cinnamon bark; of Indian 'malabathron', long pepper, white pepper, black pepper, asarabacca, plum seeds, cultivated caraway, cloves, galingale, and wild carrot, four *mithqāls* each; of pellitory, cardamon, radish seeds, and turnip seeds, two *mithqāls* each; and of hulled sesame, shelled walnuts, shelled pistachios, shelled fresh almonds, pinenuts, and sugar candy, eleven *mithqāls* each. Pulverise the ingredients, sieve vigorously, combine, and knead with honey of wild thyme, from which the froth has been skimmed, until the remedy is well mixed. Store in a vessel that is smooth on the inside, fumigated with Indian aloes. An amount the size of a walnut is to be taken before and after meals. And it will be efficacious, God willing.[12]

Pharmacology

There were two major Greek pharmaceutical sources available through Arabic translations: Dioscorides' treatise *On Medicinal Substances*, which described slightly more than 1,000 substances, and Galen's treatise *On the Powers of Simple Drugs*. In the former, Dioscorides allotted to each plant, mineral, and animal product attributes such as warming, softening, astringent, diuretical, sleep-inducing, or emetic. He structured the treatise, as he announced in his introduction, 'according to the properties of the individual drugs', grouping the substances into five books: Book I on spices, oils, salves, trees, and shrubs; Book II on animal parts and products as well as cereals and herbs; Book III on roots, juices, herbs, and seeds; Book IV on herbs and roots not discussed previously; and Book V on wines and minerals. See Figure 2.4 for an illustration from Book IV in which later readers have annotated the Greek copy with Arabic and Hebrew terms.[13]

So important was the treatise by Dioscorides that it was translated and revised several times. A Syriac version was translated into Arabic in Baghdad in the ninth century. Around 948, the emperor of Constantinople, Constantine VII, offered a beautifully illustrated copy of Dioscorides' treatise, in the original Greek language, to the Umayyad caliph at Córdoba, 'Abd al-Raḥmān al-Nāṣir (r. 912–961), along with a Latin *History of Orosius*. The caliph had to ask the Byzantine emperor to send someone to translate the treatise from the Greek, for there was no one at the court in Córdoba who could do that, though they could translate the Latin book. In 951 the monk Nicholas was sent from Constantinople, and he worked with a team of Arab and Jewish scholars to revise the earlier Arabic version, using this new manuscript and adapting terminology to

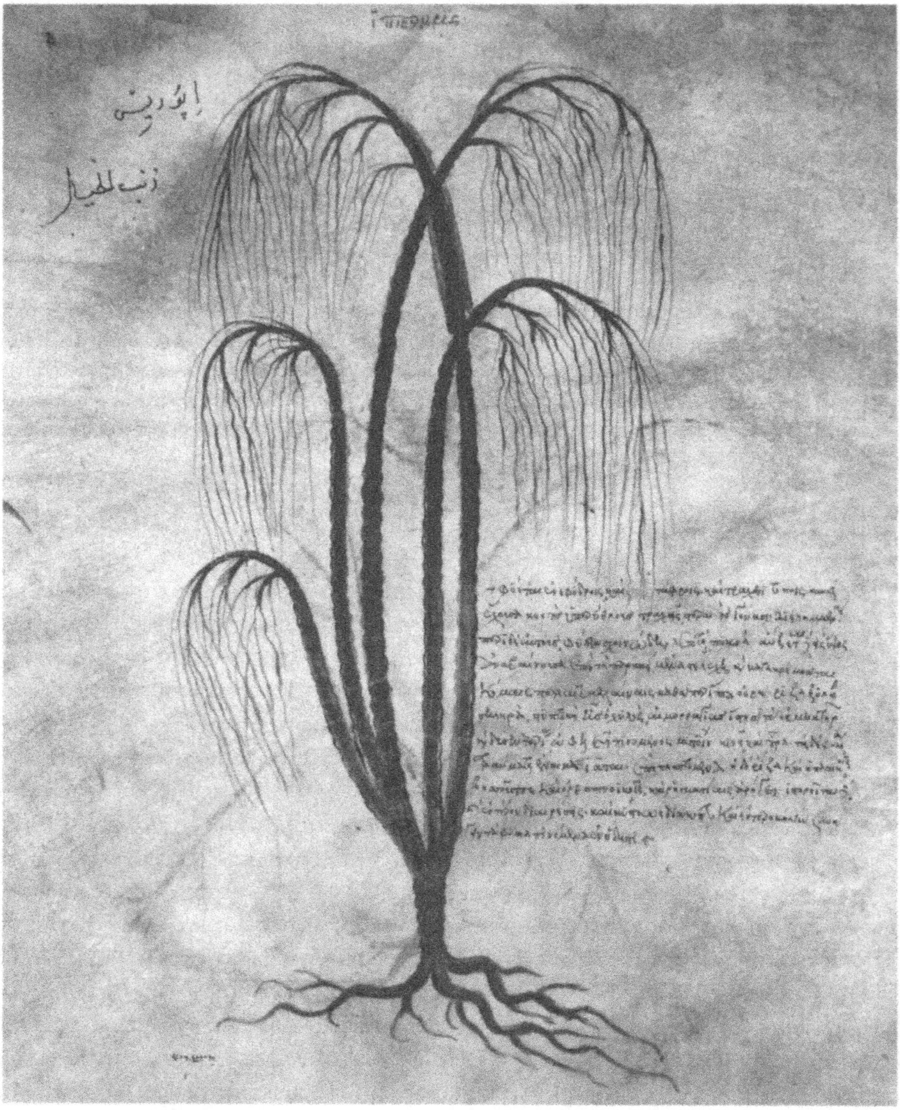

Figure 2.4 The illustration of 'horsetail', a variety of *Equisetum sylvaticum* L., from a copy made about 510 of the Greek treatise by Dioscorides on medicinal substances. The Greek name of the plant, *hippouris*, has been written in Arabic script by a later reader, along with the Arabic translation of the plant name: *dhanab al-khayl* 'the tail of the horse'. At the bottom of the page, the Greek name is transliterated into Hebrew.

reflect the Hispano-Arabic nomenclature of Muslim Spain. Later re-adaptations were made in eastern provinces of the Islamic empire.

While drawing heavily upon Dioscorides, Galen was innovative in two respects and, in doing so, set the format for most Arabic writings on the subject. First, he listed the medicinal substances in alphabetical order. Second, he fine-tuned the system of classification by assigning to each medicament a pair of the primary qualities (dry or moist, warm or cool) and grading their intensity on a scale from one (weakest) to four (strongest). Acacia, for instance, is drying in the third degree, and cooling in the first – or the second, when washed. By recognising and employing these properties, a physician could attempt to counterbalance the humours and qualities in patients.[14]

A considerable proportion of the plants described by Dioscorides and Galen would not have been known in various regions of the Middle East. The differing climatic conditions of the desert, marsh, mountain, and costal communities meant that species of medicinal plants, as well as animals and minerals, varied greatly from one region to another. Sometimes related local species and varieties could be identified as similar to those described by Dioscorides or Galen, but in other instances the substances described in the Greek sources meant little to an Arab practitioner. For this reason many Arabic and Persian authors would provide synonym lists giving equivalents in different languages such as Classical Greek (*Yūnānīyah)*, Byzantine Greek (*Rūmīyah*), Latin, Syriac, Persian, Hindi, Berber, and Spanish. These lists, however, are not very consistent in their assignments of local terms, and much of the interest appears to have been antiquarian rather than practical.[15]

The wide and varied geographic horizons of Islamic writers, however, brought them into contact with new drugs. It was for this reason that Ibn Juljul (d. c. 994), a physician of Córdoba who participated in the translation of Dioscorides, also wrote a treatise on medicaments not mentioned by Dioscorides. Traders and travellers played as important a role in the knowledge and development of medicinal substances in the Islamic world as did the treatises of Dioscorides and Galen in their Arabic dress. Because drugs from India, for example, might not be readily available in North Africa, nor those from Spain in Baghdad, and less expensive ingredients were sometimes wanted, treatises were written on substitute drugs. Greek physicians such as Paul of Aegina had previously listed medicinal substances that could be substituted one for another, but the genre expanded at the hands of Islamic physicians.[16]

Most influential of all the Arabic treatises on basic medicinal substances, *materia medica*, was the manual by Ibn al-Bayṭār (d. 1248), originally from Malaga in the kingdom of Granada. His *Comprehensive Book on Simple Drugs and Foodstuffs* was an alphabetical guide to over 1,400 medicaments in 2,324 separate entries, taken from his own observations as well as over 260 written sources which he quoted. His enormous manual formed the basis of many later guides to medicaments.

Recipes for compound remedies were recorded in formularies, called *aqrābādhīn* in Arabic from the Greek *graphidion* meaning 'prescription', and usually arranged by type or class of compound, such as eye remedies, syrups, gargles, dentifrices, emetics, suppositories, poultices, dressings, and so forth. Such formularies could form part of a medical compendium or could circulate as a separate treatise, as that by the early polymath al-Kindī (d. after 870).[17]

Formularies were also associated with hospital dispensaries. For instance, a Christian physician of Baghdad by the name of Sābūr ibn Sahl (d. 869) wrote such a pharmacopoeia which was still being used in the following century by the hospital physician al-Kaskarī in Baghdad. In fact it remained the most important medical formulary until that complied by Ibn al-Tilmīdh (d. 1165) for use in the 'Aḍudī hospital founded in Baghdad in 981. A version of Sābūr's *Formulary* adapted for the same hospital is still preserved today in a Munich manuscript. In the hospitals in Egypt and Syria, the *Hospital Formulary* by the Jewish apothecary Ibn Abī al-Bayān (d. c. 1240) was in common use. The following is a typical entry, in this instance employing one ingredient not known to Greek physicians, the plum-like fruit of a variety of myrobalan, a genus of tropical trees that came to be used extensively in compound remedies as well as in the dying and tanning industries:

> Another recipe for a confection that is a 'cordial' (*mufarriḥ*), useful for palpitations of the heart, pains of the chest (lit. heart) and stomach, and jaundice due to causes arising from the cold: mix together 5 dirhams each of cinnamon, clove, Chinese cinnamon, and hyacinth; 10 dirhams each of lichen, bugloss, wild pomegranate flower, and basil; and 3 dirhams each of saffron and [flowers of] the mastic tree. All of it is to be pounded, sifted, and then kneaded with three times its weight of honey from emblic myrobalan. Then 2 to 3 *mithqāls* of it are to be taken with a drink.[18]

The formulary of Ibn Abī al-Bayān was eventually surpassed in popularity by that compiled about 1260 by another Jewish physician, al-Kūhīn al-'Aṭṭār. Similarly, other regions had their popular formularies. In Muslim Spain, however, compilations of compound remedies seem not to have been as popular as treatises concerned with individual plants and medicinal substances.[19]

The topic of poisons was also of interest in both antiquity and in medieval Islam. Two chapters on the subject were falsely ascribed to Dioscorides. Though known by medieval Arabic writers to be not genuine works, the chapters were usually appended to Arabic copies of Dioscorides' treatise *On Medicinal Substances*. A rich Arabic literature on the topic soon developed, one of the earliest being that on poisons by Ibn Waḥshīyah (*fl.* before 912), who also composed agricultural and alchemical treatises. Snake and dog bites as well as the deleterious effects of scorpions, spiders and other animals caused much concern, while the poisonous properties of various minerals and plants, such as aconite, mandrake, and black hellebore, were exploited.

Diagnosis and prognosis

Diagnosis and prognosis involved recognising the patient's temperament and the humoral balance, whilst taking into account as well the seasonal and environmental factors, physical symptoms, and the account of the illness given by the patient. It was particularly important that a physician be able to see when a case was impossible to cure, and thus avoid undertaking to treat it. Moreover, the ability to predict if and when a patient might die was both a means of self-protection on the part of the physician and a way of demonstrating great skill in the craft.

Examination of the pulse was a basic diagnostic tool. The topic figured prominently in every medical encyclopedia, such as *Complete Book of the Medical Art* (also called *The Royal Book*) by al-Majūsī (*fl.* 983), who dedicated his compendium to ʿAḍud al-Dawlah, the ruler of Persia and Iraq from 949 to 983. *The Royal Book* was a major source for the chapter on the pulse included by al-Sulamī (d. 1208), 'chief physician' in Egypt and Syria, in his *Experts' Examination of all Physicians*, written in question-and-answer format:

> Question Sixteen: How is the pulse of someone who suffers from anxiety? Answer: This is recorded in *The Royal Book*. Slight, weak, and irregular. If it [the anxiety] continues until it consumes the [vital] faculty, the pulse becomes worm-like and then ant-like [increasingly faint] while the [vital] faculty declines and disappears.[20]

Equally important was the examination of the urine. The major monograph on the subject, cited by most subsequent writers, was the *Book on Urine* by Isḥāq ibn Sulaymān al-Isrā'īlī (d. c. 932), of an Egyptian Jewish family who migrated to Kairouan (al-Qayrawān), then capital of Ifrīqiyah (modern Tunisia). The subject was basic, however, to the earliest Arabic treatises, as well as to the earlier Greek literature. A large portion of Ḥunayn ibn Isḥāq's ninth-century *Questions on Medicine for Beginners* was devoted to diagnosis by urine, an example being:

> When there is blood and pus in the urine, what does it indicate? It indicates that without doubt there is an ulcer, although it does not localize the ulcer in a specified organ. However, it is either in the kidneys, or in the bladder, or in one of the two ureters, or in one of the organs above them.[21]

Diseases specific to one bodily part

The basic knowledge of diseases and their symptoms was derived from the Greek medical literature. Islamic physicians, however, were keen observers and in many instances they elaborated new details. In a few instances Arabic physicians described for the first time pathological conditions apparently unknown to the Greeks. The description of smallpox and measles occurs for the first time in Arabic literature. Haemophilia appears to have been unknown or unrecognised amongst the Greeks, but is described in Islamic medical treatises, perhaps prompted by the practice of circumcision. The observational acuteness of al-Rāzī in ninth-century Baghdad is evident in his description of the production of catarrh as an allergic reaction to the scent of roses – in other words, a form of hay fever. On the other hand, certain conspicuous diseases that are now endemic to the region, such as bilharzia (or schistosomiasis, a parasitic infection with trematode worms) in Egypt, escaped their attention, perhaps suggesting a reduced incidence at that time.

Diseases could be classified in various ways. Al-Majūsī in his *Complete Book of the Medical Art* grouped them into two general categories: internal and external. The causes and symptoms of internal afflictions were then discussed in order from head to toe: headache, epilepsy, and melancholy (all three thought to originate in the brain), eye diseases, ear diseases, digestive disorders, and so forth. External diseases were subdivided into three groups: those with visible external manifestations such as fevers and tumours, those occurring superficially (smallpox, leprosy, scabies, itching, lice), and those not related to certain parts of the body (wounds and lesions, animal and insect bites, poisons).[22]

Ibn Sīnā, whose *Canon of Medicine* soon dominated medical discourse, organised the material slightly differently. For him, the major division was between diseases specific to one part of the body and those not specific to any single part. For those in the first category, the causes, symptoms, and treatments were also presented in order from head to toe.

Some disorders were the subjects of monographs. Eye diseases, in particular, generated their own specialised literature that will be discussed later in more detail. Both Ibn Sīnā and his predecessor al-Rāzī wrote essays just on colic (*qawlanj*, a term that could also include intestinal obstruction). Haemorrhoids were the subject of many monographs, including an especially popular short Arabic essay composed about 1187 by the well-known Jewish philosopher and physician Ibn Maymūn, known in Europe as Moses Maimonides (d. 1204). Haemorrhoids appear to have been a particularly troublesome problem to both ancient and medieval populations around the Mediterranean, but whether that was due to diet or a sedentary lifestyle has not been established. Another of Ibn Maymūn's essays concerned asthma (*rabw*). Here the emphasis is upon regimen to be adopted by his unnamed asthmatic client rather than a complete exposition of its causes and symptoms, which, he says, are fully treated in the medical encyclopedias.[23]

Diseases not specific to one part

For Ibn Sīnā, conditions not specific to one bodily part where subdivided into (1) fevers, (2) pustules, abscesses, ulcer, swellings, leprosy, smallpox, wounds, fractures, and dislocations, (3) poisons, and animal and insect bites, and (4) obesity and emaciation, offensive body odours, and care of hair, skin, and nails.

Fevers were considered sufficiently important to merit large sections in every compendium and a number of separate monographs. The fact that malaria was endemic to the Mediterranean rim was probably a major factor in this focus upon fevers. They were classified in several ways, the basic one being by location of the causal factors: ephemeral (usually involving the pneuma), putrid (due to putrefaction of humoral residues), and hectic (occurring in a major organ). Each of these in turn had many sub-types; Ibn Sīnā, for example, listed 23 different types of ephemeral fevers (short term and not repeating), including those resulting from sun burn or bathing in water with sulphur. Recurrent fevers were classified by their periodicity: tertian (recurring every third day, counting the day of occurrence as the first day of the cycle), quartan (recurring every fourth day), and quotidian (recurring daily, day after day).

The recurring fevers reflect the patterns of febrile paroxysms characteristic of malaria. One of the most comprehensive treatises on the subject was written by Isḥāq ibn Sulaymān al-Isrā'īlī (d. c. 932), who also composed the leading discourse on diagnosis by urine. After discussing in great detail the causes, symptoms, and varieties of hectic fever (*ḥummá iqṭīqūs*) associated with consumption (*sill*), al-Isrā'īlī turns to the subject of the air surrounding the patient 'since it is with air that we are naturally in most immediate, constant, and uninterrupted contact':

> The patient's position inside the room should be in front of the opening to the ventilating window on bedding of linen or Tabaristan cloth. Rooms should be strewn with aromatic plants and mats of the sort just indicated. From one end of the house to the other the mats should all the time be kept lightly sprinkled. Running fountains should be installed in front of the patient so that he may listen to the gentle fall of water; for the splash of water, if light and gentle, will induce sleep. Continual use should be made of sandalwood and rose-water. Camphor is contra-indicated for the reason we have already given, namely that it desiccates the innate moisture and confines vapours and prevents their dissolution.[24]

Other systemic conditions were discussed in monographs and shorter sections of compendia. Qusṭā ibn Lūqā (d. c. 912), a Christian physician of Greek origin from Ba'albakk in Syria, wrote a monograph on numbness employing sources from Late Antiquity. One of the best known writings of the physician and clinician al-Rāzī (d. 925), and one showing considerable originality, is his *On Smallpox and Measles*. In it he is particularly concerned about protecting the eye, and, indeed, corneal damage caused by smallpox was a major cause of blindness until very recent times in the Middle East. Smallpox, like leprosy (*judhām*) and plague (*ṭāʿūn*), was generally considered transmissible and was greatly feared.[25]

Epidemic and pestilential diseases

The following definition of an epidemic disease was given by Ibn Riḍwān in the first half of the eleventh century:

> The meaning of an epidemic (*al-wāfidah*) illness is that it encompasses many people in one land at one time. One type is called *al-mawtān* (plague, lit. 'death'), in which the mortality rate is high. Epidemic diseases have many causes that may be grouped into four kinds: a change in the quality of the air, a change in the quality of the water, a change in the quality of the food, and a change in the quality of psychic events.[26]

The psychic events which Ibn Riḍwān says can cause epidemic disease are fear of a ruler or anxiety about a possible famine, for these can produce prolonged sleeplessness and worry that result in bad digestion. Diseases arising from polluted water can result 'when the water's course passes by a battlefield where many dead bodies are found, or the river passes by polluted swamps and it carries and mixes with this stagnant water'. Of food-related illnesses, he says:

> If blight attacks the plants, prices rise and most people are forced to change their foods. If most of the people increase their consumption of these foods at one time, as at the festivals, dyspepsia increases and people become ill. And if the pastureland and the water of the animals that we eat are corrupted, it will cause epidemic illness.[27]

When several causes occur at the same time, Ibn Riḍwān says, the result is more intense and the mortality rate higher. As an example he cites a famine and pestilence that had recently occurred in Egypt (c. 1055–62):

> Many wars took place then, killing a large number of the enemy as well as our own people. A great fear of the enemy and high prices befell the Egyptians. Furthermore, the inundation of the Nile was extraordinary in both its increase and decrease. Considerable decay from the dead mixed with the water, and the air surrounding them was contaminated by the decay of these things. Famine increased, and a high mortality occurred among the people. About a third of the people died from it.[28]

The occurrence of the 'Black Death' in 1348 formed a fault line in the history of the region. Thereafter plague tracts were composed with the purpose of collecting and interpreting *ḥadīths*, utterances of the Prophet, reporting what he and other early figures said about concepts of contagion and transmissibility of diseases as well as the proper reaction to such occurrences. The authors also attempted medical explanations and remedies for plague, and sometimes a history of plagues up to the time of composition. Amongst the numerous authors, three Andalusian figures (Ibn Khātimah, al-Shaqūrī, and Ibn al-Khaṭīb) wrote at the time of the Black Death in the fourteenth century as it struck Muslim Spain, while Ibn Ḥajar al-ʿAsqalānī wrote during the plague epidemic in Cairo in 1429–30. The authors were for the most part religious scholars, although a few were trained both as physicians and theologians.[29]

Two terms dominate the classical Arabic plague terminology: *ṭāʿūn*, usually rendered as 'plague', and *wabā'*, a more general term for pestilential disturbance or contamination of the environment. While there is inconsistency and confusion in their use by various authors, in general *wabā'* is the more inclusive term. Physicians of the Graeco-Roman tradition attributed the cause of pestilences to a *miasma* or corruption of the air. The issue of whether Muslim religious scholars allowed for a belief in the transmission of disease (*ʿadwá*) amongst humans is complex, with ambiguous and conflicting traditions. Many criticised physicians for their belief that plague was contagious, attributing its occurrence instead to *jinn* (demons whose existence was recognised in the Qur'ān) or directly to God. In support of such a view, various *ḥadīths* were cited, most famously: 'There is no transmission, no augury, no owl, and no *ṣafarah*'. The meaning of the last word in this saying is uncertain; some scholars leave it untranslated, some render it as 'yellow water', and others as 'serpent' (*ṣafar*), referring to a notion of a gastro-intestinal disorder that could spread easily from one person to another. Augury (*ṭiyarah*) here denotes omens apparent in the behaviour of birds, and the owl alludes to the spirit of a man wrongly slain who will not rest until avenged. The ideas in this *ḥadīth* apparently reflect pre-Islamic notions of divination and causation, all of which are being here rejected.[30]

Other *ḥadīths* suggest an implicit belief in the transmissibility of disease. The injunction 'flee from a leper as you would flee from a lion', immediately following the above quoted *ḥadīth* in the collection prepared by the traditionalist al-Bukhārī (d. 860), appears to contradict the statement that there is no contagion. Another says: 'If you hear that plague has broken out in a country, do not go there; if it breaks out in a country where you are staying, do not leave it.' While there is a strong element of resignation to God's will in the latter, it is also sound advice if the aim is to reduce further spreading of the pestilence.[31]

Anatomy

All the major Arabic and Persian medical encyclopedias had sections on anatomy, describing the bones, muscles, nerves, arteries, veins, and the compound organs (the eye, liver, heart, brain), as well as chapters on embryological theories. They were occasionally illustrated with schematic diagrams of the cranial sutures and the bones of the upper jaw and nasal cavity. Debates arose regarding several issues, such as the total number of bones and muscles in the human body, the male and female roles in generation, and the length of foetal development in humans and animals.

Islamic writings concerned with anatomy remained quite conservative, deviating but little from their Hellenistic models. Ibn al-Nafīs' emendation of Greek notions of the movement of the blood in the heart and lungs was one exception to this general trend. Another contribution to human anatomy was the result of chance observation. The versatile scholar and physician 'Abd al-Laṭīf al-Baghdādī (d. 1231) taught medicine in Damascus and composed various medical writings, as well as a detailed description of Egypt that included his observations on a famine that occurred there in 1200. During this latter calamity, al-Baghdādī had been able to examine a good number of skeletons, which led him to conclude that Galen had been incorrect regarding the structure of the bones in the lower jaw and in the sacrum. If al-Baghdādī had not been a physician, well-trained in anatomy as described in earlier literature, his accidental observation of skeletons during a famine would not have resulted in a refinement of our knowledge of human anatomy. These anatomical observations, however, went unnoticed in subsequent medical literature, for they were buried in a treatise on descriptive geography rather than medicine.[32]

Systematic human anatomical dissection was no more a pursuit of medieval Islamic society than it was of medieval Christendom, although it is clear from the available evidence that in neither society were there explicit legal or religious strictures banning it. Indeed, many Muslim scholars lauded the study of anatomy, primarily as a way of demonstrating the design and wisdom of God. Typical of such sentiments is the saying by Ibn Rushd quoted at the beginning of this chapter, or that associated with the theologian al-Ghazālī (d. 1111): 'Whoever does not know astronomy and anatomy is deficient in the knowledge of God.' What is meant by 'anatomy' in such statements is not the dissection of an animal in order to determine its structure, but rather the elaboration of the ideas of Galen regarding the structure and function. There are, however, some references in scholarly medical writings to dissection, though to what extent these reflect actual practice it is difficult to say.[33]

No anatomical illustrations of the entire body are known to have been produced in the Islamic world before those that accompany copies of *Manṣūr's Anatomy* by Manṣūr ibn Ilyās (*fl.* 1394–1409). This Persian-language treatise was dedicated to a Persian provincial ruler who governed from 1394 to 1409, probably a grandson of Tīmūr (known to Europeans as Tamerlane). It consists of an introduction followed by five chapters on the 'systems' of the body: bones, nerves, muscles, veins, and arteries, each illustrated by a full-page diagram with numerous labels. The anatomy presented is entirely Galenic in nature, and reflects none of the refinements introduced by Ibn al-Nafīs or 'Abd al-Laṭīf al-Baghdādī. A concluding section of *Manṣūr's Anatomy* concerns compound organs and the formation of the foetus is usually illustrated with a diagram showing a pregnant woman.[34]

A similarity has been noted between the first five illustrations accompanying *Manṣūr's Anatomy* and a set of anatomical illustrations that appeared in earlier, apparently twelfth-century, Latin medical treatises. All the figures are in a distinctive squatting posture, but the similarity is particularly evident in the diagram of the skeleton which in both the Latin and Islamic versions is viewed from behind, with the head hyperextended so that the face looks upwards. The series clearly predates the Persian treatise by Manṣūr ibn Ilyās by at least two centuries, but its origin remains a puzzle.[35]

Although anatomy at this period was primarily book-learning, most elite physicians emphasised the necessity of anatomical knowledge for successful practice. In a twelfth-century Syrian manual for the regulation of practices in the markets, the author states that a phlebotomist must know 'the anatomy of the parts, and the veins, muscles and arteries' lest he make a mistake and cut one of them, and that the phlebotomist should practice making incisions with a lancet on the veins in beetroot leaves. Similarly, according to this manual, the surgeon must 'know anatomy and the parts of the human body, and the muscles, veins, arteries, and nerves that are in them, so that they will avoid them when opening abscesses or excising haemorrhoids'. As al-Zahrāwī put it at the beginning of the eleventh century: 'For he who is not skilled in as much anatomy as we have mentioned is bound to fall into error that is destructive to life.'[36]

Surgery

Like anatomy, surgery figures in most Arabic or Persian medical encyclopedias. The most influential section on this topic was part of the encyclopedia written in Córdoba around the year 1000 by Abū al-Qāsim al-Zahrāwī (known to Europe as Albucasis) – an encyclopedia with a lengthy title translating roughly as *The Arrangement of Medical Knowledge for One Who is Not Able to Compile a Book for Himself*. Like all early Arabic writers, al-Zahrāwī based his work upon Greek authorities, but in this instance particularly upon the seventh-century Alexandrian physician Paul of Aegina. Nonetheless, al-Zahrāwī's surgical chapter has a pervading sense of personal experience on the part of the author. He also included illustrations of instrument designs – an important innovation in the history of surgical literature.[37]

A Damascene physician by the name of Ibn al-Quff (d. 1286) composed what appears to be the earliest medieval Arabic treatise intended solely for surgeons. His *Basics in the Art of Surgery* was a general medical manual covering anatomy and drug therapy as well as surgical care, concentrating on wounds and tumours. Ibn al-Quff excluded ophthalmology, which he considered to be a speciality with its own technical literature.[38]

There were various approaches to the surgery. Al-Zahrāwī's lengthy section on the subject is divided into three books: on cauterisation, on incisions, venesection and wounds, and on bone-setting. The much shorter surgical chapter by al-Rāzī (d. 925) in his *Book for al-Manṣūr* (not to be confused with *Manṣūr's Anatomy*) is overwhelmingly devoted to bone-setting and the treatment of wounds and swellings, with much shorter sections on phlebotomy, cupping, use of leeches, the excision of the guinea worm (*Dracunculus medinensis*, a parasite, mistakenly thought by medieval writers to be a moving 'vein'), the extraction of arrows, and skull fractures. The chapter by al-Rāzī is unique in ending with a description of the tricks employed by charlatans pretending to extract things from the body.

In some general surgical writings, physicians occasionally commented that no one was known actually to perform a given operation, even though at the same time they included a description of the procedure based on earlier authoritative texts. Other times they might say that they declined to operate, as when al-Zahrāwī saw a hydrocephalic child with an enlarged head due to abnormal fluid in the brain but stated 'I have preferred not to undertake operation in these cases', even while giving instructions drawn from earlier sources. Perhaps some of the procedures described in this surgical literature represented a literary tradition unrelated to the actual practice of surgery. This interpretation is encouraged by a writer's failure to mention an example of a procedure's use, or to modify the procedure or instrumentation in any way from that handed down from his authorities (for what cook cannot resist altering a recipe or artisan improving a technique?). For example, procedures for abdominal surgery for an umbilical hernia are presented in almost all surgical chapters, including that by al-Zahrāwī. Yet no Islamic physician mentions seeing it done or modifies the procedure in any way from that found in Greek treatises available in Arabic translation, and the very nature of the description is so imprecise that its applicability is dubious.[39]

Another operation included in the manuals, and of great potential risk to the patient, is a tracheotomy (an incision in the windpipe for relief of an obstruction to breathing). This procedure was earlier described by Graeco-Roman physicians, but not advocated or approved by many. Al-Zahrāwī, working in Muslim Spain, stated that he had not seen the operation performed in his day, but he did recount his experience with a slave-girl who had been wounded in the throat with a knife:

> My own experience was this: a slave-girl seized a knife and buried it in her throat and cut part of the trachea, and I was called to attend her. I found her bellowing like a sacrifice that has had its throat cut. So I laid the wound bare and found that only a little haemorrhage had come from it. I assured myself that neither an artery nor the jugular vein had been cut, but air passed out through the wound. So I hurriedly

> sutured the wound and treated it until it healed. No harm was done to the slave-girl except for a hoarseness in the voice which was not extreme, and after some days she was restored to the best of health. Hence, we may say that a tracheotomy is not dangerous.[40]

In this clinical account, we observe a physician well-versed in Graeco-Roman medical writings (through Arabic translations) who was able to apply the techniques in an emergency but who also stated that the operation was unknown in his own time. His successful treatment of his patient suggested to him that a tracheotomy or laryngotomy might be possible. In the twelfth century, also in Muslim Spain, Ibn Zuhr (d. 1162) said that he practised the procedure on a goat, in case he ever had to perform it, but that he had never seen it performed on humans.[41]

Gynaecological matters always occupied a chapter in surgical tracts, even though the treatises were written by men. Forceps were described by al-Zahrāwī, though not for use in live births, and variant designs given for a vaginal speculum, or dilator. The alleviation of a difficult birthing was discussed in nearly all general manuals, and there was great concern shown for extracting a dead foetus from the womb. Instruments were described in both the Greek and Arabic literature for cutting the foetus into parts that could then be removed. It has been questioned, however, whether such techniques were ever actually used, and pertinent to the argument is a comment made by the Egyptian oculist al-Shādhilī in the fourteenth century:

> We possess written accounts of various procedures which cannot be performed nowadays because there is no one who has actually seen them performed; an example is the instrument designed to cut up a dead foetus in the womb in order to save the mother's life. There are many such procedures: they are described in books, but in our own time we have never seen anyone perform them because the practical knowledge has been lost, and nothing remains but the written accounts.[42]

A substantial proportion of the surgical literature was devoted to the removal of tumours and growths on all parts of the body. This type of treatment involved relatively simple excision and cauterisation. An example is the removal of haemorrhoids – again, an ancient procedure for what appears to have been a very troubling problem.

According to the surgical manuals, incisions were made for the removal of stones in the neck of the bladder. This also was a procedure well described in classical antiquity. A calculus in the kidney or in the duct carrying urine from the kidney to the bladder would be inaccessible and untreatable through surgery. But a calculus impacted in the duct carrying urine *from* the bladder could be surgically removed, and al-Zahrāwī described a new technique using a fine drill inserted through the urinary passage.[43]

Al-Zahrāwī also included in his discourse a design for a concealed knife that could be used to open abscesses on the skin in a manner not to alarm the patient. This instrument, in three sizes, he called a 'deceiver', the idea being that there was a blade between two curved plates attached to a handle, and the blade could be protruded or withdrawn at will. He appears to have been concerned to reduce the anxiety of a nervous patient when the knife could not be avoided.[44]

According to the manuals, techniques for tonsillectomies were improved. With the tongue held still by a tongue depressor, the swollen tonsil was held by a hook and then, according to al-Zahrāwī, removed with a scissor-like instrument with transverse blades which apparently both cut the gland and held it for removal from the throat. Then the patient was to gargle with vinegar and water, and, if haemorrhage followed, gargle with styptics. Such procedures were quite within the surgical capabilities of the day. As recently as the early twentieth century, itinerant removers of tonsils were still practising in parts of the United States and the United Kingdom, where they successfully removed the tonsils of children in their homes, using virtually the same techniques, with little or no anaesthetic and little antisepsis.[45]

Somewhat related to the treatment of growths was the suggested treatment of enlarged or pendulous male breasts (described also in Graeco-Roman literature) by a semicircular incision on each, dissection of the fatty tissue, and suturing of the incision followed by applications of styptics. Whether such proposed therapies represent actual practice is uncertain.[46]

Other aspects of medieval surgery covered in these manuals did not involve cutting with the knife. For example, extraction of teeth was a common topic. Dental forceps of various designs are frequently illustrated, as well as other tools necessary for extraction of roots and broken pieces of the jawbone sometimes left after the removal of the tooth. Teeth that were loose or had been knocked out, or made artificially from ox-bone, could be, it was suggested, connected to sound teeth by means of gold or silver wire – continuing the Roman, and before that Etruscan and ancient Egyptian, practice.[47]

The two topics that dominate the surgical literature, however, are the setting of bones and the treatment of wounds. In fact, the two treatises devoted only to surgery – that by Ibn al-Quff (d. 1286) written in Syria and another by Muḥammad al-Shafrah (d. 1360) composed in Muslim Spain – are concerned almost exclusively with those two surgical requirements. Writers on surgery presented numerous methods of suturing wounds, and the use of animal gut for sutures is first mentioned in Arabic literature, along with the older usage of wool, linen, and silk. Reducing tables were employed to extend the limbs so as to restore dislocations and fractures. An injured limb was bandaged, and a splint was applied, made of cloths soaked in lime and egg-white. The repair of broken noses was also given much attention in the literature. Skull fractures were said to be treated by removing part of the skull with a cylindrical drill (a method known today as trepanation), but with the borer outfitted with a protruding collar to prevent it sinking into the underlying meninges (or membranes of the brain). Trepanation for any other purpose is not mentioned in the Islamic literature.[48]

Ophthalmology

While nearly every general medical compendium contained chapters on eye diseases, the most comprehensive coverage was to be found in treatises devoted solely to this topic. In ninth-century Baghdad both Yuḥannā ibn Māsawayh and his student Ḥunayn ibn Isḥāq wrote influential monographs on the subject. Though based to a large extent upon Greek sources, they already display some advancement in knowledge, including the description of previously unrecognised pathological conditions, for which intricate surgical procedures soon developed. Ocular anatomy also featured in these specialised tracts, often illustrated with diagrams of the eye or the visual system. Ḥunayn's *Ten Treatises on the Eye* contains the earliest detailed drawings of the eye preserved today, one of which is illustrated in Figure 2.5.[49]

One of the most widely-read medieval Islamic ophthalmological manuals was written by ʿAlī ibn ʿĪsá al-Kaḥḥāl ('the ophthalmologist'), who practised in Baghdad in the tenth century. His *Memorandum Book for Oculists* covered 130 eye ailments with a very systematic discussion of the symptoms, causes, and treatments of the eye disorders, presented in terms of humoral pathology. A near contemporary of his was ʿAmmār ibn ʿAlī al-Mawṣilī, originally from Iraq, who dedicated his only work, a treatise on eye diseases, to the Fāṭimid ruler of Egypt, al-Ḥākim (r. 996–1021). ʿAmmār's treatise discusses only 48 diseases, but contains some interesting clinical accounts that will be discussed later in Chapter 4.[50]

For reasons as yet unknown, interest in ophthalmology grew during the twelfth and thirteenth centuries in Spain, Egypt, and Syria, as can be seen from the unprecedented number of treatises composed on this subject. It is possible that this increased production reflected a rising incidence of ocular complaints; in any case it is paralleled by the dominance of eye diseases and fevers amongst the health concerns evident in the mostly twelfth- and thirteenth-century materials preserved in the cache of discarded documents known as the Cairo Geniza. A particularly innovative example of an ophthalmological treatise of this time period was that written by Khalīfah ibn Abī al-Maḥāsin al-Ḥalabī in Syria between 1256 and 1275. Not only did he meticulously cite previous writers on the subject, but he also included a considerable amount of novel material, such as the first recorded instance of the use of a magnet to remove a foreign object from the eye – in this case a piece of a needle that had broken while couching

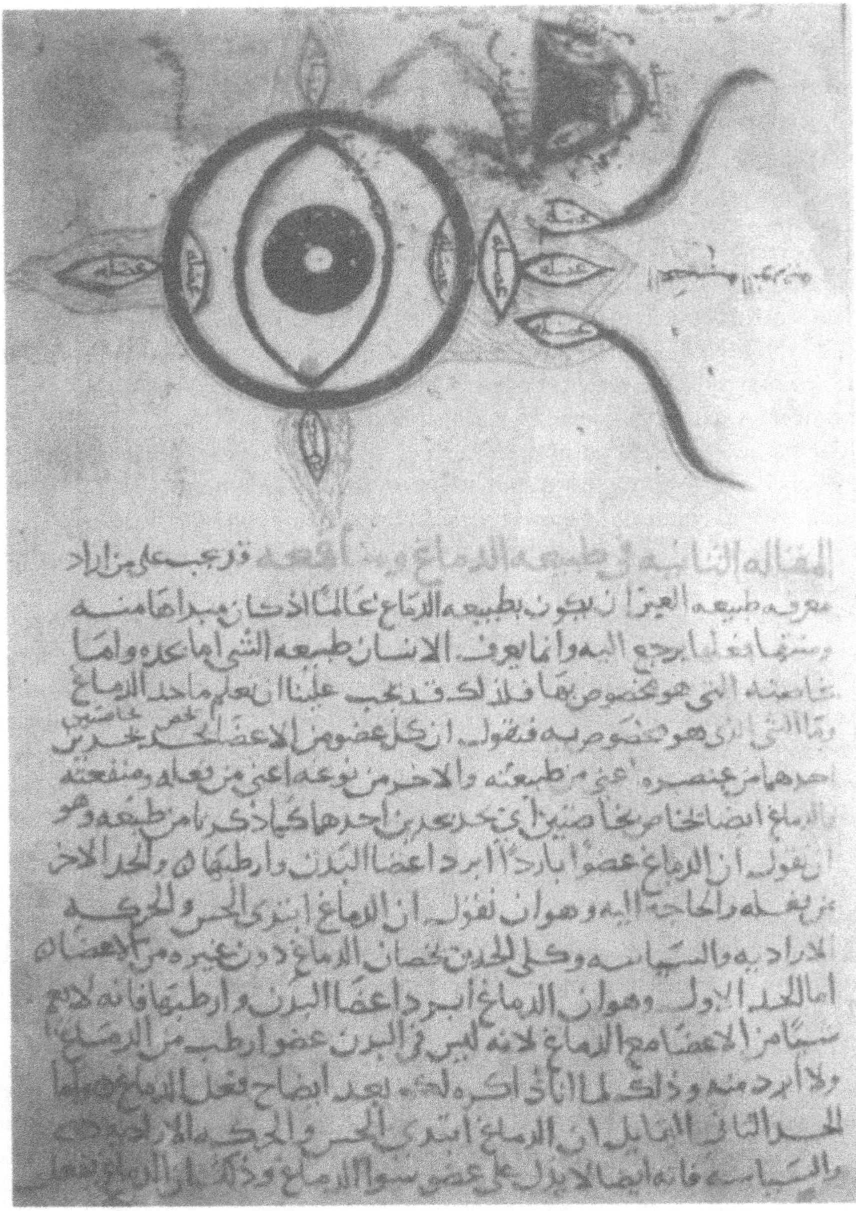

Figure 2.5 The muscles of the eye, from Ḥusayn ibn Isḥāq's *Ten Treatises on the Eye*, copied in 1197 in Syria from a manuscript made in 1003 that was in turn copied from the original composed by Ḥunayn about 860. The eyeball is depicted frontally, though the attached muscles extending [at the right] toward the brain, with two ribbon-like oculomotor nerves, are viewed in a horizontal cross-section. The separate parabolic form above represents the muscles of the upper eyelid.

a cataractous eye. His diagrammatic charts of all the instruments required by an oculist in his day, illustrated in Figure 4.2 on p. 126, are a stunning example of medical illustration.[51]

In all these ophthalmological manuals, recipes for compound remedies were given for nearly every eye disease or disorder, and the physician was instructed to begin with drug therapy and progress to surgery only when that failed. Compound ocular remedies took several forms, one of which was called a *kuḥl*. In it, the ingredients were ground to a very fine powder and applied with a probe to the eyelids. Outside the context of specialised ophthalmic care, the word *kuḥl* denoted various compound substances to enhance the beauty of the eye. The major component of these cosmetics has traditionally (but incorrectly) been identified as a type of antimony, usually antimony sulfate or antimony sulphide (stibium or stibnite). Recent research indicates that it was not a form of antimony, but probably lead, though some have suggested a kind of powdered iron. The word *kuḥl*, from which the word for oculist, *kaḥḥāl*, is derived, ultimately came to mean not just a fine eye powder but any fine essence, and, taken with the Arabic article, *al-kuḥl* eventually gave rise to the word alcohol.[52]

Much of the ophthalmic surgery described in the manuals concerns the removal of growths from the eyelids – cysts, styes, papillomas, vesicles, and tumours of various sorts. Trachoma, well-known to both Graeco-Roman and Islamic physicians, was, together with its complications, the major cause of blindness. The modern name trachoma is taken directly from the Greek term *trachōma* meaning 'roughness', while the Arabic term is *jarab* ('scabies'). It was considered a disease of the eyelid that usually progressed through four stages, though today it is viewed as a disease of the conjunctiva. From the ninth century, Islamic oculists classified four conditions as complications of trachoma. These complications are known today as trichiasis (from Greek *trichiasis*, literally 'hair disease') whose Arabic term *sha'r munqalab* ('ingrown lashes') accurately reflects the nature of the condition; entropion or ectropion, that is either the eyelid turning inward or turning outward (Greek *ektropion* 'eversion', Arabic *shatrah* 'inversion of the eyelid'); pterygium, a triangular-shaped ingrowth of the conjunctiva onto the cornea (Greek *pterugion* 'wing', Arabic *ẓafarah* 'pellicle'); and pannus, an invasion of the cornea by vessels from the limbus, a condition not described in Greek sources but called in Arabic *sabal* ('rain'). All but pterygium are still considered complications or second characteristics of trachoma. Surgical techniques were advocated and described in great detail for treating all four of these eye afflictions, which, judging from the prominence they are given in the literature, occupied much of the oculists' attention.[53]

Cataracts also caused blindness and figured prominently in the ophthalmological manuals, where various surgical procedures were presented. How these eye diseases were actually treated will be further explored in Chapter 4 below.

Types of medical discourse

Medical discourses which presented and developed these various concepts took many forms. In addition to monographs on single topics, such as eye diseases, fevers, melancholy, simple and compound remedies, medical aphorisms, or how to treat stomach disorders, a variety of formats existed.

The great translator Ḥunayn ibn Isḥāq wrote two quite similar treatises intended to provide the medical student with the most essential material: an *Introduction to Medicine* and *Questions on Medicine for Beginners*. The subject matter is the same in both treatises, but his didactic approach differed considerably. In both, he explained humoral pathology, the function of the different organs, diagnosis, and other fundamental concepts of medical theory. In the *Introduction*, however, he presented the material discursively, as running text, whilst he used the form of questions and answers, a sort of catechism, in his *Medical Questions*. The former text became, in Latin translation, the core introduction to the subject in the Latin Middle Ages. The latter, on the other hand, found greater favour in the Islamic world and established a genre of medical writing that had considerable currency in subsequent centuries.

The use of questions and answers as a didactic device continued an older Alexandrian model. In addition to his *Questions on Medicine for Beginners*, Ḥunayn ibn Isḥāq composed a small *Questions Concerning the Eye*, reflecting his particular interest in ophthalmology. Others physicians followed this model of teaching manual, including al-Sulamī (d. 1208), cited above. In the treatises themselves there are few clues as to their intended audience or purpose. On occasion commentaries were written expounding further on the questions and answers. In one instance we have a copy providing a hint as to the role in teaching that such treatises played. In a manuscript copy of a commentary written by Ibn Abī Ṣādiq al-Nīsābūrī (d. after 1048) on Ḥunayn's *Questions on Medicine for Beginners*, there is a note in which the physician Muwaffaq al-Dīn al-Sāmirī (d. 1282) certified that his student named Amīn al-Dawlah Tādruṣ had 'read it in order to investigate its questions and to understand and comprehend its contents'.[54]

Didactic medical poetry was a popular device as well, with rhyming verses that enabled the student or practitioner easily to remember the basic ideas. The *Poem on Medicine* by Ibn Sīnā was widely read and is preserved in many copies today.[55]

Synoptic tables also proved a popular means of presenting material, Ibn Buṭlān's *Almanac of Health* being the most well-known example. The format lent itself particularly well to the presentation of rules for food and drug use, but it was also used for listing diseases and aligning them with appropriate therapies. An example of the latter application is *The Almanac of Bodily Parts for the*

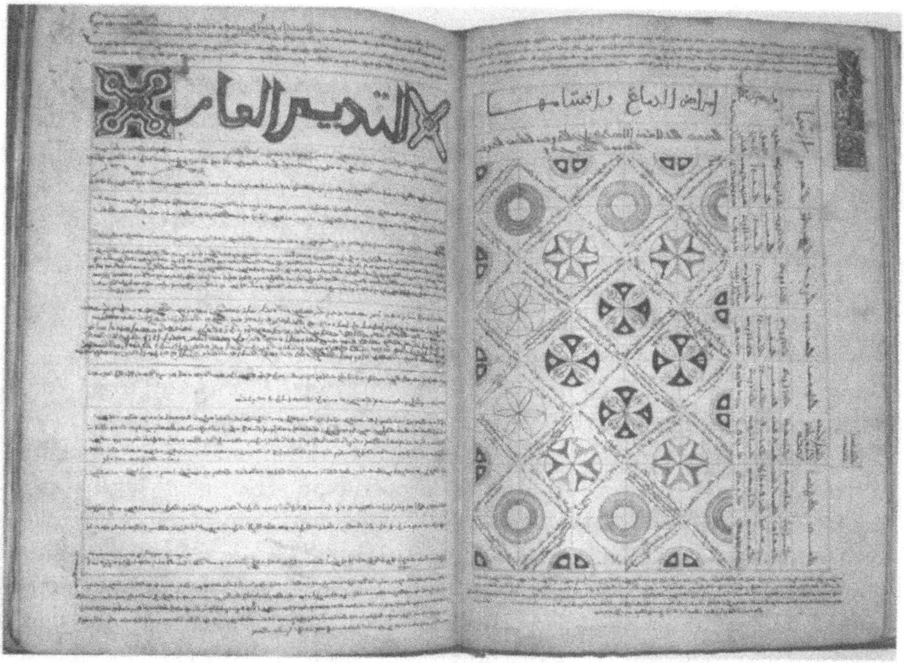

Figure 2.6 A copy made for the Syrian Christian community of *The Almanac of Bodily Parts for the Treatment of People* by Ibn Jazlah (d. 1100). The heading of this synoptic table ('diseases of the brain and their classifications') is written in Arabic script, while most of the text is written in Karshuni – that is, Arabic written in the Syriac alphabet. In some of the cells of this tabular presentation of diseases and their therapies, the information has been written diagonally and the spaces filled with geometrical decorations unrelated to the contexts of the treatise.

Treatment of People by Ibn Jazlah (d. 1100), a Christian convert to Islam who practised as a physician in his place of birth, Baghdad. Forty-four tables display information on 352 diseases, with the data for each one and its treatment set forth in twelve columns. In Figure 2.6, showing a double-page diagram written in Karshuni (Arabic text in Syriac letters), the right-hand six narrow columns give the name of the disorder, its temperament, associated age, season, country in which it frequently occurs, and its prognosis. Five square cells then give, for each condition, information on the causes, symptoms, appropriate method of evacuation, a 'royal' treatment, and a simple treatment. In this particular copy the information has been written diagonally, with the spaces filled with geometric decorations. The left-hand page contains the twelfth column giving full details on the general treatment and regimen for each disorder.[56]

Of all forms of medical writing, however, that of the medical compendium or encyclopedia proved the most enduring. The genre had developed in Late

Antiquity and proved to be particularly influential in the Islamic scholarly medical tradition.

Three Arabic compendia had the greatest impact: First, the *Book for al-Manṣūr* by al-Rāzī (d. 925). It was dedicated in 903 to a local Iranian prince named Abū Ṣāliḥ, governor of the town of Rayy near present-day Tehran – a town where al-Rāzī directed a hospital and where he was to die. Because of this association with then prominent town of Rayy, he bore the name al-Rāzī, meaning 'of Rayy'. Equally important was the *Complete Book of the Medical Art*, by al-Majūsī, working in Shiraz, due south of Rayy.[57]

The third Islamic medical compendium was the *Canon of Medicine* by Ibn Sīnā (d. 1037), whose opening was used to begin this chapter. Ibn Sīnā composed it over a lengthy period of time as he moved westward from Gurgān, at the southeast corner of the Caspian Sea, to Rayy and then to Hamadān even further southwest. This massive encyclopedia rivalled, and in many quarters surpassed, the popularity of al-Majūsī's compendium. The tight logical arrangement of material reflects Ibn Sīnā's skill in logic and philosophy. He divided it into five books: Book I consists of four parts: (1) on the elements, humours, temperaments, anatomy of homogeneous parts (bones, muscles, nerves, arteries, veins), and the three faculties; (2) the six 'non-naturals', general symptoms of diseases, and diagnosis by pulse, urine, and stools; (3) regimen for children, adults, and the aged, as well as effects of climatic change and medical advice for travellers; and (4) general methods of therapy including emetics, enemas, liniments, bloodletting, cautery, and the relief of pain. Book II is on medicinal substances arranged alphabetically, following a discourse on their general properties. Book III concerns diseases peculiar to one part of the body, and also includes its anatomy. Book IV covers conditions not specific to one bodily part, including poisonous bites, obesity, body odours, and care of the hair and skin. Book V is a formulary of compound remedies. With the exception of Books II and V, the contents of each book are further subdivided into parts (*fanns*), then into chapters (*taʿlīms*), subchapters (*jumlahs*), sections (*faṣls*), and subsections (*bābs*), thus tightly ranking and ordering the material.[58]

These attempts at systematising and synthesising the Greek medical literature succeeded in producing a coherent and orderly medical system, essentially Galenic in nature but much modified and elaborated. Their sheer size, reinforced by titles such as the *Canon*, gave them an aura of authority that was to prove stultifying rather than invigorating. After the middle of the eleventh century, few writers undertook to produce an encyclopedia on the scale of al-Majūsī or Ibn Sīnā.

The *Canon* did not meet with universal praise, however. In Muslim Spain, when Abū al-ʿAlāʾ Zuhr (d. 1131) received a copy as a gift, he so disliked it that he refused to put it in his library. He preferred to cut off its margins and use them for writing prescriptions. For, as he said, the *Canon* 'was not suitable for those beginning the study of medicine because it contains unusual terms and philosophic concepts'. Ibn Sīnā, like most Islamic physicians, wed philosophy with medicine, continuing the philosopher–physician tradition of earlier Greek physicians such as Galen.[59]

This anecdote of Abū al-'Alā' Zuhr's reaction to the *Canon* provides us with some evidence as to how long it took for a treatise written at one end of the Islamic empire to become available at the other. In this instance, it took about a century after the *Canon* was completed in Hamadān for it to become available in Muslim Spain. The hostile reaction on the part of the progenitor of a five-generation family of prominent physicians in al-Andalus also raises the question (yet to be investigated by historians) whether medicine in Muslim Spain subsequently developed with less dependence upon the ideas of Ibn Sīnā than elsewhere.

Despite this less than enthusiastic reception in Muslim Spain, it was the *Canon* of Ibn Sīnā that came to dominate in the medieval Islamic world and eventually in Europe as well. An awareness appears to have set in, however, that the compendium was really too large to be useful for ready reference. Numerous abridgements of the *Canon* were produced to make the ideas more readily accessible, as well as commentaries to clarify the contents. The earliest abridgement seems to have been written by Muḥammad ibn Yūsuf al-Īlāqī (*fl.* 1068), a pupil of Ibn Sīnā. Yet, it was not until the late twelfth century that a serious need was perceived for aids to understanding the *Canon*. The Egyptian Jewish physician Ibn Jumayʿ (d. 1198), may have composed the earliest commentary on the *Canon*. In the next two centuries, such commentaries and epitomes followed in rapid succession, and it was this industry of glossing and condensing the *Canon* that assured the encyclopedia its pre-eminent position in medieval medicine. It also reflects the expansion of the medical trade beyond the confines of royal patronage and courts.

Among the abridgements of the *Canon* of Ibn Sīnā, that entitled *The Epitome* (*al-Mūjiz*) by the Syrian physician Ibn al-Nafīs occupied the most prominent position. Both *The Epitome* and the commentaries by Ibn al-Nafīs continued to be copied and read over the following five centuries, often generating further commentaries and super-commentaries.

Prophetic Medicine

In addition to the Greek-based medical systems advocated by physicians such as al-Rāzī and Ibn Sīnā, there was also an alternative genre of medical writing called *al-ṭibb al-nabawī* or 'Prophetic Medicine'. Its authors were religious scholars rather than physicians, and their aim was to produce a guide to medical regimen and therapy that was acceptable to pious Muslims.

A primary motivation for this genre of medical literature may have been an anti-philosophical tradition – that is, an opposition to the philosophical practices and methods of earlier Greek thinkers – of which the famous Damascene theologian Ibn Taymīyah (d. 1318) was the main proponent, for two of the major authors of treatises on Prophetic Medicine (Ibn Qayyim al-Jawzīyah and al-Dhahabī) were both direct disciples of Ibn Taymīyah, while a later influential advocate of Prophetic Medicine, al-Suyūṭī, abridged Ibn Taymīyah's work against Greek philosophy and logic.

Diagnosis based on physical causes producing diseases – a feature of the rather mechanistic humoral medicine inherited from Late Antiquity – was interpreted by some Muslim scholars as being contrary to Divine Law because it allowed for causes other than God. Similarly, prognosis could be considered contrary to Divine Order because it suggests a notion of causality which would limit the omnipotence of God. Perhaps for these reasons, diagnosis and prognosis play little role in this type of literature, the emphasis being on care and cure through food and simple medicines, proper conduct, and invocations to God. There is a conscious avoidance of any claims of medicine to absoluteness.

Both plague tracts and treatises on Prophetic Medicine were especially popular from the fourteenth century onwards. In the case of plague tracts, a few were composed by writers trained both as physicians and theologians, while the composition of Prophetic Medicine treatises seems to have been the sole domain of religious scholars. A certain pessimism is also more evident in the plague tracts, where you find aphorisms such as: 'For every disease there is medicine to cure it, except for madness, plague, and old age.'[60]

All examples of Prophetic Medicine base their medical expositions upon what was known of the practices current in the days of the Prophet Muḥammad, derived from the Qur'ān itself, and from reports about the Prophet's utterances (*ḥadīths*) and custom (*sunnah*). Therapy generally consisted of diet, bloodletting, cupping, and occasional cautery, with simple drugs (especially honey) to be preferred over compound remedies. Simple drugs such as honey, of course, were both readily available and less expensive than elaborate compound medicines. 'You have two medicines: honey and the Qur'ān', was one commonly quoted *ḥadīth*.[61]

No surgery figured in the treatises, except an occasional mention of excising a cyst and circumcision (the latter not as a treatment for a disease). Specific conditions merited particular attention: fevers, leprosy, plague, poisonous bites, protection from night-flying insects, protection against the Evil Eye, and minor illnesses such as headaches, nosebleed, cough, colic, and sciatica. The treatises also provided numerous prayers and pious invocations to be used by the devout patient, with the occasional amulet and talisman.

One of the earliest tracts on the subject, *Medicine of the Imams*, had recourse to the authority of Shī'ite imams, as its title would suggest. Two brothers, Abū

'Attab Allāh and al-Ḥusayn, sons of Bisṭām ibn Sābūr, compiled the treatise, working in the eastern provinces of the Islamic world. It is a somewhat random collection of *ḥadīths*, sayings of Shīʿite imams, magical procedures, and a few compound remedies. It contains, for instance, a garlic-based drug called 'the healing one' (*al-shāfiyah*), said to be useful for coughs, tetanus, and pain in the eye, for which it supplies a history tracing its origins back to Moses.[62]

Other Prophetic Medicine treatises were composed to reconcile the traditional medicine of Arabia and the revelations of Muḥammad with ideas and terminology from the Greek-based system. Examples are the treatises by a Syrian theologian of the Ḥanbalī school of jurisprudence, Ibn Qayyim al-Jawzīyah (d. 1350), and a Damascene scholar of the Shāfiʿī school, Shams al-Dīn al-Dhahabī (d. 1348). The latter cited, in addition to numerous authorities on *ḥadīth*, the Greek writers Hippocrates, Aristotle, Plato, Dioscorides, and Galen, and the Arabic physicians al-Rāzī, Ibn Sīnā, Ibn al-Bayṭār, and 'Abd al-Laṭīf al-Baghdādī. Most of these quotations are aphoristic in nature, such as 'Ibn Sīnā said: never have a meal until the one before it has been digested.' The final section of the treatise includes some material on the proper conduct of physicians and a justification of medicine. In the opening portion, al-Dhahabī discusses the Greek concepts of humours, temperaments, faculties, and six 'non-naturals'. While there is a brief justification given for employing compound remedies, no recipes are provided (in contrast to the earlier Shīʿīte treatise) and the bulk of the work constitutes an alphabetical listing of food stuffs and medical substances. When discussing the possible origins of medicine, and praising Hippocrates and Galen as the two greatest physicians, al-Dhahabī says that the ultimate origin of medical knowledge has to be the revelation and inspiration of God, adding the statement: 'This much is certain: experiences (*al-tajārib*) and analogy (*al-qiyās*) are insufficient for it [the development of medicine].' Yet it is analogy with the folkloric behaviour of animals that is the basis for some of his medical theories, as, for example, the statement that physicians use fennel to treat weak vision because snakes emerge after winter having poor eyesight and seek out fennel to eat, with the result that their eyesight is improved.[63]

Much of the material and even phraseology of al-Dhahabī is to be found in Ibn Qayyim al-Jawzīyah's treatise, but in a different format. Ibn Qayyim, however, supports the use of cupping, cautery, magical invocations, and talismans (especially against the Evil Eye), which al-Dhahabī does not. On the other hand, Ibn Qayyim cites many more Muslim or Jewish physicians trained in the Greek-based system; in addition to al-Rāzī and Ibn Sīnā, he cites by name ten from the eastern or central areas and three from Muslim Spain.

While Ibn Qayyim and al-Dhahabī were clearly well-read in humoral medical literature, there is no evidence that either were practising physicians. Amongst the physicians cited by both authors is the name 'Abd al-Laṭīf al-Baghdadī (d. 1231), one of the physicians and scholars in the entourage of Ṣalāḥ al-Dīn (Saladin). A manuscript copy of al-Dhahabī's treatise in which the author's name is given as 'Abd al-Laṭīf, now in the library of Cambridge University, has caused considerable confusion and given rise to the false assertion that 'Abd al-Laṭīf himself composed a treatise on Prophetic Medicine.[64]

The Shāfi'ī legal scholar and polymath Jalāl al-Dīn al-Suyūṭī (d. 1505) in his book titled *The Correct Method and Refreshing Source for the Medicine of the Prophet* approached the subject rather differently. Virtually the only source he cited as representing the Greek-based system is Ibn al-Nafīs' popular epitome of the *Canon* of Ibn Sīnā. Taking topics such as anatomy, general principles of regimen, cautery, bloodletting, simple medicinal substances (honey, figs, pomegranate, etc.), and certain diseases (headache, melancholy, weakness of vision, diarrhoea, insect bites), he compared statements from the epitome of the *Canon* with legal authorities, often citing Ibn Qayyim and al-Dhahabī as authorities in the field. Amulets and magic play no role in al-Suyūṭī's discourse.[65]

Other authors on Prophetic Medicine included very little material from the Greek humoral tradition. For example, al-Ṣanawbarī (d. 1412) in his still popular *Book of Mercy on Medicine and Wisdom* devoted only a very short paragraph to the four humours and a slightly longer one to the four corresponding temperaments, with but one brief mention of Hippocrates and none of Galen. The remainder of the sizeable book is devoted to quotations of *ḥadīths*, instructions for the use of substances such as honey, and magical and talismanic procedures. The latter include the following injunctions: for a person suffering from sorrow or anxiety, you should write certain words in a spiral design, and the person will be cured upon seeing it; to cure a headache take the right leg joint of a sheep and attach it to the head of the sufferer and he will be cured, or place your hand on the head of the sufferer and say a specified pious phrase, repeating it three or seven times.[66]

From a medical standpoint, there is no comprehensive or consistent underlying theory in the prophetic medical texts, for they combine elements of Greek medical learning (in Arabic dress) and religious elements specific to Islam with pre-Islamic Arabian practices, the latter being unlikely to have ever been encompassed by a consistent medical theory or system. From a philosophical viewpoint, however, Prophetic Medicine presents a medical system based for the most part upon religious authority. The underlying belief that God would provide a cure for every ailment, however, did not mean that people were to remain passive, for they still needed to discover and employ that remedy.

This genre of medical writing flourished for centuries alongside the Greek-based humoral tradition, and many texts are still available in print. It is certainly too harsh an assessment to consider, as some have, the tracts on Prophetic Medicine to be quackery piously disguised. Quackery implies a conscious effort to defraud. Prophetic Medicine was and is believed in by its proponents. Evidence suggests that treatises on Prophetic Medicine were not considered detrimental to, or competitive with, medical practices based primarily upon Greek humoral medicine. The growth of this genre of medical literature was not a direct threat to 'scientific' or 'rational' medicine, nor was it responsible for the decline of science and medicine, but rather it was symptomatic of the frame of mind and concerns of an increasing proportion of the society. It is noteworthy that those Islamic physicians trained in the Greek-based traditions (no matter what their particular religious beliefs) did not criticise Prophetic Medicine by name, even when voicing great concern for inept and fraudulent medical practitioners or when criticising those who believed that medicine was not permissible from the religious point of view.[67]

* * *

Virtually every aspect of medicine – from the fundamental principles of humoral pathology to anatomy, surgery, ophthalmology, pharmacology, diet, regimen, and reactions to epidemics – were covered in one or more of the formal and highly theoretical treatises discussed above. Yet these written treatises provide only a limited view of the actual medical practices of the day, and on occasion they are not corroborated by other available sources. Evidence, fragmentary though it is, for the application of this scholarly medical knowledge will be the subject of Chapter 4. Before taking up the day-to-day practice of medicine, however, we will discuss the functioning of the physician within the wider context of medieval Islamic society.

Suggested reading

For the basic principles of humoral pathology, see Ullmann, *Islamic Medicine*, 55–64; Dols, *Medieval Islamic Medicine*, 10–21; and the first book of the *Canon* of Ibn Sīnā (see the English translation, made from an Urdu version, by Shah, *The General Principles*, and that made from the Latin, Gruner, *A Treatise on the Canon of Medicine of Avicenna*); the English translation of the *Introduction* (*Isagoge*) by Ḥunayn ibn Isḥāq is also useful (Cholmeley and McVaugh, 'The Galenic System'). For further explanations of digestion and fermentation, see Good, *Medicine, Rationality, and Experience*, 101–15.

For regimen and dietetics in general, see Waines, 'Dietetics in Medieval Islamic Culture'; Fahd, 'Botany and Agriculture'; and Varisco, *Medieval Agriculture*. For pharmacology, see R. Kruk, art. 'nabāt', *EI*² vii. 831a–4a; B. Lewin, art. 'adwiya', *EI*² i. 212b–214b; Levey, *Early Arabic Pharmacology* (to be used with caution). For epidemic and pestilential diseases, Dols, *Medieval Islamic Medicine;* Conrad, 'Epidemic Diseases'; Conrad and Wujastyk, *Contagion*; and Dols, *The Black Death*.

Anatomy and embryology in general is discussed by E. Savage-Smith, art. 'tashrīḥ', *EI*² x. 354b–6b; Savage-Smith 'Attitudes toward Dissection'; Weisser, *Zeugung*; Musallam, 'The Human Embryo'; and Bummel, 'Human Biological Reproduction'. Several texts with French translations were published by de Koning, *Trois traités d'anatomie arabes*. For the anatomy of Manṣūr ibn Ilyās in particular, see G. Russell, art. 'Ebn Ilyās', *Enc. Ir.*, viii. 16a–20b.

For surgery, see Savage-Smith, 'Practice of Surgery'; Sanagustin, 'La chirurgie'; Ṣādeq Sajjādī, art. 'Čašm-Pezeškī', *Enc. Ir.*, v. 39b–44b; E. Savage-Smith, art. 'Zahrāwī', *EI*² xi. 398a–9b. For ophthalmology, see Meyerhof, 'History of Trachoma'; Hirschberg, *Geschichte der Augenheilkunde*; Sezgin, *Augenheilkunde*; and Blodi, et al., *Arabian Ophthalmologists*.

The topic of Prophetic Medicine is the subject of a monograph by Perho, *The Prophet's Medicine*, and forms part of the study by Dols, *Majnūn*, 211–60; see also Rahman, *Health and Medicine*; and Bummel, 'Human Biological Reproduction'.

Notes

1 Ibn Sīnā, *Canon*, i. 3.
2 Ibn Abī Uṣaybiʿah, *Sources of Information*, i. 314, 28–9.
3 ibid., ii. 77, 13–14.
4 Dols, *Medieval Islamic Medicine*, 105–6 (with modifications) and 14 Arabic.
5 See Meyerhof, 'Ibn al-Nafīs und seine Theorie'; and Wilson, 'The Problem of the Discovery'.
6 For comparisons between Ibn al-Nafīs and Harvey implying that the discoveries were equivalent, as just one example, see a recent editorial by Azeem Majeed in the *British Medical Journal* (Majeed, 'How Islam Changed Medicine').
7 Psychosomatic cures involving various mental tricks or illusions (*wahms*) are often recounted in the literature; for examples, see Bürgel, 'Psychosomatic Methods'. See also Wilcox and Riddle, 'Qusṭā ibn Lūqā's *Physical Ligatures*', 6–9 for the concern for the congruency of mind and body and the importance of Greek ideas in establishing those of early Islamic physicians.
8 The quotation is taken from al-Rāzī, *Spiritual Medicine*, 75, 1–3; tr. Arberry, *Spiritual Physick*, 81 (the translation here is our own). For sexual intercourse as a therapeutic means, see Dols, *Majnūn*, 90; and Quṣṭā ibn Lūqā's treatise *On Sexual Intercouse and Required Regimen of the Body in order to Have It*, chapter 21 with the title 'On the diseases which reportedly benefit from sexual intercourse'; an edition and German translation of the latter was prepared by Barhoum, 'Buch über die Geschlechtlichkeit'.
9 Kahl, 'Yaʿqūb ibn Isḥāq', 32 Arabic, 52 English; translation that of Kahl, considerably amended.
10 Ibn Sīnā, *Canon*, i. 220–1 (Kitāb I, fann 4, faṣl 31).
11 Elkhadem, *Le 'Taqwīm al-ṣiḥḥa'*.
12 Bos, *Ibn al-Jazzār on Sexual Diseases*, Arabic text, 87–9. The translation is that of the present authors rather than that given by Bos on 245–6. For the subject of contraception see Musallam, *Sex and Society in Islam*.

13 See Sadek, *The Arabic Materia Medica of Dioscorides*; Riddle, *Dioscorides on Pharmacy and Medicine*; Dietrich, *Die Dioskurides-Erklärung des Ibn al-Baiṭār*.

14 For further discussion of the role of describing a drug's potency in terms of the four elemental qualities, see Langermann, 'Another Andalusian Revolt?'

15 For example, see Levey, *Substitute Drugs*.

16 See Garijo, 'Ibn Juljul's Treatise on Medicaments'. For Ibn Juljul, see Álvarez-Millán, 'Medical Anecdotes'.

17 See the translation of al-Kindī's formulary, preserved in a unique manuscript, by Martin Levey (Levey, *The Medical Formulary*); see also Tibi, *The Medicinal Use of Opium*.

18 The quotation is taken from Oxford, Bodleian Library, MS Marsh 663, fol. 279a. The adapted version of Ṣabūr's formulary is preserved in Munich, Bayerische Staatsbibliothek, MS Arab. 808/2, fols 2b–21a; unfortunately the translation of Sābūr's formulary published recently by Oliver Kahl (*Sābūr ibn Sahl. The Small Dispensatory*, based on an earlier edition by the same author) does not use this manuscript, and so it does not contain the ten recipes that are specifically marked as *'aḍūdī* (for the 'Aḍūdī hospital); see Degen and Ullmann, 'Zur Dispensatorium', 243–4 and 256–7.

19 For al-Kūhīn al-'Aṭṭār, see Chipman, *Minhāj al-dukkān*.

20 Leiser and al-Khaledy, *Questions and Answers*, 38.

21 Ḥunayn ibn Isḥāq, *Questions on Medicine for Beginners*, 329; Ghalioungui, *Questions on Medicine*, 106 (translation amended).

22 For the life and work of al-Majūsī, see L. Richter-Bernburg, art. "Alī b. 'Abbās Majūsī', *Enc. Ir.*, i. 837a–8b.

23 The treatise on colic by al-Rāzī has been edited and translated into French (Hammami, *Kitāb al-Qūlanǧ*); the treatise by Ibn Sīnā on the same topic has been edited (but not translated) and included in Hammami's volume, on 177–201. Al-Rāzī's monograph *On Gout* (*Maqālah fī al-niqris*) has recently been edited, with English translation, by Omneya Nooh and placed on the web (http://arabcivilization.com/ADHPortal/en/Manuscripts/2.asp). A new edition and translation of the treatise by Maimonides on haemorrhoids is in preparation by Gerrit Bos and others; in 1969 an English translation based on the Hebrew version was published by Rosner and Munter, *Maimonides' Treatise on Haemorrhoids*, which was then revised after comparison with an earlier edition of the Judeo-Arabic text and published by Rosner, *Maimonides' Medical Writings*), 119–52.

24 Latham and Isaacs, *Kitāb al-Ḥummayāt*, sections 29–30; the translation is that of Latham and Isaacs, slightly amended.

25 See Ambjörn, *Qusṭā ibn Lūqā, On Numbness*, and Greenhill, *A Treatise on the Small-Pox and Measles*.

26 Dols, *Medieval Islamic Medicine*, 112 and 17 Arabic.

27 ibid., 113 and 17 Arabic.

28 ibid., 114 and 18 Arabic

29 For these and other plague tracts, see Dols, *The Black Death*, and Conrad 'Arabic Plague Chronologies'.

30 The ḥadīth runs as follows in Arabic: '*Lā 'adwá wa-lā ṭiyarata wa-lā hāmata wa-lā ṣafarata*' (al-Bukhārī, *The Sound* [Book] (*Ṣaḥīh*), iv. 55, no. 19).

31 For the Arabic terminology of plague and pestilence, and the related *ḥadīths*, see Conrad '*Ṭā'ūn* and *wabā*''; Dols, 'The Leper'; and M. W. Dols, art. 'Djudhām', *EI*[2] suppl. 270–4. For resignation to disease and suffering, see Conrad, 'Medicine and

Martyrdom'; and van Ess, *Fehltritt des Gelehrten*.

32 See E. Savage-Smith, art. 'tashrīḥ', *EI*² x. 354b–6b.

33 The quotation attributed to al-Ghazālī is found in, Dublin, Chester Beatty Library, Persian MS 129, fol. 1a, where the author is given as Imām Ghazālī. The aphorism attributed to Ghazālī is written by a reader in the margin of an illuminated copy of *Manṣūr's Anatomy* by Ibn Ilyās. See Savage-Smith 'Attitudes toward Dissection'.

34 Newman, '*Tašrīḥ-i Manṣūrī*'; Maddison and Savage-Smith, *Science, Tools and Magic*, i. 14–27; and Savage-Smith 'Anatomical Illustration'.

35 See O'Neill, 'The Fünfbilderserie Reconsidered'; O'Neill 'Fünfbilderserie: A Bridge'; French, 'An Origin'.

36 The Syrian manual of market inspection in question is that by al-Shayzarī, *Utmost Authority*, the quotations occurring on 89, 3–4 and 101, paen.–102, 1 (Arabic); and 108 and 117 in Buckley's translation (the present rendering is our own); see also Savage-Smith, 'Attitudes toward Dissection', 81–2. For the quotation from al-Zahrāwī, see Spink and Lewis, *Albucasis*, 2–3.

37 The surgical chapter by al-Zahrāwī has been edited and translated into English (Spink and Lewis, *Albucasis*).

38 See Müller-Bütow and Spies, *Anatomie und Chirurgie des Schädels*. See the general study of Ibn al-Quff by Hamarneh, *The Physician, Therapist and Surgeon Ibn al-Quff* (which should however be used with caution).

39 Spink and Lewis, *Albucasis*, 170–1; see also Pormann, *Oriental Tradition*, 301–2.

40 Spink and Lewis, *Albucasis*, 338–9.

41 For the passage from Ibn Zuhr, see Ibn Zuhr, *Easy Guide*, 149, 15–150, 5.

42 The passage from al-Shādhilī is contained in a manuscript at the National Library of Medicine (NLM, MS A 29.1, fol. 118b); see Savage-Smith, *Islamic Medical Manuscripts*. For the instruments described in Arabic and Greek treatises for cutting up a dead foetus, see Spink and Lewis, *Albucasis*, 484–94, and Adams, *Seven Books of Paulus*, ii. 387–92.

43 See Spink and Lewis, *Albucasis*, 410–19; see also Kaadan, 'Albucasis and Extraction of Bladder Stone'.

44 Spink and Lewis, *Albucasis*, 354–8.

45 ibid., 300–5; for an early twentieth-century example of the technique, see Savage-Smith, 'The Practice of Surgery', 316, n. 37.

46 Spink and Lewis, *Albucasis*, 362–6.

47 ibid., 276–87 and 292–5.

48 For Muḥammad al-Shafrah, see Llavero Ruiz, 'La medicina granadina del siglo XIV'; Llavero Ruiz, *Un tratado de cirugía hispanoárabe del siglo XIV*, and McVaugh, *Medicine before the Plague*, 53.

49 For an English translation along with an edition of Ḥunayn's treatise, see Meyerhof, *The Book of the Ten Treatises on the Eye*. For knowledge of the anatomy of the eye, see also Russell, 'Anatomy of the Eye'.

50 For an annotated English translation of 'Alī ibn 'Īsá, see Wood, *Memorandum Book of a Tenth-Century Oculist*. For 'Ammār, see Meyerhof, *The Cataract Operations of 'Ammār ibn 'Alī al-Mawsilī*; and Blodi, et al., *Arabian Ophthalmologists*.

51 For the treatise by Khalīfah ibn Abī al-Maḥāsin al-Ḥalabī, see the index under his name. For the Geniza documents, see Isaacs and Baker, *Medical and Para-Medical Manuscripts*; Goitein, 'The Medical Profession in Light of the Cairo Geniza Docu-

ments', 190–1; Goitein, *A Mediterranean Society*, ii. 257–72.

52 E. Wiedemann and J. W. Allan, art. '*Kuḥl*', *EI*[2] v. 356a–7a; Ullmann, *WKAS* under *kuḥl* i. 73b21–74a37 and 549b13–39.

53 See Savage-Smith, 'Ibn al-Nafīs's *Perfected Book on Ophthalmology*'; Pormann, *Oriental Tradition*, 155–6, 158–60, 184–7; Blodi, et al., *Arabian Ophthalmologists*, 88–91, 98–9, 108–14.

54 The note by Muwaffaq al-Dīn al-Sāmirī is contained in Oxford, Bodleian Library, MS Marsh 98, fol. 208a. For Ḥunayn's *Questions Concerning the Eye*, see the edition and French translation by Sbath and Meyerhof, *Le livre des questions sur l'œil*.

55 Jahier and Noureddine, *Avicenne, Poème de la médecine*.

56 Ibn Jazlah's treatise, though popular at the time, has not been printed or translated. For Ibn Buṭlān's *Almanac*, see Elkhadem, *Le 'Taqwīm al-ṣiḥḥa'*.

57 Neither al-Rāzī's *Book for al-Manṣūr*, nor al-Majūsī's treatise have been translated into any modern European language; for the latter, see Lutz Richter-Bernburg, "Alī b. 'Abbās Majūsī', *Enc. Ir.*, i. 837a–8b.

58 For the life and writings of Ibn Sīnā, see M. Mahdi, et al., art. 'Avicenna', *Enc. Ir.*, iii. 66a–110b.

59 The reaction of Abū al-'Alā' Zuhr (d. 1131) to the *Canon* is recounted by Ibn Jumay' (d. 1198), one of the physicians to Ṣalāḥ al-Dīn (Saladin), in Oxford, Bodleian Library, MS Marsh 390, fol. 1a2–9. The anecdote is also repeated by Ibn Abī Uṣaybi'ah, *Sources of Information*, ii. 65, 2–6; see also Iskandar, *Catalogue*, 36–7.

60 Shihāb al-Manṣūrī (d. 1492); Cairo, Dār al-Kutub MS *majāmi' mīm* 102, fol. 201b; translation by Dols, *Black Death*, 109. For plague tracts in general, see Dols, *Black Death*.

61 See, for example in al-Ṣanawbarī, *Book of Mercy*, 12.

62 See Ispahany and Newman, *Islamic Medical Wisdom*, 165–9. At about the same time as this treatise was composed in the east, Ibn Ḥabīb (d. c. 853) composed in Muslim Spain an essay on medicine also drawing upon *ḥadīths* as a major source; see Álvarez de Morales and Girón Irueste, *Mujtaṣar fī l-ṭibb* for a Spanish translation.

63 Two English translations have been published of Shams al-Din al-Dhahabī's treatise, both of them incorrectly attributed to al-Suyūṭī (d. 1505); see Elgood, '*Ṭibb-ul-Nabbi*' and Thomson, *As-Suyuti's Medicine of the Prophet*. For the authorship by al-Dhahabī, see Savage-Smith, 'Attitudes toward Dissection', 73–4; and Perho, *The Prophet's Medicine*, 36–40. For the quotations cited here see al-Dhahabī, *Prophetic Medicine*, 12 and 234; tr. 12, 130.

64 The Cambridge University Library manuscript (MS Qq. 161) has even been edited and published under 'Abd al-Laṭīf's name; for the arguments against it being a composition by 'Abd al-Laṭīf, see Perho, *The Prophet's Medicine*, 37–8.

65 For the text of Suyūṭī's treatise, see the index under his name; no translation has been published. The English translations of a treatise on Prophetic Medicine that are under his name are in fact translations of the treatise by Shams al-Dīn al-Dhāhabī.

66 al-Ṣanawbarī, *Book of Mercy*, 33 and 37.

67 For discussions of the 'myth' of great opposition to Greek sciences on the part of Islamic scholars, see Gutas, *Greek Thought*, 166–75.

3

Physicians and society

> He [Abū l-Ḥārith Asad ibn Jānī] was a physician. Once business was slow, so someone said to him: 'It is a plague year, disease rampant everywhere, and you are a knowledgeable man with steadfastness, experience, and clear understanding. How does it come about that you have this dearth [of patients]?' To which he replied: 'For one thing, people know me to be a Muslim, and they have held the belief, even before I began to practice medicine, no indeed even before I was born, that Muslims are not successful in medicine. Moreover, my name is Asad, when it ought to have been Ṣalīb, Jibrā'īl, Yuḥannā, and Bīrā [that is, Christian or Jewish names]. My surname [*kunyah*] is Abū l-Ḥārith, but it ought to have been Abū 'Īsá, Abū Zakarīyā', and Abū Ibrāhīm [that is, Christian or Jewish surnames]. I wear a shoulder mantle of white cotton, yet my shoulder mantle ought to be of black silk. My pronunciation is that of an Arab, when my dialect ought to be that of the people of Gondēshāpūr [a city famous for its Christian physicians].'
> – al-Jāḥiẓ (d. 868/9), *Book of Misers*[1]

When asking the question how physicians operated within a larger social context, it is important to remember that the different Islamic societies could vary greatly. Situations must have been considerably at odds with each other from country to country, from culture to culture: the social setting of medical practice in Muslim Spain in the eleventh century, for instance, varied from that in Eastern Afghanistan at the same period, even if the learned medical theory did not differ greatly at these two poles of the Islamic world. Moreover, even in the same locality, conditions changed tremendously over time. Baghdad, for example, at the beginning of the ninth century, was the capital of the vast 'Abbāsid empire and a political and economic powerhouse, second to none in the world at that moment. Some four centuries later, however, even before the Mongols sacked it, the Muslim travel-writer Ibn Jubayr (d. 1217) qualified Baghdad in dispiriting terms:

> Most of its outline has disappeared, and all that remains is its famous name … It resembles … obliterated ruins and erased traces, or the spectre of a disappearing ghost. No beauty is in it which could catch the eye … except the River Tigris …[2]

The reasons for Baghdad's decline were manifold: its might and prosperity waned as new centres emerged in the wake of geopolitical fragmentation, and the recurrent inundations of the Tigris and Euphrates did their share to deface its former beauty, with particularly devastating floods in 1074, 1159, and 1217. Hence, the situation regarding medical practice was quite different in the early thirteenth century from that in the ninth, as many physicians now preferred Damascus and Cairo to the erstwhile capital of the Islamic world. Additionally, even at the same time and in the same region, the differences between urban and rural localities could be immense. A great complexity of social life existed in the medieval Islamic world, within which physicians and other providers of medical care occupied various roles. Yet, because of the lack of adequate documentation, we can only offer glimpses at what it might have been like to be a patient or practitioner in the period discussed here.

The choice of example is dictated to a large extent by the sources which have been the object of scholarly attention. For urban physicians, the best available evidence deals with Baghdad, Damascus, and Cairo, all three at some stage important capitals of different Islamic dynasties. To investigate solely the elite health care within a metropolitan setting is, however, unsatisfactory. We have therefore endeavoured to highlight some other elements, such as provisions for the poor, competition in the medical market place, and women as patients and practitioners. Certain trends and tendencies regarding the position of the physician within the various societies will emerge. It is likely that this preliminary picture reflects the situation at other times and in other urban or rural settings within the confines of medieval Islam.

Medical education

> One of the requirements for the student of this art is that he should be in attendance at the hospitals [*bīmāristāns*] and the places of the sick; that he consult extensively with the most skilled teachers among the physicians about their [the patients'] situations and circumstances; and that he examine frequently the conditions of the patients and the symptoms apparent in them, calling to mind what he has read about these conditions and what they indicate of good and ill. If he does this, he will reach a high degree of perfection in this art.
> – al-Majūsī, *Complete Book of the Medical Art*[3]

> The best and most excellent way [to train medical students] is in the hospitals, as they are the places where the doctors and the sick gather and where students can perfectly train themselves in the practice of this art under the supervision of teachers skilled in it.
> – Ibn Jumay' (d. 1198), *Treatise to Salāḥ al-Dīn (Saladin) on the Revival of the Art of Medicine*[4]

How did one become a doctor? The answer to this question will reveal a great deal about the position of the physician within society. The issue of medical education will in turn lead to another related topic, namely the definition of good medical practice: who was considered to be a 'physician', what did it mean to be one, and how did physicians differentiate themselves from other medical practitioners in the marketplace.

As with any field of study, the potential pupil had two basic choices: either to learn from a master, or to teach himself. There are some famous examples of the latter technique. The celebrated Ibn Sīnā (Avicenna, d. 1037) boastfully claimed in his autobiography to have mastered the art of medicine by the age of sixteen through independent study. Recent scholarship, however, has cast doubts about Ibn Sīnā's veracity in the matter of his being a medical autodidact.[5] Another self-taught physician was the Egyptian Ibn Riḍwān (d. c. 1068), who allegedly was too poor to afford to study medicine with a teacher and wrote a tract defending the method of self-education.

It seems likely, however, that these famous cases (true or not) of medical autodidacts are the exception rather than the norm, and students would generally have striven to be instructed by someone with both theoretical skills and practical experience. The *Hippocratic Oath* was well known in the Islamic world through its Arabic translation (which we had occasion to discuss in Chapter 1). It advocated medical teaching in a family-like context, in which the pupil was to consider the children of his master as his own siblings, and, if the opportunity arose, to teach them medicine free of charge. Many physicians handed down medical knowledge to their own offspring, thereby creating some famous lineages. The Bukhtīshū', a Nestorian family hailing from the famous city of Gondēshāpūr, for instance, served as court physicians to caliphs in Baghdad for nearly three centuries. The Ibn Zuhr family, five generations of physicians in Muslim Spain, are another example.

One could also be the apprentice to a physician who was not a relative, for which a fee would generally be required. Al-Rāzī, for instance, tells the interesting story (to be cited in full shortly) of a Cairene physician who had a pupil staying with him. The master sends his pupil packing upon discovering that the pupil deceived a client. Al-Rāzī himself had many pupils, and he even composed an *Epistle to One [ba'ḍ] of His Students*, in which he addresses the problem of serving as a physician to royalty and high society in general. His students recorded case notes during his consultations, which are still extant in the *Book of Experiences*. Moreover, they posthumously edited his notes on various medical matters and published them as the *Comprehensive Book*.[6]

A third avenue towards medical education lay in the hospitals, which, by the first half of the tenth century, had become important centres of medical learning. Many of the best physicians practised and trained their students there. The opening quotations of this section illustrate that some prominent physicians regarded hospitals as the best place to receive medical instruction from the tenth century onwards.

Finally, the *majlis* (literally 'session') provided an opportunity for medical education. Throughout the Islamic world, it was (and sometimes still is) a custom for a teacher to sit in a public place such as a mosque, market, or the court of a palace, with students gathered around him in circles. He would lecture on his subject, ask questions, and answer queries from the audience. One doctor who acquired a reputation for repartee and a sharp wit in these sessions was Yuḥannā ibn Māsawayh (d. 857), personal physician to four successive caliphs in Baghdad and the teacher of Ḥunayn ibn Isḥāq. Another physician who held such sessions was al-Dakhwār, a famous teacher of medicine in Damascus who was charged with the 'supervision (*ri'āsah*) of physicians in all of Egypt and Syria'. Two years before his death in 1230, the Ayyūbid ruler of Damascus al-Malik al-Ashrāf 'created (*ja'ala*) for him a *majlis* for instruction in the art of medicine', as we are told in a near contemporaneous source. This would suggest that on occasion such venues were underwritten by rulers, though it is unclear what form the support took.[7]

Al-Dakhwār is important in another respect, for he was the first to establish a school (*madrasah*) devoted exclusively to teaching medicine. He bequeathed as a charitable trust (*waqf*) his house in the old goldsmiths' quarter east of the date-sellers' market in Damascus to establish this school. It opened, with considerable ceremony, on 12 January 1231 (8 Rabīʿ I 628), and we learn from other sources that it was still in existence in 1417, when it underwent some repairs. Al-Dakhwār established his school in the classic form of a *madrasah* in that he provided endowments for its maintenance, the teacher's salary, and student stipends, but gave it the unusual purpose of teaching medicine rather than Islamic law (*fiqh*). Al-Dakhwār's initiative, although singular in terms of medical teaching, was in line with general trends in the late twelfth and early thirteenth centuries which saw the founding of many *madrasahs* and other measures responsible for a gradual institutionalisation of knowledge. Generally speaking, *fiqh* was the primary focus of *madrasahs*, though occasionally instruction in a few ancillary subjects such as medicine would be offered. Shortly after al-Dakhwār's foundation, according to a sixteenth-century source, there were also in Damascus two additional *madrasahs* where medicine was taught, though not as the sole subject.[8]

In conclusion, it is therefore fair to say that the four most important avenues for studying the medical art consisted of familial tuition, apprenticeship, attendance at *majlises*, and hospital training, while *madrasahs* constituted venues for medical education only occasionally and not before the thirteenth century. These different forms of learning were not, to be sure, mutually exclusive. Al-Rāzī's students, for instance, accompanied him to the hospital, as well as his home.

What then did students learn? Which texts did they have to master? And what exams (if any) did they have to pass? In the ninth century, Ḥunayn ibn Isḥāq makes the following remark about the medical education of his day:

> Those [the *Sixteen Books of Galen*] are the books which were read exclusively at the place of instruction in Alexandria. [...] They used to gather each day to read and interpret one major work just as our Christian friends nowadays gather at the places of instruction which are known as '*uskūl*' [from Greek *scholē*, 'school'] to read a major work from among those for beginners.[9]

This quotation illustrates the great importance of Galen's *Sixteen Books*, as well as the influence of Alexandria on medical teaching in Baghdad. Some two centuries later, the Muslim author Ibn Riḍwān (d. 1068), one of the medical autodidacts mentioned above, shared the view that Galen's works should form the core curriculum. He did, however, criticise severely the medical teaching of his day, which, in his mind, relied too much on commentaries and abridgements, and neglected the Galenic and Hippocratic originals:

> Summaries and commentaries of Galen's books do not make the latter superfluous. Summaries fail to encompass all of Galen's ideas, while commentaries increase the length of the art, and distract [students] from studying, since, of necessity, these would have to be read for verification together with their [original] medical works.[10]

Ibn Riḍwān himself advocated the following educational ideal:

> I divide the teaching of medicine into two parts: one is theory, which is to be studied either from the books of Hippocrates or those of Galen, without resorting to any other books – if you wish to, consult them together, for this is the perfect and clearest [method]. The other is practice, by which I mean the study of bone-setting, the restoration of dislocations, incision, suturing, cautery, lancing [*baṭṭ*], [application of] of eye remedies (*kuḥl*), and all other manual procedures.[11]

To be sure, we do not know to what extent this ideal was realised in practice. His condemnation of current educational practices, however, provides us with an interesting insight into how medical students were actually taught at his time.

Commentaries and summaries were not the only medical genres which incurred Ibn Riḍwān's scathing criticism. He equally lamented the increased reliance on compendia, the origins of which he saw in Late Antiquity. In all these medical genres, great emphasis is placed on division and systematic organisation of knowledge. These expository techniques are especially evident in Ibn Sīnā's *Canon of Medicine*, which in its turn became a manual used in teaching medicine both in Islamic lands and in medieval and early modern Europe.

Thus, Galenic and Hippocratic treatises remained central to the medical curricula from the ninth century onwards, both in full and abridged Arabic versions, with commentaries as aids for their understanding. Moreover, as the Arabic medical encyclopaedias that digested and expanded the earlier material became increasingly available, they too became part of medical teaching. These tendencies not only continued in Arabic-speaking circles, but also penetrated Persian ones. The twelfth-century Persian writer in Samarqand, Niẓāmī-i ʿArūḍī, provided the following account of a proper medical education in his day:

> On the science of medicine the student should procure and read the *Aphorisms* of Hippocrates, ... Then he should take up one of the more detailed treatises, such as the *Sixteen Books* of Galen, the *Comprehensive Book* of Muḥammad ibn Zakarīyā' al-Rāzī; the *Complete Book of the Medical Art* [by al-Majūsī]; the *Hundred Books* of Abū Sahl al-Masīḥī (d 1010); the *Canon* of Abū 'Alī ibn Sīnā; and the *Treasure Book for Khwārazmshāh* [a widely-read Persian medical compendium by al-Jurjānī, d. c. 1136].[12]

Over time, the earlier educational inclinations to begin with Galen and Hippocrates were complemented by using compendia and encyclopedias. These patterns were perpetuated for centuries in both the Islamic world and the West. Moreover, the move towards a greater reliance upon compendia and commentaries in medical teaching was paralleled in other areas of knowledge such as jurisprudence (*fiqh*).[13]

From the thirteenth century, we possess a few examples of a physician certifying that a particular student had read a text with him. In a copy made in 1269 of a commentary written by Ibn al-Nafīs on Hippocrates' *On the Nature of Man*, Ibn al-Nafīs certified in his own handwriting that a Christian student by the name of Shams al-Dawlah Abū Faḍl ibn Abī al-Ḥasan 'demonstrated clarity of intellect' by having thoroughly studied the entire treatise with this illustrious master. Here we see an example of a prominent Muslim physician, who was educated in Damascus but spent much of his working life in Cairo, instructing a Christian pupil on an Arabic commentary expounding a Hippocratic treatise. Such documents at the end of a particular medical book, certifying that it has been read and mastered by a certain individual, are regrettably rare, but there are a few other examples. While they provide useful information regarding the teaching methods employed by prominent and learned physicians, they are not equivalent to a document licensing physicians upon completion of an approved programme of training.[14]

Medical regulation

Documents such as the one just mentioned, written by Ibn al-Nafīs, did not constitute a universal system for vetting physicians. Nor was there ever, before the Ottoman period, some central authority which could grant licences to practise. There are, however, two main sources for our knowledge of topics and texts on which medical students might be tested: (1) injunctions by physicians themselves, usually presented in treatises and chapters having titles such as *On Examining the Physician* (*fī miḥnat al-ṭabīb*) or in treatises having a question-and-answer format, and (2) procedures provided in manuals of market inspection (*ḥisbah*).

Following Greek models, Yūḥannā ibn Māsawayh (d. 857), Ḥunayn ibn Isḥāq (d. c. 873), and al-Rāzī (d. 925) all composed treatises on the examination of physicians, though regrettably the first two are now lost. Moreover, in treatises on medical ethics, to be discussed more fully in the next section, doctors included chapters titled 'On Examining Physicians' in which they gave directions as to what questions to ask in order to assess practitioners. The general picture emerging from this literature is the following: students needed to master a canon of Greek medical texts expounding the principles of humoral pathology. Al-Rāzī's treatise *On Examining the Physician*, for instance, contains many quotations from treatises by Galen, such as *That the Best Physician is Also a Philosopher* and *On Examinations by Which the Best Physicians are Recognised*, the latter forming the model for al-Rāzī's own work of a similar title. Hippocrates is the second authority whom al-Rāzī invokes.

The question now arises to what extent this literature reflects examination practice. Some treatises, such as the one which al-Sulamī composed in question-and-answer format and titled *The Experts' Examination of all Physicians*, contain extremely complicated and longwinded answers to questions which the students could hardly have been expected to answer. Others, as R. Kruk has persuasively argued, show a real concern for the technicalities of how to test a potential practitioner. To the modern reader the latter type therefore appear to be more likely candidates for having actually been employed as examination manuals. To give just two examples: al-Rāzī urges his readers not to rely on uroscopy when examining potential physicians; whether a candidate can distinguish between animal and human urine, for instance, is not always a valid criterion for knowing whether he would be a good doctor. Secondly, in his treatise on medical ethics, Ṣā'id ibn al-Ḥasan included certain questions which seem to lend themselves well for examination purposes, such as the following:

> What is the difference between the symptoms of pleurisy (*dhāt al-janb*) and those of a swelling of the liver; and how are they indicated? [...]
> What is the difference between the symptoms of a colic (*qawlanj*) and those of a stone formed in the kidneys or bladder?[15]

These questions deal with differential diagnostics – that is to say, the problem of distinguishing between different diseases with somewhat similar symptoms. Sā'id does not, however, provide answers to these questions.

Another genre of medical literature, that of the question-and-answer treatises discussed in the previous chapter, is relevant to our knowledge about the content of examinations. There is a natural overlap between the subjects covered in the works titled 'On Examining the Physician' and those in question-and-answer format. If students memorised the latter, they may well have been expected to be examined on their content. Indeed, the first question quoted above from Ṣā'id ibn al-Ḥasan regarding the difference between pleurisy and liver swelling occurs in a very similar form in a treatise on differential diagnosis organised as a catechism. In the latter case, however, the author also provided an answer. We can only speculate which questions – whether from the examination manuals or the question-and-answer treatises – the medical examiner might have asked.[16]

No less puzzling a problem is the identity of those who held medical examinations, and the frequency with which they occurred. Market inspectors (*muḥtasibs*) appear at times to have carried out this task, at least if we can trust the manuals of market inspection (*ḥisbah*) written from the twelfth century onwards. The latter laid down standards for merchants, traders, and artisans operating in markets – a group that included druggists, surgeons, and physicians. The ideas expounded in the examination handbooks filtered down into some of these manuals, suggesting that the former did not merely constitute a literary tradition with no bearing on actual reality.

One of the earliest and most influential of these manuals was written by al-Shayzarī, who worked in Syria during the reign of Ṣalāḥ al-Dīn (Saladin, r. 1169–93). It is entitled *The Utmost Authority in the Pursuit of Market Inspection* and contains a number of chapters specifically concerned with how to regulate the different medical practitioners in the market. Al-Shayzarī directed that physicians be tested in compliance with the guidelines given by Ḥunayn ibn Isḥāq in his treatise *The Examination of the Physician* (now lost); ophthalmologists be examined on the content of *The Ten Treatises on the Eye* by the same Ḥunayn; bone-setters, on the sixth book of Paul of Aegina's *Compendium*; and surgeons, on Galen's *On the Composition of Drugs according to Place* [*in the Body*]. Again, to fulfil these requirements, one needed to be conversant in Greek medical theory in its Arabic garb, although al-Shayzarī added that Galen's book on examining physicians was to be avoided since no physician could be expected to perform what was required in it.

Another person potentially involved in examining physicians was the chief physician (*ra'īs al-aṭibbā'*). As early as the ninth century we hear that Ḥunayn ibn Isḥāq was appointed chief physician by the caliph al-Mutawakkil. Others such as Ibn Tilmīdh (d. 1165) in Baghdad and al-Dakhwār (d. 1230) in Damascus served in this function. The legal scholar and secretary al-Qalqashandī (d. 1418), the author of a monumental chancery manual, classes the chief physician – together with the chief architect, the chief oculist (*ra'īs al-kaḥḥālīn*), and the chief surgeon (*ra'īs al-jarrāḥīyah*) – under the title 'master of office (*rabb al-waẓīfah*)' 'from among the people of the arts (*ahl al-ṣinā'āt*)'. He provides the following description:

> The second ['master of office'] is the chief physician. He rules over the class (*ṭā'ifah*) of physicians, grants permission [*ya'dhanu*] for medical practice, and the like. [...]
>
> The chief physician is appointed to supervise his class, and to know their conditions. He orders the person carrying out treatment first of all to know the true [nature] of the illness, and its causes and symptoms; [...] He [this person] ought

> not to deviate from the common practice [*'ādah*] of the physicians. [...] He should avoid medication when treatment through food is possible; [avoid] compound drugs when one can apply simple ones; and resort to analogy [*qiyās*] only if the procedure is confirmed through the experience of others, such as people who have previously employed it.[17]

This description would suggest quite a sophisticated regulatory framework for medical practice in early fifteenth-century Mamluk Egypt. Corroborating evidence providing details of how these chief physicians carried out their tasks is unfortunately relatively rare.

We know of four concrete examples when the political authorities set up control mechanisms to stamp out medical malpractice, two of which involved chief physicians. First, in ninth-century Baghdad, druggists who were unable to recognise the falseness of a deliberately incorrect prescription were banned from continuing their trade. Second, in 931 the 'Abbāsid vizier 'Alī ibn 'Īsá (d. 946) instructed Sinān ibn Thābit (d. 942), a polymath and prominent practitioner, to examine the physicians in Iraq. We are told that only those who passed the test or had an impeccable reputation could carry on practising, but, apart from some anecdotal evidence, exact details are lacking. Third, later in Baghdad the chief physician Ibn Tilmīdh (d. 1165) examined a doctor who had practical experience, but lacked theoretical knowledge. The fourth instance occurred in Damascus where the Ayyubid ruler al-Malik al-'Ādil I charged al-Dakhwār (d. 1230) with looking into the practice of oculists. Here again, specifics are absent, and it is recorded simply that 'for those oculists who produced benefit through the treatment of eye diseases and satisfied him, al-Dakhwār wrote a statement (*khaṭṭ*) by which he acknowledged this, thereby discharging his duty.'[18]

These different pieces of evidence, taken together, appear to suggest that the call of physicians to regulate medical practice was at least occasionally heeded by the powers that be. Yet, whatever the efforts of the authorities might have been to make practitioners adhere to certain standards, they were largely unsuccessful in excluding those who did not conform to the ideal developed in the literature on medical ethics, as we shall see shortly.

Medical ethics

> He [the physician] should frequently enter and serve in hospitals; he can study rare diseases which he encounters [there]. One often witnesses in such places diseases which are unheard of and which one does not see [discussed] in the written [medical literature]. [...] If he sees any such rare condition, he should record it in his notebook and thus preserve it so that he and others can benefit from it. When he comes to the hospital, he should sit in the place which behoves and befits him. He should clothe himself in calm and dignity, and be attentive and listen with benevolence to the complaints of the patients. [...]
>
> – Ṣā'id ibn al-Ḥasan (d. 1072), *Stimulating a Yearning for Medicine*[19]

To have mastered a set canon of medical knowledge was – at least according to the theoretical medical literature just discussed – one requirement to be a physician. Yet, in order to be a fully-fledged doctor, one also needed to adhere to certain ethical standards and customs discussed in the many treatises on medical ethics. For instance, the quotation given above by Ṣāʿid ibn al-Ḥasan, a Christian doctor, illustrates that outer appearance and bedside manner were important elements in the conduct of clinicians. Physicians needed to treat patients kindly and win their confidence. To this end, they were required to appear dignified, which they achieved by dressing and speaking in a specified or customary manner. When al-Jāḥiẓ relates the anecdote – cited at the beginning of this chapter – of the physician Asad ibn Jānī not being able to attract enough patients because he neither speaks nor dresses like his Christian or Jewish competitors, he indirectly confirms that patients had a notion of a physician's appropriate accent and attire.

But physical appearance was not the only important factor. Through his bedside manner, the physician ought to inspire confidence (as can also be seen from the quotation by al-Rāzī opening Chapter 2). For instance, the physician should deduce as much as possible himself through observation, and only then ask the patient pertinent questions, in this way demonstrating his diagnostic skills. Al-Ruhāwī (*fl.* mid 9th century) gives the following example of how to proceed in his *Ethics of the Physician:*

> A physician visits a patient and finds him coughing and suffering from difficulty in breathing. He feels his arteries and concludes that he has a fever. The physician knows that the specific symptoms indicating pleurisy are four, namely the three which he encountered in this particular patient, with the fourth being a pricking pain [*nakhas*] which the patient feels in his side. Since this pricking is not detectable by sense-perception [on the part of the physician], and since he cannot be absolutely certain from these three indicators just mentioned that it is pleurisy – for they could be symptoms of a different disease – the physician must necessarily ask the patient whether he feels the pricking or not. If pricking of the side is accompanied by coughing, difficulty in breathing, and fever, it is correct that the patient suffers form pleurisy. Then the physician ought to begin searching for the cause that brought about this disease in order to establish which type of pleurisy it is.[20]

Such an approach to questioning would make the patient have confidence in his doctor, and al-Ruhāwī is concerned that the patient's trust should not be undermined in any way. In general, he should behave in a dignified, but also gentle, manner. It was not, however, enough just to be knowledgeable, dress and speak properly, and behave kindly towards the patient. As in the *Hippocratic Oath*, certain moral imperatives should also guide the practitioner: firstly, to employ medicine for the benefit of the patients, and not to harm them; and secondly, not to violate the patient's confidences.

The ideal physician is therefore competent, well-spoken, properly dressed, kind, righteous, and discrete – at least in the view of the doctors who laid down the guidelines in writings on medical ethics. It is easy to agree to these norms and to applaud the physicians who codified them. After all, they had the interest of the patient at heart. There may well have been other motives, however. Rules served to legitimise certain practitioners to the exclusion of others. A specified code of conduct distinguished – at least theoretically – those who could provide proper health care from those who could not. Take the example of medical knowledge. On the one hand, the canon of Greek-derived theory which one should master certainly stood the medical practitioner in good stead when treating his patients, as shown in the example above of the patient suffering from pleurisy. Yet, display of one's knowledge of medical literature was also a powerful means to advertise one's skills. By partaking of the medically orthodox discourse, the doctor demonstrated that he was educationally sound, regardless of whether or not he really needed all the theoretical learning to treat the patient. Islamic as well as Greek physicians displayed their erudition through writing learned medical treatises in order to promote themselves at the expense of the competition. Maintaining certain standards in other respects – dress, speech, bedside manner – also assisted the community of physicians in defining acceptable practice, thereby excluding potential rivals, often labelled as charlatans.[21]

Charlatans

Charlatans are, so to speak, the other side of the coin: defining correct medical practice implies a notion of what is incorrect. Physicians have always tried to delineate themselves from quacks and mountebanks, and it is therefore not surprising that we find a whole host of efforts by the medical establishment to denigrate the medical other. A good example is al-Rāzī. Not only did he write a treatise on *Examining Physicians* (as we have seen above), but also an *Epistle on the Reason Why the Ignorant Physicians, the Common People, and the Women in the Cities Are More Successful than Men of Learning in Treating Certain Diseases, and the Physician's Excuse for This*, now unfortunately lost, and a *Treatise on the Causes Why Most People Turn Away from Excellent Physicians towards the Worst Ones*, which survives in a Hebrew translation. As these titles indicate, competition was a major concern for al-Rāzī. 'Ignorant physicians, common people and women', as he put it, operated in the medical arena and took away his own and his colleagues' potential patients. He therefore denounced their practices. In his *Book for al-Manṣūr*, he lists a number of common tricks which charlatans used to fleece people out of their money. They include surreptitiously putting worms into people's mouths and then removing them in order to make the patient believe that a worm was extracted from the tooth.[22]

Much of this literature appears to be of a conventional type – decrying the decline of standards and promoting one's own practices. On the other hand, it is clear that the underworld of charlatans and tricksters did purposely defraud those who were ill, and that there was genuine concern about exposing their ruses. The extent to which this practice of medical charlatanry was a serious problem is difficult to judge at this distance. An insight into some of these stratagems is provided by the thirteenth-century Syrian reformed mountebank al-Jawbarī, who had first-hand experience. He explains this subterfuge, amongst others, in some detail:

> Another trick is the following. If they want to make a spectacle showing that they administer a drug which expels worms, they take the sinews of camels and give them the shape of the worm. Then they take some laxative plant and put these sinews into it without the idiot noticing it. When he eats it, his bowels are moved and nature secretes something which is like water, and in which these sinews similar to worms are present. The patient does not notice anything. Pay attention to this. Know that if I were to explain all that I have insight into, then it would be a long book. But a part of something exemplifies the whole.[23]

Such fraudulent practices must therefore have occurred frequently in the market. Physicians' attitudes towards them, however, were not always unambiguous. The same al-Rāzī who warned patients against possible deceit also thought that the great Galen did right in tricking patients when it was for their benefit. Al-Ruhāwī also approved of Galen's curing through cunning a patient who thought that he had swallowed a snake. When, despite all efforts of persuasion, the patient still stubbornly believed that a snake was in his belly, Galen had him blind-folded, gave him an emetic, and threw a snake into the basin into which the patient vomited. This cured the patient.[24]

In the same vein, the Muslim theologian al-Ghazālī (d. 1111) told the following story:

> Someone complained to a physician about his wife being infertile and not bearing [him] any children. He [the physician] felt her pulse and said: 'No need to worry about infertility treatment, for you are going to die in forty days, as is indicated by your pulse.' The woman was overcome with fear and lost all appetite for life; she took out her money, divided it and bequeathed it. She remained without eating and drinking, but the [allotted] time passed without her dying. The husband went to the physician and said: 'She did not die.' He replied: 'I know that. Have sex with her now, and she will give birth.' The husband retorted: 'How so?' The physician explained: 'I saw that she was overweight, and that fat had collected at the orifice of the womb. Moreover, I knew that she would only lose weight if she were afraid of dying, so I put this fear into her. Thus she lost weight, and the obstacle against conception has disappeared.'[25]

Here, too, we see the physician using deceit, as Galen did, but for the benefit of the patient; at least this is how he would justify his actions.

The path between right and wrong behaviour could, however, be arduous to tread. Al-Rāzī reports the story, alluded to earlier, of a physician who had taken an apprentice. It is interesting for a number of reasons, and therefore deserves to be cited here in full:

> A great and learned physician in Cairo had a young pupil. A woman came to him with a vessel filled with urine. The young man went down to see who knocked on the door and to know who was at the gate. He found her and asked her to show him the urine. After he inspected it, he said: 'The urine is that of a Christian; yesterday, he ate lentils, and he lives in such and such a neighbourhood.' She answered that all this was true, paid him, and left. The physician saw this from the window and heard what was said. When the pupil came back upstairs, he [the physician] inquired: 'You said this and that to the woman. Now tell me truly how you knew what I myself could not have known.'
>
> He began to beat the apprentice with whips until he confessed and replied: 'I said that he was one of the Christians, because the cloth in which the vessel was carried had a picture of the hanged one [Christ] on it. I surmised that he ate lentils yesterday, since it is the habit of the Christians to eat lentils on Friday. I declared that he was living in such and such a neighbourhood because of the red mud that she had at her hem, for in the whole city there is red mud only in this neighbourhood.' The physician said to him: 'Do no longer come before me, for in the art of medicine, which is a noble science, it does not behove one to employ tricks [*taḥbūlōt* in the Hebrew translation].'[26]

This anecdote is one of many with which al-Rāzī strove to illustrate medical fraud. The deception here lies in the pupil's successful attempt to make the woman believe that he could infer the diet, location, and even religious affiliation of the patient from his urine, while in fact he deduces these things in a Sherlock-Holmes-like fashion from other clues. Remarkably, he provides neither a diagnosis of the illness nor any instructions for treatment. Al-Rāzī might have neglected these medical details to focus on his main point, the deceptive behaviour, for otherwise it is curious that the woman departs content with just having been told what she already knew. The master physician's anger may well have been motivated by two different, and somewhat conflicting, considerations. On the one hand, he states clearly that he dismisses his apprentice for using tricks. Yet, he also seems to resent his pupil's knowing what he did not; the latter was too clever by half and had to pay the penalty.

Let us briefly turn to another aspect of the medical 'other'. Rivalling physicians sometimes accused each other of incompetence. A famous example is the quarrel between the Christian physician Ibn Buṭlān of Baghdad (d. after 1063) and the Egyptian Muslim doctor Ibn Riḍwān (d. c. 1068). Evidence for it survives in the form of an exchange of epistles on the major and momentous problem whether 'the chicken has a warmer nature than a young bird'. In it they accused each other of medical incompetence, and Ibn Riḍwān went so far as to deny that Ibn Buṭlān should be called a physician ('*ṭabīb*').[27] The frame of reference in this exchange by which it was established whether or not someone was a proper physician was a canon of Greek learning, and so Greek theory is again the touchstone used to distinguish between 'proper' physicians and 'the other'.

The two stories by al-Ghazālī and al-Rāzī just quoted also highlight a number of other points – for instance, that Muslim physicians had Christian patients, and that they could see women as well as men. But before turning to the question of intercommunal relations and that of women as patients and practitioners, let us first consider the place of the physician, both in the sense of his station in society and the locus of medical practice.

Status of physicians

Doctor 'Īsá, please show pity! You are Noah's deadly deluge;
Separating soul from body is your treatment's only purpose.
Doctor 'Īsá, the physician, and Christ, 'Īsá the Messiah, have indeed nothing in common.
While the latter, Scripture tells us, had the dead restored to new life,
You are quite a different 'Īsá. You are here to kill the healthy.
– Anonymous poet (note that "Īsá' is the Arabic form of 'Jesus')[28]

History often only remembers the conquerors, not the conquered. One is therefore scarcely astonished that our sources record the names of distinguished doctors and recount stories of success while usually avoiding to mention their failures. Similarly, when physicians talk about their own profession, it comes as no surprise that they depict it as noble and elevated. This picture can be supplemented, however, by some other, more critical and often satirical, accounts of medical practice. An example is the one presented in the verses quoted above.

The life of Ḥunayn ibn Isḥāq (d. c. 873), even though extraordinary in many respects, is typical for that of an elite physician. Born into a family of Nestorian Christians in southern Iraq, he moved to Baghdad to study medicine. He ultimately became not only the chief instigator of a huge translation movement, but also the court physician to the caliph al-Mutawakkil. During his lifetime Ḥunayn managed to accumulate an enormous fortune, as well as an extensive library. Disaster struck him, however, in two different guises: first, his library was tragically lost, and then he fell into disgrace with the caliph al-Mutawakkil. The latter seized his estate and threw him into prison because of a religious imbroglio over Christian icons. Yet Ḥunayn was later returned to favour, and remained main court physician until his death.

There were many other physicians throughout the medieval Islamic world who enjoyed close associations with the ruling elite, accumulated considerable wealth, and built extensive personal libraries. An interesting case is the Jewish physician Ifrā'īm ibn al-Ḥasan, who lived in eleventh-century Cairo, and about whom Ibn Abī Uṣaybi'ah says:

> He was in the service of the caliphs of his time, and received from them a very great amount of money and favours. He had studied the art of medicine with … ʿAlī ibn Riḍwān and was his most illustrious pupil. He had an acute interest in acquiring and copying books, so that he accumulated large scores of them on medicine and other subjects.[29]

Ibn Abī Uṣaybiʿah goes on to relate how there were always scribes in Ifrāʾīm's employ, working frantically, and that he travelled far and wide to purchase more works. These efforts resulted in a library boasting 20,000 volumes and being of such quality that different individuals attempted to buy it. Another example is Ibn al-Muṭrān, a Christian who lived in Syria, converted to Islam, and found in Ṣalāḥ al-Dīn (Saladin) a generous patron. His book collection reportedly numbered 10,000 volumes at the time of his death in 1191.[30]

This glorified image of the physician as an extremely learned and wealthy individual is vividly painted in the bio-bibliographic works. The deontological literature also underlines the great intellectual culture and wisdom of physicians, but is more ambivalent about the economic aspects of medical practice.

On the one hand, certain authors on medical ethics urged physicians not to strive after financial gain, but rather to be guided by higher ideals. In Iraq, Ṣāʿid ibn al-Ḥasan, for instance, enjoined that the true physician should not be driven by greed: if a patient is unable to pay, the doctor ought to have mercy on him and treat him free of charge. Likewise, the Egyptian author Ibn Riḍwān warns against the pleasures of this world, which might distract the physician from what he ought to do: become more learned in the medical art. He proclaims:

> Oh doctor, beware of occupying yourself with the pleasures of brute beasts such as eating, drinking, intercourse, accumulating riches, vanity, love of bragging about mounts, clothing, and other things in which one takes pride. You deceive the common people by associating with those who have wealth, letting your beard grow long, and having grey hair. Being obsessed by all of these things prevents you from completing your education in the art of medicine. These things are what Galen and other philosophers and doctors rebuke.[31]

This general topos in the medical literature, that the doctor should have contempt for worldly possessions, continues certain Greek precepts regarding the correct comportment.[32]

It is, however, clear that these lofty ideals of disregarding money were not universally shared nor always adhered to. For instance, the Jewish physician Isḥāq ibn Sulaymān al-Isrāʾīlī advised his colleagues to collect their fee before the cure is complete. He states in his *Ethics of the Physician*:

> Fix your fee with the patient when his illness is increasing and most virulent, for once he is cured he will forget what you have done for him.[33]

This short passage highlights the financial aspects of the physician's occupation as well. The most wealthy practitioners could easily afford to be generous with their services, but there are others who depended on their fees to make a living.

The tension between the need to live, the wish to prosper, and the imperative to have the patients' well-being as one's first priority – regardless of their financial means – is therefore well illustrated in these few examples. In real life, some practitioners did need to charge a fee, and others were at least perceived as being motivated by avarice not only by their colleagues (as in the case of Ibn Riḍwān), but also by the non-medical public. An eloquent example of the latter is al-Jāḥiẓ's portrayal of the Muslim doctor Asad ibn Jānī (quoted at the opening of this chapter) as greedy, and wanting to profit from the general bad health in the country. It is a thinly veiled criticism of the medical establishment in general. Yet, doctors were not only the target of mockery because of their perceived rapacity, but also their presumed incompetence, as shown by the verses of the anonymous poet, quoted at the beginning of this section. A physician called 'Īsá (Jesus) is ridiculed because, unlike the Jesus of the New Testament and the Qur'ān (5:110), he kills rather than cures those who come to him.

In any case, the status of physicians differed greatly. The best and the brightest could certainly rise to considerable esteem and wealth. Others may have belonged to the 'upper middle class', as scholars have argued on the basis of documents from the Geniza (a storage space in a Cairo synagogue from which much firsthand material has been recovered). Yet, not all doctors belonged to this middle class, and there must have been many who struggled to make a living. They are those whom history often forgets, who disappeared as if they never existed, and about whom we know very little. Unlike their illustrious colleagues, they may well have practised in the market rather than the palace or the hospital.[34]

Places of medical practice: between the hospital and the market

Where did physicians treat their patients? There are four main places where caring and curing could take place: the markets, about which we have already had occasion to talk, the home of the patient, the home of the physician, and the hospital. In al-Rāzī's *Book of Experiences*, it is evident that patients often visited him. Similarly, the Christian woman, in the anecdote about the deceitful medical pupil quoted above, came to the practitioner's home. Moreover, al-Rāzī himself mentioned on numerous occasions in his *Doubts about Galen* that he treated patients 'in my home (*fī manzilī*)'. He also referred quite frequently to his hospital practice and observations both in his *Doubts about Galen* and his *Comprehensive Book*. He was, after all, a hospital director, and therefore practised there as well as in his home. A near contemporary of al-Rāzī, the physician al-Kaskarī, also treated patients in various hospitals, but specifically says that he made house calls to the palaces of the powerful, as did some of his colleagues. This chimes well with al-Rāzī's activity, since we know that he too went to the palace in Khurāsān to treat the sultan.[35]

The market or *sūq* appears to have been the arena of less respectable (yet still hugely successful and important) medical practitioners such as cuppers, bone-setters and oculists. Some of these may have been itinerant, although the manuals of market inspection do give guidelines on how to test physicians and surgeons. This suggests that some of them set up shop there as well. Regarding medical practitioners in markets, not only the manuals of market inspection, but also Arabic *belles-lettres* (or *adab* in Arabic) provide interesting information, for the latter contain depictions of real-life scenes in the market, even if they are fictional. A case in point is al-Ḥarīrī's popular *Maqāmāt* ('Assemblies'), written in late-eleventh century Baghdad. They contain one episode where the mountebank Abū Zayd poses as a cupper to fleece onlookers out of their money. At the beginning of the story, the narrator, Ḥārith ibn Hammām, sends his slave to find a cupper to come to his house; when the latter fails to do so, Ḥārith himself goes to the market, and encounters Abū Zayd. The scene is illustrated in many of the medieval copies of al-Ḥarīrī's masterpiece, and a particularly attractive example can be seen in Figure 3.1; the painting, however, is as satirical as the story itself and cannot be taken as a reliable guide to medical practice or medical equipment. As in the case of al-Rāzī and al-Kaskarī visiting their powerful patients, might and market forces determined whether Ḥārith received treatment at home or elsewhere.[36]

Islamic hospitals

Hospitals provided another venue for medical practice. In the Fielding H. Garrison lecture of 1972, entitled 'The Physician in Medieval Muslim Society', Franz Rosenthal characterises Islamic hospitals as follows:

> The noblest expression of the deep concern of medieval Muslim society with matters of public health was a highly developed hospital system, a network of urban institutions with large staffs, providing numerous services and frequently having teaching facilities attached to them.[37]

Where is the origin of this Islamic hospital system? How did it create such advanced institutions of medical provision and education? And how did they differ from hospitals in other cultures? Just as historians have asked themselves when the so-called 'first hospital' was founded, the question of which was the first Islamic one has occupied the minds of many scholars. Others regard this search for 'the first' hospital or 'the first Islamic' hospital to be of antiquarian rather than historical interest. Be that as it may, Michael Dols has argued that the Islamic hospital emerged in the late eighth or early ninth century in Iraq and

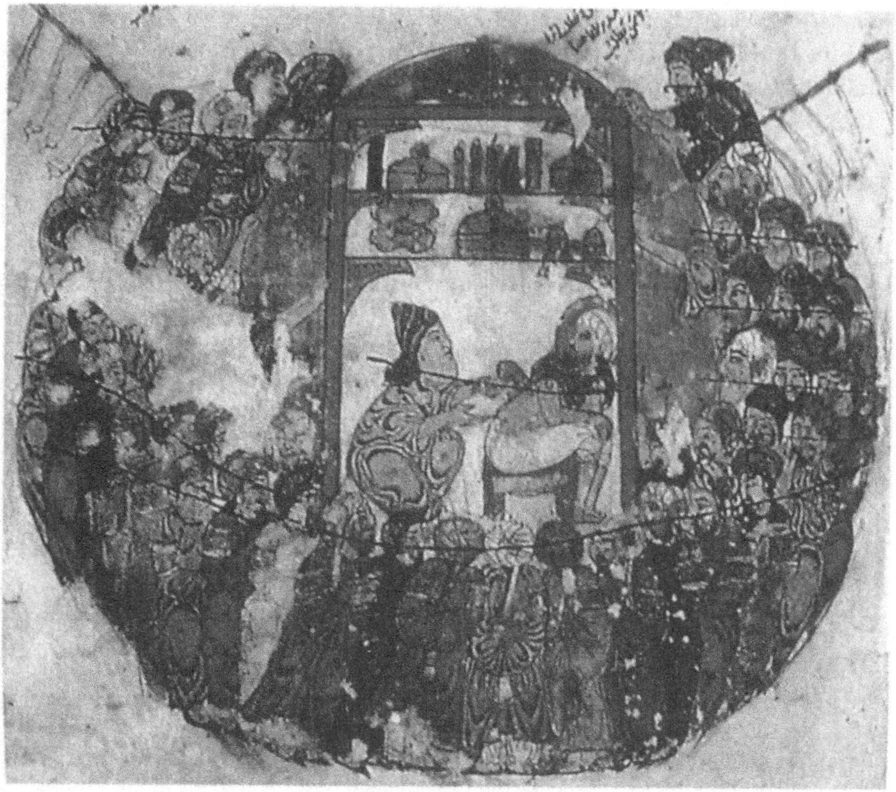

Figure 3.1 Cupping, as depicted in a thirteenth-century copy of the *Assemblies* (*Maqāmāt*) by al-Ḥarīrī (d. 1122), where the trickster and wit Abū Zayd teams up with his son to fleece onlookers of their money.

continued a Nestorian Christian tradition. This influence of Christian charitable ideals and institutions on the development of the Islamic hospital should be stressed here again. However, precious little is known about *bīmāristāns* (as they were called, see pp. 20–1 above) in these earlier days.

From the early tenth century we have much more detailed sources not only for the outer history of the hospital, but also for the inner workings. The caliph al-Muqtadir (r. 908–32), his mother Shaghab (d. 932) and his 'good vizier' 'Alī ibn 'Īsá (d. 946) were all involved in the establishment of hospitals in Baghdad in the 910s and 920s. These, as well as earlier and later, hospitals were generally paid for out of a charitable trust or endowment (*waqf*) set up for this purpose, but some received a monthly grant directly out of the coffers of the caliph. The endowment donated for a *waqf* could consist of shops, mills, caravanserais, or even entire villages. The revenue from these properties went towards building and maintaining the hospital, and sometimes (particularly later) could supply a small stipend to the patient upon dismissal. The people entrusted to oversee the running of these early institutions were often elite physicians such as Sinān ibn Thābit and al-Rāzī, who also counted high-ranking dignitaries amongst their patients. The most important of the Baghdad hospitals was that established in 982 by the local ruler ʿAḍud al-Dawlah (r. 949–83), after whom it was named. When this ʿAḍudī hospital was founded it reportedly boasted twenty-five doctors, including oculists, surgeons, and bone-setters. It was partially destroyed in a flood of 1045, but rebuilt 23 years later, at which time it employed twenty-eight physicians. Two centuries later the traveller Ibn Jubayr, when describing the general ruin of Baghdad in 1184, remarked that the famous hospital was still 'a large structure having many chambers and rooms and all the appurtenances of a royal residence'. He also reported that physicians visited twice a week to prescribe treatment. The fact that they were not in attendance all the time is probably to be interpreted as a sign of decline.[38]

For the twelfth- and thirteenth-century hospitals, a number of documents relating to their endowments and administrative costs are preserved. We know that by the end of the twelfth century there were at least two hospitals active in Damascus. In 1184 Ibn Jubayr observed that there was an old one and a new one:

> The new one is the most frequented and the largest of the two, and its daily budget is about 15 *dīnār*. It has an overseer in whose hands is the maintenance of registers giving the names of the patients and the expenditures for the required medicaments, foodstuffs, and similar things. The physicians come early in the morning to examine the ill and to order the preparation of beneficial drugs and foods as are suitable for each patient.
>
> The older hospital is of this format, but the attendance in the new one is greater. This old hospital lies west of the venerable mosque. In addition, for the insane (*majnūns*) who are interned, there is a special form of treatment, that is, they are chained in fetters.[39]

The new hospital mentioned by Ibn Jubayr is the famous Nūrī *bīmāristān*, founded by Nūr al-Dīn ibn Zangī, a Turkish prince and ruler of Syria from 1146 to 1174. About half a century before the Nūrī hospital was established, a hospital had been founded west of the Great Mosque of the Umayyads, and it is likely that this was the older hospital referred to by Ibn Jubayr. In 1165, when Ibn al-Tilmīdh, then head of the ʿAḍudī hospital in Baghdad, died at the advanced age of 95, many of his students as well as other prominent physicians left Baghdad for Damascus and the Nūrī hospital, which by then had been in operation for about ten years. This emigration of physicians from Iraq into Syria was a major stimulus to the medical activity in Damascus, for which the Nūrī hospital became the major centre in the thirteenth century. It was expanded in 1242, renovated in 1285 and again in 1410. It continued to function as a hospital, though in an increasing state of decline, into the nineteenth century; today it is a museum of medical history.

In Egypt, Ṣalāḥ al-Dīn (Saladin) established a hospital in 1171, but the most splendid one was certainly the Manṣūrī hospital in Cairo, completed in 1284 and named after its founder, the Mamluk ruler al-Malik al-Manṣūr (the victorious king) Qalāwūn. It formed part of a larger complex containing the founder's mausoleum, as well as a school. The Manṣūrī hospital remained the primary medical centre in Cairo until the fifteenth century, and continued to function as a hospital well into the nineteenth century when the Frenchman Pascal Coste (d. 1879) drew a detailed architectural sketch of its plan at that time, reproduced in Figure 3.2.

The great Syro-Egyptian hospitals were built around a central courtyard

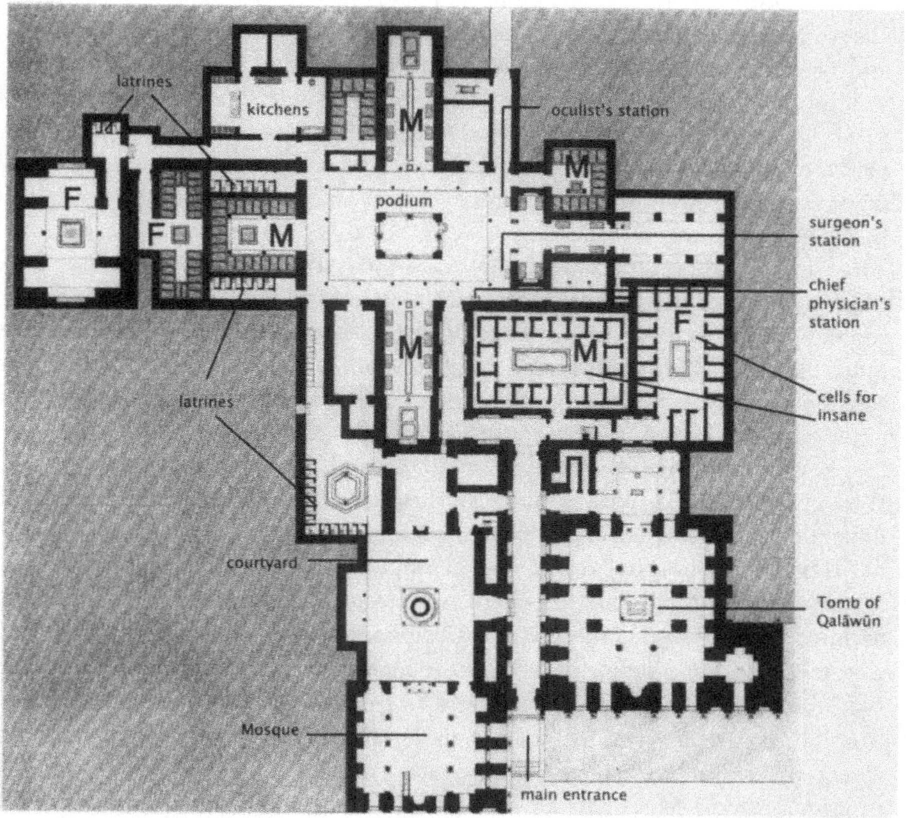

Figure 3.2 The Manṣūrī hospital, with attached funerary complex and mosque, built in Cairo in 1284–5 by Sultan al-Manṣūr Qalāwūn, after whom it was named. This plan shows it as it was functioning in the 19th century when Pascal Coste illustrated the major Cairene architectural structures of his day. F and M indicate areas designated for female and male patients respectively.

surrounded by four *īwāns* (vaulted halls with arched openings). It is evident from inscriptions and book niches that the largest of the *īwāns* often served as a lecture hall. Large rectangular pools of fresh water occupied the centre of the courtyard or were placed in each *īwān*. Adjacent rooms functioned as wards for patients, and there were a number of smaller rooms, including kitchens, storage areas, a pharmacy, living quarters for staff, latrines, and sometimes a library. Separate halls accommodated female patients, and special wards were set aside for the mentally ill and for those recuperating from surgery. Other areas were reserved for particular conditions such as gastrointestinal complaints (especially dysentery and diarrhoea), eye ailments, fevers, and even occasionally for rheumatics and cold sufferers (*mabrūds*). Sometimes there was an out-patient clinic with a free dispensary of medicaments.

The staff of these large hospitals included pharmacists and a roster of physicians who were required at appointed times to be in attendance, make the rounds, and prescribe medication. Stewards and orderlies (*mubāshirs* and *mushārifs*), as well as male and female attendants (*farrāsh/ahs*) catered for the basic needs of those in their care. An administrator (*nāẓir*), who was not usually trained in medicine, oversaw the entire staff and was responsible for the general management of the hospital. In most instances he was a political appointment, subject to the unpredictable fluctuations of favour, for this position was a lucrative one. The chief of staff, on the other hand, was a medical man, and in the case of the Manṣūrī hospital, he had his own quarters there and gave lectures in a special room. For a physician to have a position in one of these hospitals was apparently quite desirable. This is illustrated by a petition, written about 1240 for such a salaried post at the Nāṣirī hospital built by Ṣalāḥ al-Dīn; it has been preserved amongst documents in the Cairo Geniza.[40]

Besides those in Baghdad, Damascus, and Cairo, hospitals were built throughout Islamic lands. Hospitals in Muslim Spain, however, were established comparatively late, the earliest possibly being that built in Granada in 1397.

The Islamic hospital served several purposes: a centre of medical treatment, a convalescent home for those recovering from illness or accidents, an insane asylum, a retirement home giving basic maintenance needs for the aged and infirm who lacked a family to care for them, and a venue for medical education. Not all these activities, of course, were to be found in every medieval Islamic hospital. In the first two instances, admission would be for a limited period of time, with the view of curing a particular disorder. As for those using it as a retirement home, it is unclear how many, if any, were of the truly indigent and uneducated classes. On the other hand, it is unlikely that any truly wealthy person would have gone to a hospital for any purpose unless taken ill while travelling, for the medical needs of the wealthy and powerful would have been administered in the home or palace.

It is therefore evident that the medieval Islamic hospital was a more elaborate institution with a wider range of functions than the earlier poor and sick relief facilities offered by some Christian monasteries and hospices. The care for the insane in hospitals was unprecedented and an important part of even the earliest Islamic hospitals. Although early Islamic hospitals drew on Christian models, there are some things which make them unique. First, unlike their Christian counterparts, the medicine practised there was secular in character, insofar as it was based on the principles of humoral pathology rather than religion. Treatment in Christian institutions before the eighth century would customarily begin with a confession, and be carried out by monks or priests – that is to say, by Christians for Christians through Christian ritual (although of course not limited to it). In contrast, there were no mosques or places for religious ritual associated with Islamic hospitals, though in a few instances mosques were attached at a later date. In Islamic hospitals from the tenth century onwards (as far as we know), Muslim, Jewish, Christian, and even pagan doctors worked together, treating not only patients of their own community, but also those of other communities. Secondly, elite medical theory and practice came together in Islamic hospitals in a way that they had not done so before. This is illustrated by the fact that some of the best physicians of the time worked in hospitals and produced there some of their most advanced and innovative research. Thirdly, over time hospitals became centres for the teaching of medicine, in which students were encouraged to obtain their medical education. Finally, hospitals were part of wider public health efforts promoted by the ruling elite.

Muslims, Jews, and Christians: between cooperation and competition

The example of the hospital has shown that Jews, Christians, and Muslims did cooperate as physicians. When looking at education, we saw that the Jewish doctor Ifrā'īm ibn al-Ḥasan was the star pupil of the Muslim practitioner Ibn Riḍwān, while Ibn al-Nafīs had a Christian student whose studious accomplishments he commended. Even in the case of Ibn Riḍwān quarrelling by letter with the Christian physician Ibn Buṭlān, religion did not enter the debate. In theory, it would have been easy for the former to attack the latter for his trinitarian beliefs, often depicted as polytheistic in Islamic polemical literature. This general tolerance led Shlomo D. Goitein to extol the members of the Mediterranean medical milieu as the 'torchbearers of secular erudition, the professional expounders of philosophy and the sciences [...], disciples of the Greeks, heirs to a universal tradition, a spiritual brotherhood which transcended the barriers of religion, language, and countries.' While it is certainly true that there was great tolerance and mutual respect between intellectuals of the different confessions, the golden age of boundless tolerance, often ascribed to the medieval Islamic world, never existed in such pure and undiluted terms. Generally speaking, Jews fared much better under Islam in medieval times than they did in Christendom. Yet inter-communal tensions did exist, and, despite the general climate of tolerance, frictions occurred.[41]

In the quotation from Jāḥiẓ's *Book of Misers* which opened this chapter, the Muslim physician Asad ibn Jānī complains about the non-Muslim competition. The caliph al-Muqtadir, who set up hospitals and whose vizier had a keen interest in public health provision, also barred Jews and Christians from public office – with two exceptions: medicine and tax administration. It is evident from these and other examples that Christians and Jews dominated the medical scene, at least until the mid-tenth century, at which time the hospital physician al-Kaskarī exaggerated the situation and vented his spleen, saying: 'The physicians of the land were mostly Jews, fond of using falsehood and deceit.'[42]

Although it is impossible to compile accurate statistics for this time period, the later medieval histories of famous physicians do give us a rough idea about the distribution over time of the different denominations within the medical profession. In the ninth and tenth centuries, so it would seem, Christians constituted the majority of physicians; Jews were less frequent, and Muslims rather the exception. This picture changes from the eleventh century onwards, when the latter entered the profession in much greater numbers and came eventually to dominate it.[43]

Another author who shows clear anti-Semitic tendencies is al-Jawbarī (*fl.* 1240s), the former fraudster whom we have encountered earlier. He has a chapter on Jews in which he attacks them in a particularly vile fashion. For instance, he insinuates that most Jewish physicians cannot be trusted and may try to murder their patients. To illustrate his point, he tells the story of a Jewish quack who is asked by a wife to kill her husband through his treatment. Not only does he agree to do this, but he also forces the wife to have sex with him, pretending that the sperm is needed to produce the lethal drug.[44]

The picture of the relationship between the different confessional communities is therefore a composite and complex one. On the one hand, because the theoretical framework for medical practice was not linked to a specific faith, Muslims as well as Christians and Jews could accept it and partake in a secular scientific discourse. In many instances, physicians from various communities collaborated and treated patients regardless of their particular religious allegiance. Yet, on the other hand, tensions between Muslims, Christians, and Jews did exist, as can be seen from the examples of al-Kaskarī and al-Jawbarī. Religion, however, was not the only criterion used to single out and criticise a certain group within a complex health network. Women, too, often had to bear the brunt of vilification.

Female practitioners

> How amazing it is [that patients are cured at all], considering that they hand over their lives to senile old women! For most people, at the onset of illness, use as their physicians either their wives, mothers or aunts, or some [other] member of their family or one of their neighbours. He [the patient] acquiesces to whatever extravagant measure she might order, consumes whatever she prepares for him, and listens to what she says and obeys her commands more than he obeys the physician. He believes that this woman, despite her lack of intelligence, is more knowledgeable and of sounder opinion than the physician.
> – Ṣāʿid ibn al-Ḥasan (d. 1072), *Stimulating a Yearning for Medicine*[45]

It can be argued that health care, both in the medieval Islamic and in early modern European societies, was for the most part provided by women. Within the family they looked after the medical needs of the children, as well as after those of their husbands and other members of the extended family. As nurses and midwives, as carers and curers, they contributed fundamentally to the health of the wider society. Earlier we observed that in pre-Islamic times it was often women who acted as healers, and the tradition continued in one way or another throughout the medieval Islamic period.

Yet when we look at the learned medical discourse, we find that it was largely dominated by men. No medical handbooks by medieval Islamic women have come down to us, and female physicians are only rarely mentioned in the bio-bibliographical and medical literature. There is, however, one exception: medical men frequently reviled women and warned against them in the starkest terms. Such physicians would bemoan the fact that their patients might turn to women rather then themselves, and Ṣāʿid ibn al-Ḥasan, quoted above, is amongst them. His general attitude is crystal clear: he thinks that patients should consult professional physicians like himself, and not 'senile women'.

Female practitioners clearly constituted potentially powerful competition for their male counterparts. Like Ṣāʿid ibn al-Ḥasan, al-Rāzī (d. 925) had talked of women poaching his patients, and gave concrete examples. There is, for instance, the case of someone suffering from bladder stones who consulted al-Rāzī and received treatment from him extending over a period of time. Yet, when his ailment did not improve, the patient gave up on al-Rāzī, turned to a woman, and was cured shortly thereafter. Al-Rāzī explained this in terms of *his* treatment being responsible for the cure – it only took longer than the patient was willing to give it; what the woman did was irrelevant.[46] In another case, one of al-Rāzī's own hospital employees looked for cures elsewhere. Al-Rāzī describes the incident in the following manner:

> One of the employees in the hospital once complained that he had difficulties moving one of the joints in his finger because of a boil on his index finger, which

> resisted for some time the softening remedies tried by him. He cursed and abused the physicians publicly, saying: 'If their attempts to cure a small boil on a finger appear to be deceptive and insufficient, then what about broken ribs or arms?' He looked for treatment amongst women and the populace [*hā-'ām*].[47]

This episode illustrates two aspects of the physician's frustration. First, when he cannot immediately cure the patient, or when the treatment takes time, the patient grows impatient, loses trust in him, and publicly mocks him. Second, when orthodox medicine was perceived not to work, people turned to alternative practitioners, many of whom were female.

We possess sporadic information about female physicians and oculists from a variety of disparate sources. There is, for instance, the legendary Zaynab, the physician (*ṭabībah*) of the Banū Awd, who is alleged to have been famous for her skills as an oculist.[48] Some Geniza documents refer to female oculists (*kaḥḥālahs*); one such person, for instance, is mentioned in a list of people receiving alms, suggesting that she belonged to the lower strata of society.[49] The thirteenth-century Italian ophthalmologist Benvenutus Grassus reported that in North Africa women treated trachoma (rather unsuccessfully) by scraping the eyelids with fig-tree twigs and sugar.[50] There are in fact a comparatively high number of instances where the female practitioners mentioned in our sources worked as oculists. What precisely they did, and what procedures they performed, is unclear. Nor do we know whether they would have been aware of, or employed, the sophisticated manuals on ophthalmology. It is possible that the level of medical care provided by these oculists was such that it did not require much formal training in the sense that is represented by the ophthalmological manuals discussed in the previous chapter.

It is also evident that women practised other branches of the medical art as well. A *fatwah* (legal advice) by the judge (*qāḍī*) Ibn Ziyād (d. 924) refers to the practice of a female physician (*ṭabībah*). She had treated the daughter of another woman who disputed the amount of the fee.[51] Female physicians seem to have been relatively rare, however, at least in Muslim Spain in the tenth and early eleventh centuries, if we can believe al-Zahrāwī, who makes the following remark when discussing the surgical treatment of bladder stones:

> The treatment [of women suffering this complaint] is indeed difficult and is hindered by a number of things. One is that the woman may be a virgin. Another is that you will not find a woman who will expose herself to a [male] doctor if she be modest or married. A third is that you will not find a woman competent in this art, particularly not in surgery. [...] If necessity compels you to undertake this kind of case, you should take with you a competent woman doctor. As these are very uncommon, if you are without one, then seek a eunuch doctor as a colleague, or bring a midwife experienced in women's ailments or a woman to whom you may give some instruction in this art. Have her with you and bid her to do all that you instruct.[52]

Another important aspect of health care in which women were often involved was the establishment of hospitals and other structures providing care and shelter. A number of female patrons, often closely connected with the family of the caliph or ruler, not only set up various charitable institutions, such as wells and shelters for pilgrims, but also endowed hospitals. Shujāʿ, the mother of the caliph al-Mutawakkil (r. 847–61), for example, increased the endowment of the Badrī hospital in Baghdad, and thereby assured that it could continue to function and grow. Shaghab, the caliph al-Muqtadir's (r. 908–32) mother – who wielded tremendous power and influence in the court, so much so that she was simply known as 'the Lady (*al-Sayyidah*)' – founded a hospital named after her, which opened on 14 June 918 in the area of 'John's Market (Sūq Yaḥyá)' in Baghdad. These and other initiatives resulting from female patronage improved the medical care available to the wider community, and thereby constituted a considerable contribution to public health.[53]

Women patients

The quotation from al-Zahrāwī in the last section illustrates that in certain situations female patients could be embarrassed to expose themselves, and especially their private parts, to male physicians. The question therefore arises whether there were any coherent guidelines which ruled the doctor-patient relationship in this respect. An anecdote in the *Tabletalk* by al-Tanūkhī (d. 994), a work of *belles-lettres*, illustrates the shame which a female patient could feel at certain disorders. The daughter of a rural magnate concealed a pain in her vagina. The father, however, found out about it, but was at first uneasy to let a physician examine her. When she was 'at death's door', he reluctantly consulted an experienced [male] practitioner who discovered that a tick nesting in that region was the cause of the trouble and removed it.[54]

According to the Arab historian and theologian Shams al-Dīn al-Dhahabī (d. 1348), who also wrote a manual on Prophetic Medicine, neither father nor daughter should have been wary to consult a doctor. Quoting *ḥadīth* and legal authorities such as the famous Ḥanbalī scholar al-Marwazī (d. 945), he argued that a female patient can receive treatment from a male physician not belonging to her family (*ajnabī*). The latter may even examine her genitalia, provided there is a medical need for this, just as women can see male genitals under similar circumstances.[55]

In general it seems that women did occasionally consult male doctors. They went to their surgeries, as in the case of the woman whom the physician's pupil duped (see above p. 92). We have also many instances of female patients being mentioned in the case histories recorded by al-Rāzī's students. One instance where al-Rāzī examined the patient's breasts is the following:

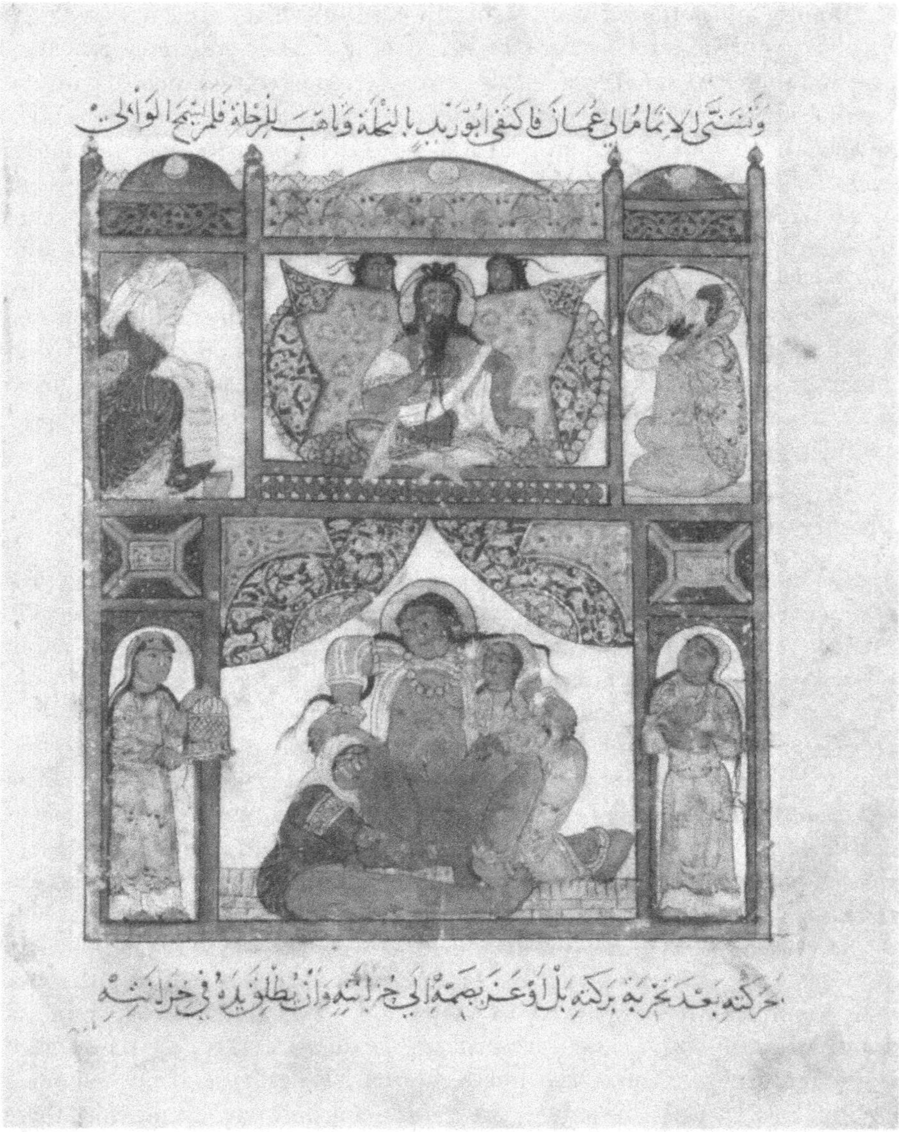

Figure 3.3 The hour of birth, painted by Yaḥyá ibn Maḥmūd al-Wāsiṭī in 1237, probably in Baghdad, in a copy of the *Assemblies* (*Maqāmāt*) by al-Ḥarīrī (d. 1122). In the mansion of an eastern ruler (rendered as an Indian seated in the upper storey), the wife is in the throes of giving birth. She is assisted by a midwife and an attendant supporting her. Two servants in the wings standby, one with an incense burner. Also in the upper storey, an Arab astrologer employs an astrolabe to make a horoscope, while on the left another Arab writes on a scroll, presumably an amulet to assure a successful birthing.

> A woman presented with one breast … [? *ṭufisat*], whilst the other breast had become hard like a movable and protruding knot. He [al-Rāzī] said: 'This is a serious matter, since it is constantly hot, so that the heat overpowers her and has consumed the moisture [in the body]. One might imagine that this tumour is a cancer. A cancer, however, does not protrude, for otherwise it could be cut.'[56]

There were, to be sure, certain issues which concerned only women: menstruation, pregnancy, childbirth, and breastfeeding, for instance. Yet these topics were discussed in detail in the scholarly medical tradition, whose authors (at least those we know about) were all men. However, many of these male writers, such as Ibn Sarābiyūn (*fl.* c. 870s), for the most part repeated the descriptions and medications which they found in their Greek sources. A case in point is the monograph by the Damascene physician al-Baladī (*fl.* c. 970s), called *Book on the Regimen of Pregnant Women and Children*, which draws almost exclusively on previous sources. On the other hand, al-Rāzī makes practical observations, confronting medical theory with experience in his *Comprehensive Book*. One example is the following remark:

> I read in another book that sexual intercourse with a pregnant woman makes it easier for her to give birth. This is easily understood, since sexual intercourse moves the menstrual blood a lot, and brings it down. A friend of mine told me that he slept with a pregnant woman whose delivery was overdue. Her labour began the moment he had finished, and thereafter she gave birth with ease.[57]

In the same context of difficult delivery, al-Rāzī gives detailed instructions how to introduce an abortive drug into the womb 'according to what I have seen' as he puts it.[58] Moreover, al-Zahrāwī introduced some new procedures to help with birthing, such as forceps and vaginal specula to be used in the extraction of dead foetuses. It can, however, be assumed that in general a midwife, not a physician, would assist with childbirth. The scene in Figure 3.3 depicts how a wealthy woman gave birth. No physician is present, and she is assisted only by a midwife and an additional attendant.

In many matters of health, particularly those concerned with childbirth and child-rearing, women consulted women and sought the counsel of members of their own sex. The practicalities of breastfeeding, for example, remained in the female domain. And this was so despite the fact that male physicians and jurists gave directions about the diet and regimen of the woman nourishing the newborn, and discussed the benefits of having a wetnurse, how to choose her, and when to wean the child.[59]

From ninth-century Egypt we have preserved today a letter from a mother to her daughter, giving medical advice:

> I have written to you, my beloved daughter, a letter before this one, and sent with it a paper containing a remedy for your stomach. Write to me that you have received

> [it] and that my letter has reached you, that you have drunk it [the remedy], and benefited from it. Write to me, so that I can be in good spirits [again], for I am extremely worried about you. I ask God to grant me relief.[60]

Even if this ailment was not a gynaecological one but a stomach complaint, the letter well illustrates that women would naturally help each other in medical matters, providing remedies and recipes when needed. The stereotypical female figure offering medical advice to all was, of course, the 'old woman' (*'ajūz*), omniscient of all traditional cures but inept in the eyes of the 'professional' physician.

Medicine in rural settings

That medical care available in remote and rural areas differed greatly from that in urban settings seems rather self-evident. The point is well illustrated, however, by two specific incidences, one reported in Arabic *belles-lettres* and the other in a historical account. In the first, recorded in Tanūkhī's *Tabletalk*, someone tells the story of how he resorted to the medical care of an old woman, since he was in the countryside and no other therapy was available. This is his account:

> 'Alī Muḥammad al-Anṣārī stated: I had pustules on my leg ... I went out to a village close to Mabrawān, the district of [the city of] al-Anbār. I stayed with a farmer whose name was Ibrāhīm ibn Sham'ūn. Seeing my pustules, he said: 'There is an old woman who uses magic to cure them'. I had her brought in, and she said: 'This is a disease called *al-dukūk* and I can cure it for you'. She wrote out a lengthy talisman and then spread ... ointments and said: 'Do not remove it before three days'. Three days later, I removed it and was cured.[61]

Al-Anṣārī found himself in a rural area of Iraq where there were no sophisticated medical institutions, nor even, it appears, a regular physician who could treat his skin condition. In the absence of orthodox medical care, he accepted treatment by an old woman (*'ajūz*) who, as well as an ointment, employed a variety of strategies belonging to the popular medical register, such as amulets and invocations. As will be evident in Chapter 5, magical practices were not restricted to rural areas or untrained practitioners. On the other hand, in the Iraqi countryside as elsewhere, self-taught and traditional practitioners were often the only people to whom the ill and infirm could turn for treatment.

The lack of trained physicians in rural areas was of great concern to the Baghdad vizier 'Alī ibn 'Īsá (d. 946), so much so that he instructed Sinān ibn Thābit (d. 942) to remedy the situation around the year 920. In an edict (*tawqī'*) which 'Alī sent to Sinān, he describes the situation as follows:

> I have thought about those people who live in the Sawād [the alluvial plain of the Tigris and Euphrates in central Iraq]. It is possible that there are patients to whom

> no practitioner is close by, because the Sawād is far away from physicians. Therefore, order – may God prolong your life – that practitioners be recruited who have stores of drugs and potions at their disposal. They should make the rounds in the Sawād, and stay at each place as long as is necessary, treating the patients there. Then they should travel to the next place.[62]

'Alī ibn 'Īsá defines the problem succinctly: in remote areas, potential patients do not have access to physicians, and his solution is to set up a system of itinerant doctors who would cater to the medical needs of the rural community. The son of the man instructed to organise these provisions, Thābit ibn Sinān (in whose *History* this edict is preserved), stated that his father 'carried out this order'. It is, however, important to note that this is the only campaign of its kind mentioned in our sources, and that, even if successful at the time, it must have remained an extraordinary measure. What this edict does confirm, however, is the fact that formally-trained medical care was scarce in the countryside, and that its inhabitants often had to fend for themselves.

Public health care

The measures undertaken by 'Alī ibn 'Īsá to provide medical care to rural Iraq would, in today's terms, without doubt fall within the remit of a public health policy. Rulers, high-ranking officials, and female patrons at the courts of the caliphs also set up many of the great hospitals in the Islamic world. Moreover, there were at least sporadic attempts on behalf of the authorities to regulate medical practice. The office of the inspector of the market (*muḥtasib*) is an example, as are the incidents of medical supervision detailed earlier. In light of this, some scholars have characterised public health initiatives in medieval Islam as sophisticated and comprehensive, akin to modern medical provision. This picture, however, is extrapolated from a variety of disparate sources describing events at different times and places, and those painting it were often uncritical or overly optimistic in accepting prescriptive texts as describing actual historical realities. [63]

In reaction to this excessively enthusiastic interpretation, other scholars have viewed these events as exceptional, denying that they had much influence on ordinary people's lives. Lawrence Conrad, for instance, stated that hospitals 'were established and funded as acts of personal charity and not as matters of state policy, though the founders were most often rulers or highly placed administrators', and that 'they were in all cases extremely limited compared to the vast size of the populations they served [...], and that their function must always have been rather to demonstrate and promote ideals of compassion and charity and to serve as foci for the activities and expansion of the medical profession.'[64]

In order to assess these various claims, let us first look at what we know of the hospitals. A good criterion for evaluating the relevance of hospitals for the wider population would be to know how many hospital beds per capita were available at a given time and place. Statistics for medieval societies, however, are notoriously difficult to compile. Nonetheless, it is worthwhile at least to speculate about the role which these institutions might have played in the framework of public health provision. The following comparison is thought-provoking, though some historians may consider it naïve or lacking statistical rigor. According to figures published by the World Health Organisation, there were 0.68 beds per 1,000 inhabitants in Pakistan in 1998. Baghdad in the tenth century had an approximate population of 300,000 to 500,000. Let us, for argument's sake, assume that the population was approximately 400,000. In that case, there would have to have been 272 beds in tenth-century Baghdad to have the same hospital coverage as in Pakistan as a whole in 1998. We know of twelve hospitals in Baghdad by the eleventh century, and there may well have been others about which our sources are silent. Between them, they probably had at least that number of beds, given the large size of the structures and the great number of physicians in attendance at some of the hospitals (25 at 'Aḍudī mentioned earlier, for example). While exact, or even approximate, figures are not available, it would seem that the number of hospital beds per capita in medieval Baghdad and modern Pakistan might not have been completely dissimilar. Likewise, the population of Damascus in the thirteenth century can be estimated at about 60,000, and we know that there were two hospitals in operation during this time, one of them the very large Nūrī hospital. The number of beds provided by these two hospitals must have well surpassed the number required (40.8) to equate to the same hospital provision as is currently available in Pakistan.[65]

These numerical considerations must of course be considered highly speculative for a variety of reasons: lack of accurate statistical data, difference in the definition of a 'hospital bed' then and now, and geographic variation. They do provide, however, a sense of the magnitude of institutional medical provision within a metropolitan context. Moreover, when the travel writer Ibn Jubayr visited Syria in the 1183–5, he remarked that there was hardly a city without a hospital. It therefore seems that their presence must have made a difference to a considerable number of people who would otherwise have struggled to receive medical care.[66]

At times, there was also a clear political will behind the establishment of hospitals as charitable institutions. 'Alī ibn 'Īsá certainly pursued public health objectives through numerous initiatives, and the grand hospitals of Baghdad, Cairo, and Damascus were anything but private affairs. It is true, however, that the distinction between the public and the private sphere in the case of the political elite was not always clearly drawn. The public purse, for instance, was the coffers of the caliph. Money paid from them for hospital expenses, for instance, may therefore be viewed as both private and public. This said, the spread of hospitals throughout the Islamic heartlands was often nourished by concerns about public health on behalf of the ruling elite, and in that sense, it should not be relegated to the domain of the purely private.

Hospitals were, moreover, not the only provision with which the authorities strove to improve the general health of the population. Fresh water supplies, sanitation systems, and public baths (*ḥammāms*) were other important elements maintained by governmental authorities.[67]

In conclusion then, it is fair to say that the authorities adopted certain measures and initiatives to improve public health. Even if these efforts varied greatly over time and place and were not always sustained, certain public institutions became established for which the medieval Islamic world became deservedly renowned – in particular the steam baths and hospitals – which played an important role within the framework of metropolitan societies. Rural areas, it is true, had much more restricted access to these provisions, though even here there were sporadic efforts on the part of the authorities to improve rural medical care.

The nature of the medical care that might have been available within urban institutions such as hospitals and public baths, as well as the supervised market places where medical treatment could also be sought, will be the subject of the following chapter.

Suggested reading

For medical education, see Leiser, 'Medical Education in Islamic Lands'; for medical regulation and ethics, Levey, *Medical Ethics of Medieval Islam*; and the Index of names and works under Sāʿid ibn al-Ḥasan and al-Sulamī; for charlatans, see Pormann, 'Physician and the Other'.

For the status of physicians, see Rosenthal, 'Physician'; for hospitals, Horden, 'Earliest Hospitals', Pormann, 'Islamic Hospitals', and Tabbaa, 'Functional Aspects'.

For women, see the recent survey by Green, 'History of Science'. See also Gilʿadi, *Infants, Parents and Wet Nurses*.

For public health and the poor, see Benkheira, '"La maison de Satan"'; Sabra, *Poverty and Charity*; and Cohen, *Poverty and Charity*.

Notes

1 tr. Serjeant, 86 (slightly altered); Arabic, 109–10/103.
2 Arabic text: Ibn Jubayr, *Travels*, 218, 16–20; translation by Broadhurst, *Travels of Ibn Jubayr*, 226; the present translation is our own.
3 al-Majūsī, *Complete Book*, i. 9.

4 Fähndrich, *Treatise to Ṣalāh ad-Dīn*, §120.
5 Gutas, *Avicenna and the Aristotelian Tradition*, 27 and n. 18.
6 Al-Rāzī's *Epistle* is preserved in a unique manuscript (Cairo, Dār al-Kutub, MS Ṭibb Taymūr 119/6), of which the great medical historian Max Meyerhof had a copy made; the latter, containing many annotations by Meyerhof, is now kept in the Alexandrian municipal library. The Arabic title of the treatise is ambiguous: it could also mean 'to some of his students'.
7 Quotation from Ibn Abī Uṣaybi'ah, *Sources of Information*, ii. 244, 12.
8 For al-Dakhwār's establishment of the school, see Ibn Abī Uṣaybi'ah, *Sources of Information*, ii. 244, 20–7, and al-Nu'aymī, *A Study of the History of Colleges*, ii. 127–33; for later repairs and additional *madrasahs*: al-Nu'aymī, *A Study*, ii. 133–8 and Ibn Shaddād, *Great Goods concerning the History of Syria and Arabia*, 266. For the teaching of medicine by the physician-jurist in *madrasahs* where the purpose of the school was primarily the study of *fiqh*, see Makdisi, *Rise of Colleges*, 11, 78, 87, 168, and 285. See also Leiser, 'Medical Education', esp. 57–9.
9 Bergsträsser, *Ḥunain ibn Isḥāq*, no. 20, pp. 18, 19–23.
10 Ibn Riḍwān, *Useful Book*, 90, 6–10 (ed. Sāmarrā'ī; the text in this edition is corrupt); the translation is by Iskandar, 'Attempted Reconstruction', 242, with slight modifications.
11 Ibn Riḍwān, *Useful Book*, 103, 5–9 (ed. Sāmarrā'ī); translation, with many modifications, Iskandar, 'Attempted Reconstruction', 243.
12 Niẓāmī-i 'Arūḍī, *Chahār maqālah*, 4th discourse. The translation is that (slightly amended) of Browne, *Revised Translation of the Chahār Maqála*, 78–9.
13 See also Berkey, *Transmission of Knowledge*; and Chamberlain, *Knowledge and Social Practice*.
14 For Ibn al-Nafīs' note, see Pormann, 'Physician and the Other', 207; for other examples of this type, Savage-Smith, 'Medicine', 942; and above p. 68.
15 Sā'id, *Stimulating a Yearning for Medicine*, ed. Spies, fol. 38a9–10, 13–14; German tr. Taschkandi, *Übersetzung und Bearbeitung*, 131. See Kruk, '*De Goede arts*'; for al-Rāzī's scepticism about uroscopy and European parallels, see Pormann, 'Physician and the Other', 203–4.
16 The treatise survives under a number of titles, one of which is *Discourse on the Differences of Diseases*, and was wrongly attributed to al-Rāzi (see Richter-Bernburg, 'Abū Bakr Muḥammad Al Rāzī's (Rhazes) Medical Works', 391). The question and answer on pleurisy and liver swelling is found on 127, 6–15.
17 al-Qalqashandī, *Dawn of the Blind*, v. 467 and xi. 98, 15–99, 1.
18 Ibn Abī Uṣaybi'ah, *Sources of Information*, ii. 242, 7–8.
19 Ed. Spies, fols. 22b12–23a11; German tr. Taschkandi, *Übersetzung und Bearbeitung*, 102.
20 al-Ruhāwī, *Ethics of the Physician*, facs. 135, 1–8; tr. Levey, *Medical Ethics*, 62; this is our translation.
21 See Álvarez-Millán, 'Graeco-Roman Case Histories'; Álvarez-Millán, 'Practice versus Theory'.
22 For a translation of al-Rāzī's critique of medical charlatans, see Savage-Smith, 'Medicine', 937–8.
23 al-Jawbarī, *The Choicest Part*; quoted according to Pormann, 'Physician and the Other', 218–19.

24 al-Ruhāwī, *Ethics of the Physician*, facs. 209, 9–paen.; tr. Levey, *Medical Ethics*, p. 90.
25 al-Ghazāli, *Revival of Religious Sciences*, i. 30, 7–31, 6 (bk. 1, bāb 3).
26 al-Rāzī, *Treatise on the Causes Why Most People Turn Away from Excellent Physicians towards the Worst Ones*, quoted according to Pormann, 'Physician and the Other', 202 (with slight modifications).
27 Meyerhof and Schacht, *Medico-Philosophical Controversy*; see Pormann, 'Physician and the Other', 215–17.
28 tr. Rosenthal, 'Physician', 485 [Ṯa'āl., *Yatīma*, i. 218, 2–5 according to Ullmann, *WKAS*].
29 Ibn Abī Uṣaybi'ah, *Sources of Information*, ii. 105, 18–21.
30 Makdisi, *Humanism*, 74–5; Ibn Abī Uṣaybi'ah, *Sources of Information*, ii. 105, 17–106, 6.
31 Ibn Riḍwān, *On the Prevention of Bodily Ills in Egypt*, 122 in Dols translation (reproduced here with substantial modifications); Arabic, 23, 1–6. See also, Ṣā'id ibn al-Ḥasan, *Stimulating a Yearning for Medicine*, chs 2 and 3.
32 Biesterfeldt, 'Some Opinions'.
33 §39; see Bar-Sela and Hoff, 'Isaac Israeli's Fifty Admonitions'; tr. [with modifications] Lewis, *Islam: From the Prophet*, ii. 187.
34 For the 'upper middle class' in the Geniza documents, see, for instance, A. L. Motzkin, 'A thirteenth-century Jewish Physician in Jerusalem (a Geniza Portrait)' *The Muslim World*, 60 (1970) 344–9.
35 'In my home (*fī manzilī*)', e.g., al-Rāzī, *Doubts about Galen*, 63, 10; 75, 1; hospitals, e.g., al-Rāzī, *Doubts about Galen*, 63, 9–10; 75, 1; al-Rāzī, *Comprehensive Book*, xix. 416, 8; for al-Kaskarī, see Pormann, 'Islamic Hospitals'. In his *Epistle to One of His Students* (see n. 6 above), al-Rāzī refers specifically to some patients of royal extraction whom he treated.
36 The episode occurs in al-Ḥarīrī's 47th *Assembly*. For arguments against viewing the picture in Fig 3.1 as an illustration of how cupping was done, see Maddison and Savage-Smith, *Science, Tools and Magic*, i. 42–7.
37 Rosenthal, 'Physician', 490.
38 Ibn Jubayr, *Travels*, 225, 16–20; tr. Broadhurst, *Travels of Ibn Jubayr*, 234; the translation here is our own. Strohmaier, 'Ärztliche Ausbildung', 522/394, first suggested that this was a sign of decline.
39 Ibn Jubayr, *Travels*, 283, 9–16; tr. Broadhurst, *Travels of Ibn Jubayr*, 296.
40 Richards, 'A Doctor's Petition'.
41 Goitein's quotation is taken from his 'The Medical Profession', 177; also cited by Rosenthal, 'Physician', 477; for the topic in general, see Cohen, *Under Crescent and Cross*.
42 Quoted according to Pormann, 'Physician and the Other', 212.
43 Ibid., 213.
44 Ibid., 221.
45 Ed. O. Spies, fol. 27b8–16; German tr. Taschkandi, *Übersetzung und Bearbeitung*, 109.
46 Pormann, 'Physician and the Other', 204–5.
47 al-Rāzī, *Treatise on the Causes Why Most People Turn Away from Excellent Physicians towards the Worst Ones*; Munich Bayerische Staatsbibliothek, MS hebr. 43 fol. 100a7–15; MS hebr. 280 fol. 51b1–8; see Steinschneider, 'Wissenschaft und Charlatanerie', 581 for an earlier German version.

48 Ibn Abī Uṣaybi'ah, *Sources of Information*, i. 123, 13–20.
49 Goitein, *Mediterranean Society*, i. 127–8.
50 See Eldredge, *Benvenutus Grassus*, 69–70.
51 Aguirre de Carcer, 'Sobre el ejercicio'.
52 Spink and Lewis, *Albucasis*, 420–1.
53 Pormann, 'Islamic Hospitals'.
54 Bray, 'Physical World and the Writer's Eye', 224–6.
55 al-Dhahabī, *Prophetic Medicine*, 242, 4–243, 2; tr. Elgood, '*Ṭibb-ul-Nabbi*', 133.
56 Istanbul, Topkapı Saray, Ahmed III MS 1975, fol. 49a. This passage from al-Rāzī's *Book of Experiences* has been previously translated by Álvarez-Millán, 'Practice versus Theory', 297. The present rendering is, for the most part, our own.
57 al-Rāzī, *Comprehensive Book*, ix. 129, 12–15. For Ibn Sarābiyūn, see Pormann, *Oriental Tradition*, 45–6; for al-Baladī, Weisser, *Zeugung*, 24.
58 al-Rāzī, *Comprehensive Book*, ix. 1 36, 5–14.
59 Gil'adi, *Infants, Parents and Wet Nurses*; see also Rapoport, *Marriage, Money and Divorce*.
60 Rāghib, *Marchands d'étoffes*, vol. 2, no. 28, lines 3–5. Cf. Kraemer, 'Women Speak for Themselves', 180, n. 10.
61 Tanūkhī, *Tabletalk*, ii. 94; translation with modifications by El Cheikh, 'Women's History', 140–1; Arabic; Anbār is a town on the Euphrates just opposite Baghdad; Mabrawān is a district (or ward) of Anbār.
62 Ibn Abī Uṣaybi'ah, *Sources of Information*, i. 221.
63 See, for instance, Hamarneh, *Health Sciences*.
64 Conrad, 'The Arab-Islamic Medical Tradition', 136–7.
65 For population numbers in Baghdad, see Lapidus, *History of Islamic Societies*, 56; for modern statistics see http://data.euro.who.int/hfadb/. For an alternative interpretation of the impact of Islamic hospitals (with further literature), see Tabbaa, 'Functional Aspects', 106–7.
66 Pormann, 'Islamic Hospitals'; Ibn Jubayr, *Travels*, 258, 18–20 (Arabic); tr. Broadhurst, *Travels of Ibn Jubayr*, 268.
67 See below, pp. 135–7 for a more extensive discussion of public baths.

4

Practice

If the physician is able to treat with foodstuffs, not medication, then he has succeeded. If, however, he must use medication, then it should be simple remedies and not compound ones.
– al-Rāzī (d. 925)[1]

Not every smoke comes from cooking, often it is the smoke of cauterising.
– Persian proverb, recorded by al-Karkhī (d. c. 956)[2]

The usefulness of surgery is very great, but the practice of it is less certain than its theory.
– Ḥajjī Khalīfah (Kātip Çelebī, d. 1657)[3]

Finding reliable evidence regarding the actual practice of medicine is fraught with difficulties. Medieval medical treatises seldom mention specific patients or tell us how often, if ever, they actually carried out their carefully formulated instructions and with what success. Unfortunately, few sources are preserved that might provide pertinent evidence, such as hospital records or administrative and legal documents. Only a handful of surgical instruments survive today that can be assigned to the medieval Islamic world. Virtually no palaeopathological studies have been undertaken of excavated human remains from Muslim burial sites of the period to determine the incidence of diseases leaving skeletal traces or evidence of bone surgery.[4]

Case histories and clinical notes

We do, however, possess some useful evidence – namely, collections of therapeutic procedures, usually recorded by students, and occasional case histories inserted into formal treatises. A comparison of such case histories and personal accounts with the formal and largely theoretical medical literature reveals the ways in which physicians applied medical theory in particular cases. It also provides at least a small insight into what may have been the day-to-day practice of learned Islamic physicians at that time, particularly in Iraq and Muslim Spain.

Throughout his working life, al-Rāzī recorded passages from all the medical authors he had read, copying and sorting them under topical headings such as eye diseases or gastro-intestinal complaints, occasionally adding his own comments. These working files were known to his contemporaries to be voluminous and important, so much so that, following his death in 925, his students assembled and disseminated them under the title *The Comprehensive Book* (*al-Kitāb al-Ḥāwī*).

Amongst these massive files of working notes (23 volumes in a modern printing) are to be found the occasional case history as well as a glimpse of al-Rāzī as a practising clinician. We can see him, for example, trying to determine how best to treat patients he thought might develop meningitis. He begins by describing conditions that precede meningitis: dullness and pain in the head and neck continuing for three to five days, insomnia, exhaustion, and the avoidance of bright light. He then states that he once treated two sets of such patients, the first with bloodletting, while intentionally neglecting to bleed a second. He remarks: 'By doing that, I wished to reach a conclusion; and indeed all those of the latter group contracted meningitis'. Such an approach to the refinement of therapeutics surprisingly foreshadows later experimental methods, though of course today we do not recognise a relationship of cause and effect between bloodletting and the onset of meningitis.[5]

Often al-Rāzī's comments are expansions or refinements of statements from early authorities, such as:

> Galen says that 'if you crack and sip an egg, it is useful for coughing up blood'. I, however, say that if something viscous and drying, such as yellow amber, or astringents such as wild pomegranate flower, poppy seed, and henbane seed are added, the preparation is useful when the condition is severe.[6]

or

> I have heard some amazing accounts, amongst which is the following: The physician Sa'īd ibn Baksī prescribed for gout a potion prepared with two mithqāls of colchicum, half a dirham of opium and three dirhams of sugar. The drug is to alleviate pain within the hour, but I need to verify this.[7]

It is interesting to note in this context that colchicine, the active ingredient of colchicum, is used today to treat acute attacks of gout.

Scattered throughout the *Comprehensive Book* are descriptions of particular cases encountered by al-Rāzī, such as:

> My experience: There was with us in the hospital one such man [suffering from rabies] who barked during the night and then died. Another did not drink water, but when some water was brought to him, he was not afraid of it, but said: 'It stinks, and the stomachs of dogs and cats are in it'. Yet another patient, when he saw water, shuddered, shivered, and trembled until it was taken away from him.[8]

Grouped together in these working notes are thirty-four case reports more detailed than most and apparently written with the intention that they be read alongside the case histories found in the Hippocratic book *Epidemics*. The following case was recorded by al-Rāzī to illustrate the possible dangers of using medicaments which suppress coughing, the patient apparently suffering from consumption:

> A consumptive elder came to us. He had been repeatedly coughing up much blood over a long period of time. Then it became much more distressing for him, so he took hazelnuts with water which stopped the cough. He got relief each time he did it, and he [apparently] recovered completely. Then he died ... Consequently, one should avoid remedies which suppress expectoration, except in cases where the matter flows down from the head.[9]

Al-Rāzī also included seven clinical histories of a more rhetorical style, some of them relating to the ruler of Tabaristan, in his treatise *Secret of the Medical Art*. Most importantly, there is a collection of over 900 examples of al-Rāzī's therapeutic practice, recorded by some of his students under the title *The Book of Experiences*. The following are typical examples of the collection as a whole:

> He [al-Rāzī] was told of a young woman who had been coughing for five months and had now been vomiting a foamy blood for the last three days. He was presented with this in a bowl, and it looked like pulmonary tissue. He said: 'This comes from the lung and was easily expelled'. He asked: 'Is she in pain?' He was told that she felt pain on the right side. He prescribed pastilles of poppy for her and barley-water without sugar.[10]

or

> A man complained of spasms in his right hand when he was washing with cold water. He [al-Rāzī] directed that he rub the vertebrae of his neck, as well as the rest of his body, with costus oil, that he have rose-honey [*julanjubīn*] every day, and that his diet consist of chick-pea-water and red meat fried in oil.[11]

Writing slightly later in Baghdad, al-Kaskarī (*fl.* c. 930s) included in his *Compendium* a number of therapeutic procedures that he carried out on specific patients. For example, 'I used to treat al-Qarārīṭī during his office as vizier when he became hard of hearing by putting into his ear 'nard oil' for which the recipe is in the formulary, and he was cured'. From the end of the same century, but from Muslim Spain, we have more than eighteen accounts of particular cases of his own experience mentioned by al-Zahrāwī in his encyclopedia composed in Córdoba.[12]

The *Canon of Medicine* by Ibn Sīnā (d. 1037), on the other hand, is strikingly devoid of personal experiences and case notes, nor do any case histories occur in his other medical writings. In fact there is little evidence to suggest that Ibn Sīnā had much practical experience as a physician, outside of his boastful autobiography and some entertaining stories of the twelfth century included in a Persian *adab*-treatise devoted to tales demonstrating proper conduct. His student, al-Juzjānī (*fl.* c. 1020s) , however, said that Ibn Sīnā had recorded some medical experiences which he intended to put into the *Canon*, but that the paper on which they were written was lost before the completion of the work.[13]

About twenty years after the death of Ibn Sīnā, another group of case histories was assembled in Muslim Spain by al-Hāshimī. These are medical consultations with patients conducted by two of his teachers around 1056, such as the following:

> A man came and reported that he suffered from a pain all over his head, a nosebleed, and a dry, sweet taste in his mouth. [My teacher] said to him: How is your sleep? The man replied: Heavy. My teacher asked: How are you when you get up, energetic or tired? The man said: Tired.
>
> The doctor said: Cut the cephalic vein and draw ten ounces of blood and rub your temples with caltrop mixed with oil of violets and wetnurse's milk. The man was cured.
>
> I said: Shall we record it? My teacher replied: Yes, [for use] in the spring and in youth. And I asked: What about diet? He replied: Poultry cooked with vinegar for the young, and endive and coriander for the adults.[14]

The cephalic vein mentioned in this account runs the length of the arm and is visible along the outer edges of the biceps; it was the favoured location for phlebotomy to cure headaches and nosebleeds – hence its name 'cephalic' or head vein.[15]

A century later the students of Abū al-ʿAlāʾ Zuhr (d. 1131) in Muslim Spain also recorded his therapeutic procedures, an example being the following:

> For a man who suffered from pain and roughness in his throat and who had developed catarrh, he prescribed: On an empty stomach he must gargle with this: one ounce of mulberry syrup and half-ounce of walnut syrup, mixing it all with three and a half ounces of rose-water. He must gargle it hot.[16]

The tradition of students recording their teachers' therapeutic practices was apparently widespread. Not only did al-Rāzī's students record his cases in the early tenth century, and the students of Abū al-ʿAlāʾ Zuhr followed suit in the twelfth century, but we know that a student of the Egyptian physician al-ʿAyn-zarbī (d. 1153) recorded his teacher's therapeutic practices in a treatise entitled 'Medical Experiences (*Mujarrabāt fī al-ṭibb*)', though it is not preserved today.[17]

Abū Marwān ibn Zuhr (d. 1162), the son of Abū al-ʿAlāʾ Zuhr, included a few of his own cases in his treatise *Book of Moderation Regarding the Restoration [of the Health] of Souls and Bodies*. In this he was largely motivated it would seem by a desire to promote his own skills at the expense of his competitors. Half a century later the Egyptian Jewish physician Yaʿqūb ibn Isḥāq (d. c. 1208) included occasional first-hand accounts of care in his diatribe against Damascene physicians written shortly after 1202, mostly to display the superiority of his technique. An example is the following:

> One day, I came to see a sick man from Alexandria who stayed at the inn nearby the house of Ibn Qawām [situated in the middle of the old quarter of Damascus, next to covered markets]. I found him in distress, and I asked him: 'How long have you been like this?' He replied: 'This is the seventh day'. So I surmised that it was a crisis ... I suspected the crisis would come about with diarrhoea, and I said to him: 'Do not take anything!' At the close of the day I returned and found that his discomfort was greater. I asked him: 'When did you get into this state?' He said: 'The fourth day, for on that day I ate a quince'. I prescribed an enema for him, but that he refused. I then made a suppository for him, but that did not work. So I gave him some gum tragacanth with hot rose-water and almond oil, which can act as a laxative. Ten sessions [doses ?, Arabic *majālis*] later, he had got rid of it on that day, and the affliction did not return. I only gave him this because, after he said he had eaten a quince, I guessed that he must have swallowed filth together with that quince which, then, caused a constipation ...[18]

From Muslim Spain, but the fourteenth century, we have first-hand accounts recorded in the *Book of Investigation and Confirmation Regarding the Treatment of Wounds and Tumours* by Muḥammad al-Shafrah (d. 1360). Born about 1280 in Crevillent, a Muslim enclave surrounded by Christian Spain, he studied surgery with a Christian named Bernat. He eventually moved to Granada and then in 1344 to Fez. Muḥammad al-Shafrah criticised Muslim surgery of the day as being in the hands of the uneducated. Although al-Shafrah's name means 'the knife', it was pharmacological therapy that determined virtually all of his care. Similarly, Ibn Zuhr and his father employed only diet and medicaments.[19]

As is evident from the case accounts quoted above – and these are entirely typical of the lot – drug therapy, diet, and bloodletting dominate. Surgery plays little role.

Drug therapy

In the *Book of Experiences*, it is evident that al-Rāzī's therapy concentrated on evacuation (by phlebotomy, cupping, or purgatives), regimen, medicaments, and diet, with great reliance on rose-honey and barley water. Surgery is nowhere to be seen, not even the scraping of the eyelids in chronic trachoma – a procedure advocated in all his formal writings concerned with eye diseases. Moreover, compared with the recipes for compound remedies that he recorded in his working notes and recommended in his treatises, the *Book of Experiences* shows him using a more limited range of both simple and compound drugs. In that volume, for example, ophthalmia is treated with a simple decoction of myrobalan mixed with egg white, oil of roses, and wetnurse's milk, while in his formal treatises an application is recommended that combined several collyria of multiple ingredients that are then to be further mixed with mucilage of quince seed or other ingredients.[20]

Many of the substances known to earlier Greek physicians continued to be employed by Islamic druggists, often with expanded uses. Balsam, for example, was known to Greek physicians as an aromatic resin produced only in Egypt, and it continued to be so highly valued for its medicinal and other properties, that the Egyptian chronicler Ibn Ilyās (d. c. 1523) claimed it could fetch its weight in gold. In medieval Islamic sources it is a ubiquitous component of compound remedies. Because of its warming and drying qualities, it was considered specific for diseases associated with cold – so much so that, according to the Egyptian historian al-'Umarī (d. 1347), a Mamluk sultan sent balsam from Egypt 'to the castles of Syria, and to hospitals [there] for the treatment of those suffering from illnesses of cold (*li-mu'ālajat al-mabrūdīn*).' Another example is wormwood (a species of artemisia), considered by both Greek and Arabic writers to be good for the liver and spleen. Islamic physicians added new applications such as its role as an antidote to opium poisoning. The use of this herb for spleen and liver complaints is noteworthy in light of recent interest in artemisia as a treatment for malaria, an ailment endemic to the Mediterranean basin and one characterised by an enlarged spleen.[21]

Islamic physicians brought into the pharmacopoeias new medicinal substances unknown to Greek physicians, including camphor, musk, senna, myrobalan, and sal ammoniac [chloride of ammonia]. Moreover, they introduced into medical practice the commodity of cotton, previously unknown to Europe, resulting in its fundamental role in medical dressings. Techniques such as distillation were developed that became important in the preparation of inorganic and organic acids, while the distillation of rose-water and 'essential oils (*duhns*)' from plants and flowers became a flourishing industry. New equipment was developed both for chemical preparations and for pharmaceutics. As early as the twelfth century, if not earlier, a distinctive form of drug jar was produced in Syria, one having a contracted waist, allowing them to be placed closely together on shelves but easily removed.[22]

The recipes in pharmacopoeias often contained many ingredients, but their effectiveness has not been seriously examined by modern scholars or scientists. A recent study has shown that the recipes for coughs in Kūhīn al-'Aṭṭār's formulary included fennel, hyssop, liquorice, and poppy, all of which functioned as expectorants or cough suppressants in modern medicine. Opium was a common ingredient in recipes for gastro-intestinal complaints and diarrhoea. Crude extracts were used, however, and not highly purified materials. Moreover, these substances were not employed singly, but rather were part of a recipe with many ingredients, whose effect may have been much greater – or less – than the sum of its parts.[23]

Bloodletting and cauterisation

Both bloodletting and cauterisation were old techniques indigenous to the pre-Islamic Near East as well as Ancient Greece and were basic components of any Islamic physician's armory. Cauterisation employed caustics or a heated metal rod, not just to stop bleeding, but as a treatment in itself. Bloodletting was a generally accepted way of restoring an imbalance of humours considered detrimental to health. A phlebotomist bled directly from the veins. Cuppers, on the other hand, employed much less hazardous procedures than phlebotomists, for they lightly scarified the skin and drew blood more gently to the surface by applying a heated cupping glass. They also practised 'dry cupping', in which no blood was extracted but the heated cupping glass was placed on the skin to relieve pain, itching, or other complaints. There is little evidence that leeches were much used, if at all, for the extraction of blood, despite the fact that they were common in Greek medicine and later European practice. Arabic medical writers, such as al-Zahrāwī and Ibn Sīnā, included short paragraphs on leeches, but the material is derived from the translated Greek writings.

Both phlebotomy and cupping were considered generally beneficial when ill. Documents exist indicating that phlebotomists sometimes had to pay compensation in the event of injury or death resulting from a careless incision. Though the techniques used by cuppers were slightly less fearsome than those of phlebotomists (severe blistering being preferable to bleeding to death when an artery is mistakenly cut), cuppers were nonetheless considered to be of a lower social status, frequently satirised in popular literature. For an example, see Figure 3.1, p. 97. Al-Zahrāwī implies that cuppers also undertook tooth pulling and 'often bring great troubles upon people, the least of which is to break the tooth off short, leaving the whole or part of the root behind; or to remove the tooth together with a piece of the jawbone, as I have often seen'.[24]

The predilection of medieval Islamic physicians for bloodletting was often mocked. The Syrian writer Ibn al-'Ibrī (Bar Hebraeus d. 1286) included the following anecdote in his collection of *Laughable Stories*: A physician sees a man running stark naked out of a public bath. The man tells the physician that someone has stolen his clothes and he is chasing after them. The physician prevents him from going further and insists on drawing blood from him, as a remedy for excessive excitement.[25]

Surgery and the division of labour

There is ample evidence that certain types of surgery were undertaken, and that some people, at least by the tenth century, specialised in that activity. In al-Rāzī's *Book of Experiences*, however, as well as those portions of the *Comprehensive*

Book that have been closely analysed by scholars, surgery is not mentioned as a practice that al-Rāzī undertook himself though the implication is that others performed it. Al-Kaskarī supplies us with the name of a surgeon, one Sulaymān, who treated al-Muwaffaq (the son of the caliph al-Mutawakkil, d. 891) in Basra when an arrow hit his throat during battle. In the case of Muslim Spain, we have the following explicit statement of Abū Marwān ibn Zuhr that physicians did not undertake surgery themselves:

> As for the handling of these matters with surgery, that is a function of some of the assistants to the physician. The same is true for bloodletting, cautery, and phlebotomy. What is very highly regarded amongst this class of person is something like the lifting and excision of pannus [a complication of trachoma], while the highest acclaim amongst the class of assistants is given to the successful performance of cataract couching. All of these are functions of the physician's attendants. As for the physician, he should be concerned with treating the patient by means of diet and medicaments and he should not include manual techniques [that is, surgery]. Similarly, he should not be concerned with compounding electuaries except when absolutely necessary.[26]

This division of labour advocated by Ibn Zuhr is reflected throughout his medical writings, but not always corroborated by other evidence. For example, 'Umar ibn 'Abd al-Raḥmān al-Qurṭubī (d. 1066) travelled from Córdoba to upper Mesopotamia where he studied mathematics and medicine. Returning to Muslim Spain, he settled in Saragossa and became known for his skill in 'cauterising, cutting, making incisions, and using a lancet.' Furthermore, in the case of the tenth-century physician al-Zahrāwī, it would seem that another learned Arab physician in Muslim Spain also engaged in surgery himself.[27]

In other regions, clear-cut divisions of labour may have occurred later. In the late twelfth century, the 'chief physician' in Egypt and Syria, al-Sulamī (d. 1208) clearly distinguishes ophthalmologists, surgeons, and bone-setters from general physicians in his *Experts' Examination of all Physicians*. In his treatise on Prophetic Medicine written in Damascus in the early fourteenth century, Ibn Qayyim al-Jawzīyah states specifically that the classification of physicians into the following eight specialities was a recent development in his day:

> The [term] physician in this report includes all those who give medical treatment either by medical prescriptions or practice as specialists. If [he uses] an eye-probe [*mirwad*], then he is an oculist; if a scalpel [*mubdi'*] and ointments then he is a surgeon; if a straight-razor [*mūsá*], then a circumciser [*khātin*]; if a lancet [*rīshah*], then a phlebotomist; if cupping glasses and a scarifier [*mishraṭ*], then a cupper; if dislocation [*khal'*], realignment, and bandaging [*ribāṭ*], then a bone-setter [*mujabbir*]; if cautery iron [*mikwāh*] and fire, then a cauteriser [*kawwā'*]; and if a waterskin-bag, then one who administers enemas ... Specialisation [*takhṣīṣ al-nās*] as applied to types of physicians is a recent custom [*'urf ḥadīth*].[28]

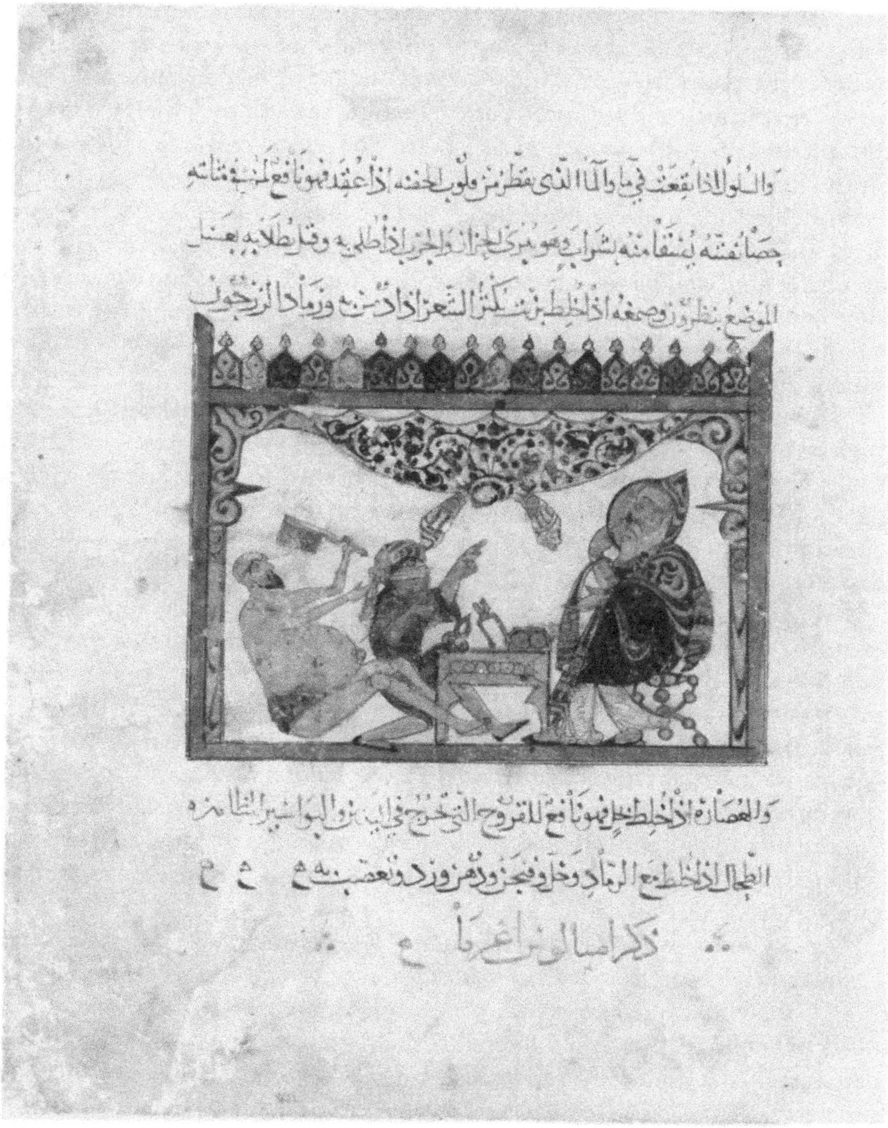

Figure 4.1 A physician with two patients, illustrating a now dispersed copy made in Baghdad in 1224 of the Arabic translation of Dioscorides' treatise on medicinal substances. The image occurs in the opening chapter of the fifth book ('On vines and wines'), where the text is describing the medicinal uses of the leaves, fruit, and juice of the cultivated grape. The illustration, however, appears unrelated to the text.

Precisely what these surgeons were doing, and how frequently they were doing it, is a puzzle. An unknown artist of Baghdad in the year 1224 painted a rather frightening scene of a blindfolded patient sitting before a surgeon (Figure 4.1). The turbaned and red-robed patient gestures towards the physician, who in turn points to his own nose or upper mouth. The nature of the two instruments on the table between them (small forceps and clamps or scissors) suggests that tooth-pulling might be contemplated. The bald and bearded figure at the left of this scene is most curious, however, for he is seated on the ground, naked except for underpants, and has an enormous swollen stomach suggesting a grotesquely large umbilical hernia or severe dropsy. He also gestures with one hand towards the physician, while holding in his left hand a fan to cool himself. Is he, too, a patient awaiting surgery?

Formal treatises provide only a limited view of the actual medical practices of the day, and on occasion they are not corroborated by other available evidence. In the scholarly surgical literature outlined in Chapter 2, physicians occasionally commented that no one was known actually to perform a given operation, even though they may have included a description of the procedure based on earlier authoritative texts.

When the surgical instructions represent a change in the usual techniques or are accompanied by a case history, our confidence is increased that the procedure was actually undertaken. For example, al-Zahrāwī described surgery for the treatment of abdominal wounds resulting in protrusion of the intestines. He modified, however, earlier methods for suturing and also presented a case history of a man wounded in the abdomen with a knife. Consequently, we can conclude that physicians did attempt on occasion to treat abdominal wounds surgically. On the other hand, instructions for surgically treating an umbilical hernia are repeated, unchanged, from earlier texts, therefore suggesting the operation was rarely, if ever, undertaken.[29]

While most major or invasive surgery was scarcely ever attempted, one traumatic operation that was the subject of every surgical manual was amputation. Gangrene was the most common reason for undertaking it, in many cases no doubt following multiple fractures. Only amputation of lower joints was performed. Al-Zahrāwī, in fact, warns against attempting amputation when the gangrene has spread above the elbow or the knee, and indeed such surgery could not have been successfully performed at that time. According to the manuals, the limb was ligatured below and above the site, the site was cauterised following and sometimes during the operation, and styptics were applied.[30]

A rather depressing success rate of recovery, however, is suggested by the following observation of al-Kaskarī in a tenth-century Baghdad hospital:

> I once saw a group of thieves in the hospital whose hands and feet had been cut off. Their limbs became spasmodic because of the amputation, and not a single one of them escaped death.[31]

A similar unhappy outcome is suggested by an account of the death in 1249 of the ruler of Egypt, sultan al-Ṣāliḥ Ayyūb. According to Ibn al-ʿIbrī (Barhebraeus), himself a physician, the sultan suffered gangrene in his thigh at the crucial moment when the delta city of Damietta had just fallen in the Seventh Crusade led by Louis IX of France, thereby threatening the rest of Egypt. The physicians amputated 'while he was [still] alive', but he died the next day. This version, however, has been shown to be unreliable, for two reasons. It was unlikely that an amputation at the thigh would have been undertaken, and a more immediate witness who was deputy to the sultan himself, Ibn Wāṣil (d. 1298 aged 93), strongly suggests the cause of the sultan's death to have been a respiratory infection with coughing up of blood and pus.[32]

On the other hand, al-Zahrāwī reported that he examined a man in Muslim Spain who had amputated his own foot, after gangrene had attacked it. Moreover, he requested al-Zahrāwī to amputate his hand when the disease appeared in that organ. Al-Zahrāwī, however, refused to perform the operation, 'fearing the man would die at the amputation of his hand', though later he heard that the patient had himself cut off his entire hand and had recovered.[33]

Most surgical procedures were far less traumatic, consisting of small incisions of boils, abscesses, and various growths. The methods of suturing wounds are numerous and described in great detail, though the actual use of these techniques is difficult to assess and the rate of success was probably quite low given that infection from the wounding implement would probably have been present.

Trachoma and eye surgery

Surgery was also employed in treating one of the complications of trachoma. Medieval Islamic physicians recognised a vascularisation which invades the cornea (called today pannus, *sabal* in Arabic) to be a complication of trachoma, considering it to be transmissible, just as trachoma was. It was treated surgically with a technique known today as peritomy, employing an instrument for keeping the eye open during surgery, a number of very small hooks for lifting, and a very thin scalpel for excision. While this procedure was first developed in the medieval Islamic world, in Europe it was 'reinvented' in 1862 by Salvatore Furnari in Palermo under the name of *tonsura conjunctivalis*, and variations of the procedure continued to be practised until after the First World War.

A similar surgical technique was available to remove pterygium, a triangular-shaped encroachment of the bulbar conjunctiva onto the cornea, usually on the nasal side. This condition, and the technique of excising it, was described by Graeco-Roman physicians and continued by Islamic oculists. The growth was lifted with small hooks and cut with a small lancet, using the same instruments as in pannus.

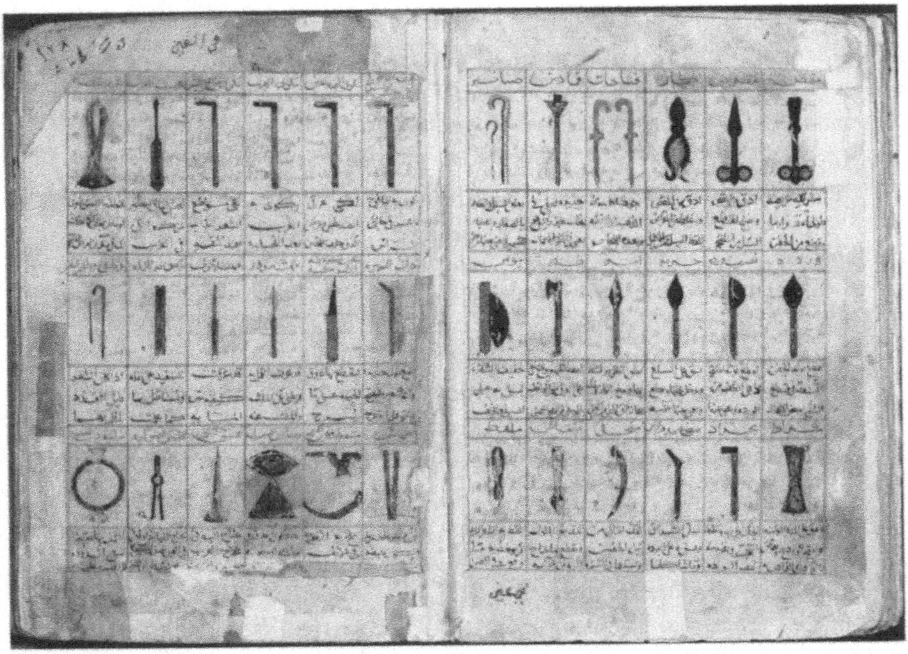

Figure 4.2 The instruments required by a thirteenth-century ophthalmologist, as illustrated in *The Sufficient Book on Ophthalmology*, written in Syria between 1256 and 1275 by Khalīfah ibn Abī al-Maḥāsin al-Ḥalabī. The top row (right to left) illustrates three types of scissors, two tools for keeping the eyelids open, a sheathed scalpel, various hooks, four cauterising tools, a probe, and small forceps. The middle row contains four instruments for excising cysts and other growths, a small hatchet for phlebotomy, a razor knife, two lancets, a round and a hollow cataract needle, a narrow tube for uprooting tumours, and a hook and needle. The bottom row includes additional forms of lancets and scrapers, along with tweezers for removing foreign bodies, and various tools for dispensing eye medicaments. The excision of the eye ailments known today as pterygium and pannus are the uses most often specified for the instruments.

Both surgical procedures – that for pterygium and that for pannus – were intricate and painstaking. They caused considerable pain to the patient, yet both appear to have been at least occasionally performed in the medieval Islamic world, as is illustrated by Ibn Zuhr's comment quoted earlier regarding the physician's assistants who specialised in lifting and excising pannus. In the chart of thirty-six ophthalmic instruments provided in the thirteenth-century Syrian manual by Khalīfah, the excision of pterygium and pannus are the uses most often specified for the instruments (see Figure 4.2).

Cataract surgery

Another common cause of blindness was the occurrence of cataracts. Today the condition is known to be due to an opaque lens, but in medieval literature it was said that a membrane or opaque fluid was interposed between the lens and pupil. Various tests were advocated for determining whether a case was operable, and fish-eating was particularly associated with the formation of cataracts.[34]

When treating cataracts, the technique commonly used was an ancient one, known to classical antiquity and possibly originating in India. In English the technique is called couching, and in it the opaque lens (or 'crystalline humour', as it was then called) was not removed but rather pushed to one side. A small incision with a lancet was made in the sclera, or white of the eye, near the limbus (edge of the cornea) and then, after the lancet was removed, a cataract needle or probe was inserted and used to depress the lens. Some oculists advocated only a needle without the preliminary incision with a lancet. The oculist was to operate on the left eye with the right hand, and the right eye with the left hand. Following the operation, the eye was to be washed with salt-water and then bandaged with cotton-wool soaked in oil of roses and egg-white. There was great concern that the cataract, once depressed, would then re-ascend, and consequently the patient was instructed to lie on his back for seven days following the operation. Concerning this operation, al-Zahrāwī observed: 'But you should know that in the case of depression of a cataract, the student cannot manage without having seen that operation performed many times; [only] then may he perform it himself.'[35]

To put the activities of these tenth-century physicians in some perspective, it seems that there is no reliable evidence for cataracts being diagnosed and treated surgically in medieval Latin Europe before the thirteenth century, despite the antique origin of the technique.[36]

It is evident that in some locales certain people did nothing but couch cataracts. In many instances, they were probably itinerant and not highly trained in other medical matters. The physician Quṭb al-Dīn al-Shīrāzī in his commentary on Ibn Sīnā's *Canon of Medicine* written in Shiraz in 1283 said: 'I practised manual techniques appertaining to medicine and ophthalmology, such as blood-letting, suturing and fastening, everting [the eyelid] and removal of pterygium and pannus, and other things, all except the couching operation which was not befitting that I should perform.'[37]

An unflattering portrayal of cataract couchers motivated only by greed is given by the physician and biographer Ibn Juljul, who in 987 recorded a brief life of Ibn Waṣīf, a specialist in couching cataracts in Muslim Spain. After Ibn Waṣīf had agreed on a given fee for the operation, he discovered that the patient was carrying more money than he under oath had sworn to have with him at the time. So Ibn Waṣīf accused the man of perjury and refused to perform the operation, but kept the 80 dirhams he had been given as payment.[38]

In many societies the practice of couching continued into the twentieth century, and may well still be practised in some remote areas. A study of over 700 cases of couching in India during the first decade of the twentieth century found the success rate to be approximately four in ten – if one counts being able to finger-count at a distance of two feet or less. Cataract couching in Senegal had an 81 per cent failure rate according to another recent anthropological study. Infection and glaucoma were the major causes for failure. Techniques for couching of cataracts in recent centuries, however, differed from those in medieval Islamic manuals. Medieval oculists used a posterior approach, behind the limbus, to depress the lens into the vitreous, while more recent couchers, from at least the beginning of the eighteenth century, used an anterior approach through the cornea. Since untreated cataracts inevitably result in blindness and the medieval world afforded few means of livelihood for a blind person, it is perhaps not surprising that couching found widespread acceptance despite its less than encouraging success rate and evident pain.[39]

On the other hand, medieval biographers relate that when al-Rāzī himself grew blind with cataracts, he declined to have them couched. It is reported that, not long before he died in 925, he told an oculist who had come to operate on his eyes:

> I acknowledge that you are the most learned of oculists. You know, however, that this operation is not without pain, which the soul loathes, and long-drawn-out discomfort, which men find wearying. And perhaps [my] life may be cut short and the time of death be near; in which case it is repugnant to someone like myself at the end of his days to choose pain and discomfort over repose. So depart, with thanks for what you intended to do.[40]

Thus, if al-Rāzī's attitude towards couching is representative, most people probably avoided the operation if at all possible.

Anaesthesia and antisepsis

For medieval Islamic physicians, the lack of antisepsis as well as deep and dose-controlled anaesthesia were indeed significant limitations on all types of surgery, though to what extent is uncertain. The vast majority of operations – other than eye surgery – followed accidents or battle wounds, in which case infection may have already set in. Only occasionally is it suggested that the patient be washed before treatment. Following the procedure, however, the area was frequently cleaned or dressed with wine, wine mixed with oil of roses, oil of roses alone, salt-water, or vinegar and water, all of which have varying antiseptic properties. Various aromatic herbs and resins, such as frankincense, myrrh, cassia, and members of the laurel family, were used as medicaments. These also have some antiseptic properties, as do the doses of lead and copper salts, alum, mercury, and borax which were mixed with resins, oils, and vinegar to make many of the recommended plasters and ointments. The efficacy of such items versus the numerous sources of infection is, of course, impossible to evaluate at this distance.

Certain drugs (henbane, hemlock, soporific black nightshade, lettuce seeds, but particularly opium) were recognised as being soporific (*muraqqid*) and analgesic (*mukhaddir*), and arguments have been put forward by modern scholars that such items were used to cause a person to lose complete consciousness before an operation. However, there is no unambiguous reference to the use of deep analgesics in the Islamic medical literature prior to the sixteenth-century. Moreover, the margin of safety in using such crude drugs as opium, hemlock, and black nightshade is dangerously low. Yet the pain-killing attributes of opium (as well as its other medicinal qualities) were certainly exploited by even early Islamic physicians.[41]

Interestingly, soporifics or analgesics are not mentioned in connection with amputations in the Islamic surgical manuals, despite their association in the popular mind with such treatment. An example of the latter is a report that in 704 an amputation of a foot was performed on the legal scholar 'Urwah ibn al-Zubayr of Medina (d. 712) who 'suffered from gangrene in his foot while in Syria with al-Walīd' (shortly to become the Umayyad caliph al-Walīd I). With each subsequent century the account was elaborated so as to better demonstrate 'Urwah's piety. The administration of a soporific is not mentioned in the early accounts. In fact, it was not introduced into the story until the twelfth century, when it was related that 'Urwah was not only offered a soporific to drink but that after the amputation he took the leg from the hands of the physicians and, addressing the leg, said: 'What makes me feel good about you is that I never moved you to disobey God'. These changing accounts of the amputation illustrate the difficulties for the medical historian. Because they were recorded to illustrate dignity and piety rather than medical care, the only evidence for therapeutics to be extracted from them is that later generations viewed the Umayyad court as supporting physicians capable of performing amputations and administering soporifics to relieve pain. Little can be said on the basis of these reports regarding what actually transpired in Syria in the year 704.[42]

Prior to the development of these two important technologies – general anaesthesia and antisepsis – surgical therapy was inevitably limited to superficial conditions, fractures, dislocations, traumatic injuries and urinary disorders.

Frequency of surgical practice

As we have seen above, it is often unclear whether the procedural instructions in manuals reflect actual practice or whether they are a repetition of an earlier written account or even simply a 'thought experiment' in which the writer guesses at what he might do were the occasion ever to arise. Case histories are crucial in providing us with some evidence for the nature and frequency of surgical interventions, as well as medical practice in general.

Al-Zahrāwī provides eighteen 'case histories' in his chapter on surgery. In two instances, he did not operate himself, one being the account of a man who had amputated his own foot and hand, mentioned above. The second is an account of a woman who had two foetuses die *in utero* followed by a swollen umbilicus which opened and produced bones. Of al-Zahrāwī's personal undertakings, four involved removing tumours or growths (a woman with a tumour in her throat, an elderly woman with one on her head, a thirty-year-old man with a tumour on his leg, and a man with two large warts on his belly). Eleven cases involved treating wounds: a young girl with a knife in her throat; a male wounded in the belly; another wounded in the throat by a spear; four instances of men struck by arrows (one in the eye, two near the nose, one in the throat) from which al-Zahrāwī extracted the arrowhead; and four instances of arrow wounds (two in the abdomen, one in the back, one in the face) where no extraction was attempted and the wound healed with the arrowhead in place. Finally, there is an obscure case of a woman with a severely inflated cephalic vein whose treatment he leaves unspecified.[43]

In the mid-eleventh century, also in Muslim Spain, the physician al-Hāshimī recorded five surgical procedures undertaken by his teachers: three for inguinal hernias or hydroceles and two for haemorrhoids or anal fistulas. In the fourteenth century, again in Muslim Spain, Muḥammad al-Shafrah presented a case in which a cupper – and not he – wields the knife (unsuccessfully, it should be noted) on a woman suffering from four boils on the right side of her head. And in another instance he even enjoins physicians to avoid instructions in manuals, for when talking about ulcerous cancer he said:

> … and you, my son, do not touch such difficult tumours like cancer, and other ulcerous, weeping, and shrivelled areas, and do not follow what therapy is given for them in books, for they will be of no use to you, since only in God is there successful recovery.[44]

When we turn to ophthalmological surgery, there is slightly more evidence of actual practice. Al-Rāzī recorded in his working notes that he observed the removal of ptergyium in a hospital (neither the hospital nor the operator are specified), and he mentioned a patient who came to him to have his eye couched, but whom he sent away to eat fish (considered an important cause) until it matured, giving no subsequent record of surgery in the case. The ophthalmological manuals of 'Ammār in the tenth century and Khalīfah in the thirteenth provide us with six clinical cases of couching – all described as difficult but successful in the end.[45]

A thirteenth-century historian recorded the following account of an Egyptian scholar and man-of-letters by the name of al-Tīfāshī, most often remembered today for his treatises on sexual hygiene and the magical uses of stones. Of al-Tīfāshī, whom he knew personally, the historian Ibn al-'Adīm (d. 1262) said:

> It has been reported to me that a cataract descended in his eyes, so that he was blind. So both [eyes] were couched, and he could see and write and was free of it. But then he drank a purgative medicine and his end came quickly, for he died 13 Muḥarram 651 H [= AD 15 March 1253].[46]

From the same century we have a legal document of about 1250 in which a physician by the name of Makārim ibn Isḥāq undertook to remove pus from the eye (*kumnah*); it was agreed that, if successful, he would be paid a fee of two *dirhams*, and if not successful, the fee would be adjusted and he would remain free of liability. The outcome of the operation is unrecorded.[47]

One century later, this time in Syria, an eyewitness testified to the skill of an oculist named 'Alā' al-Dīn ibn al-Barqa'īdī al-Kaḥḥāl (d. 1360) who worked in the Nūrī hospital in Damascus. The Mamluk historian al-Ṣafadī (d. 1363) records the following first-hand account of the oculist's skill in treating a hydatid cyst (*shirānīq* in Arabic):

> I saw an example of his surgery with the knife. In my presence, on one of my sisters, he cut a cyst on her eyelid in one single thrust, as quickly as could possibly be done. He slit the upper eyelid and expressed from it something that resembled yellow fat. He did not use the technique that others employ of lifting the eyelids with hooks and rubbing the cyst with sugar cane, because that would protract the ailment and make it more painful.[48]

Problems of evidence

Interpreting the evidence, however, is not always easy or certain. Even when medieval 'case histories' exist, they cannot always provide credible evidence for practice. As an example, there are several accounts of oculists *removing* a cataract (as opposed to employing the traditional technique of 'couching' or displacement). The Cairene oculist 'Ammār ibn 'Alī al-Mawṣilī claimed to have designed a hollow cataract needle for the removal of a cataract by suction. He states that he did not actually use the instrument until he was in Tiberias, in Greater Syria, where he operated successfully on a Christian male who had told him beforehand that he could not remain lying in bed at rest for many days. 'Ammār gives no details of the operation, but says that the patient could see immediately and that he did not need to go to bed. 'Ammār then makes the statement: '[since then] I have operated with it [the hollow needle] on a number of patients in Cairo and elsewhere, and they have recovered their sight.'[49]

Earlier, al-Rāzī had briefly described the procedure and the hollow instrument, attributing its invention to the Greek physician Antyllus of the second century. Meanwhile, in Spain, 'Ammār's contemporary al-Zahrāwī stated:

> I have heard that a certain Iraqi has said that in Iraq he makes a hollow needle by which the humour is sucked out. In our land I have never seen anyone do it in this fashion, nor have I read of it described in any of the books of the Ancients. Perhaps it is newly invented.[50]

Yet the oculist 'Alī ibn 'Īsá, working in Baghdad at this time, does not mention it. A treatise titled *The Book of Vision and Perception* was composed not long after 930, but falsely attributed to a ninth-century scholar and near contemporary of al-Rāzī, Thābit ibn Qurrah (d. 901). The unknown author of this *Book of Vision* said that the operation with a hollow needle was an illusion, that it could not be performed, and that a person should avoid anyone who says he can do it, even if he calls himself an oculist (*kaḥḥāl*).[51]

Later writers repeated 'Ammār's description of the instrument and technique but gave no further evidence of experience with it. The 'hollow needle' was also included in the chart of instruments presented in the Syrian ophthalmological manual by Khalīfah next to the conventional couching needle, though one copy has the phrase 'but God knows best' following the description of its employment – a caveat not used for any of the other illustrated instruments and clearly indicating a doubt in the copyist's (if not the author's) mind regarding its efficacy. See Figure 4.2.

In the fourteenth century the Egyptian oculist al-Shādhilī provided an interesting account of hollow cataract needles. He stated that in the Cairo markets of his day one could still buy two types of hollow cataract needles, one like a thick sewing needle and the other with a screw to replace suction by the mouth, though he said he had never seen them used or heard of anyone using them. Al-Shādhilī then tested some of these hollow needles in water and in a mucilaginous solution and found that they would draw up only pure water, not slightly thickened water which he argued was nearer the consistency of a cataract. He stated that he once observed a surgeon trying to operate with such an instrument, unsuccessfully. He asked him if he had ever seen anyone else operate with it, and he said he had not. Later al-Shādhilī discussed this instrument with one Yūsuf ibn al-Labbān, who he says was a celebrated and widely travelled surgeon. Ibn al-Labbān said that he had seen numerous surgeons in many lands with such instruments in their possession, adding 'I never saw any of them actually use one. I used to ask them to show me how the operation was performed, but to a man they declined on the grounds that they had never seen it performed either. They said that they had used the needle experimentally to see what the outcome would be, but that their operations had not succeeded because of their ignorance of the procedure.' Al-Shādhilī then concluded his discussion with ten logical reasons why such a hollow needle could not remove a cataract successfully, followed by a second-hand case history:

> A friend of mine who had travelled widely once told me that in the country of the Russians, which lies somewhere in the Byzantine lands, he saw a Christian surgeon who had a hollow cataract-needle of red brass, the point of which was made of gold and was soldered into place. In the tip of the point there was a hole like that of a syringe, as described earlier. The length [of the instrument] was greater than the span of a hand, and its thicker part was bent and curved like the curved section of a cupping-glass, except that the curved part was long and turned back on itself, with another bend at the end of it where the mouth was placed and suction applied. The length [of this curved part] was four closed fingers, adequate to enable the operator to observe the cataract. The operator would hold the needle in one hand and hold the patient's eye with the other, with the end of the curving section of the instrument in his mouth, without harming the cataract with it. In practice, however, he [this Christian surgeon] performed cataract operations only with the conventional instrument.
>
> [My friend] said: I asked him [the Christian surgeon] to use the hollow needle, but he answered that operations with the hollow needle were rarely successful. 'In that case,' [al-Shādhilī's friend in Russia] continued, 'why did you make one?' 'I did not make it,' [the Christian physician] replied; 'I was associated with a Turkoman surgeon, here in our country, and when he died this instrument was part of his estate, and I bought it.' Al-Shādhilī's friend then said to him 'Did you ever see him perform an operation with it?' 'No,' said [the Christian physician], 'I never saw him operate on a cataract with anything but a conventional triangular needle, but he would always place this one in front of him with the rest of the equipment. For some time I entertained the thought of testing it myself, and finally, although I knew nothing of the proper procedure, I undertook a trial. I found that it would loosen and shift the cataract and sometimes cause it to swirl turbulently and fulminate, with the result that the couching would be unsuccessful. Accordingly, I have given up operating with it.' Then al-Shādhilī's friend asked: 'Have you ever had a successful outcome with it at all?' 'No,' said [the Christian physician], 'but there was one case in which I used it in operating on a woman; the cataract came loose and swirled turbulently, and [the patient's eye] was inflamed for many days, but in the end her vision cleared. So I concluded that while the cataract had been loosened [as a result of the use of the needle], in the last analysis it had been Nature that had done as she wished.'
>
> [Al-Shādhilī adds:] As to the truth of this account, God the Exalted knows best ... I have related these things to you only so that you might be prepared for what you may hear about exotic procedures performed by various skilled operators. But as to the truth of what is said about the success of such procedures, God knows best, for He is the supremely excellent source of inspiration and the glorious Creator.[52]

The picture becomes even more complicated, for recently in the river Saône in southern France, five cataract needles in a cylindrical container were found at a Roman site dating from the first or second century AD. Three of them are standard needles for couching or displacement of a cataract, but two are hollow, with a tiny hole near the tip and a narrow plunger inside which could be raised to produce a slight vacuum. These hollow instruments are unique amongst Roman artefacts, and the question arises, whether they might represent a variant of the 'hollow' cataract needle that 'Ammār claimed to have invented in the tenth century and that al-Shādhilī later dismissed as unusable.[53]

Such conflicting evidence regarding the removal of cataracts by a hollow needle is difficult to interpret, but at the very least we can say that the operation was rarely, if ever, undertaken and then probably unsuccessfully. Yet if that interpretation is accepted, then we must dismiss as credible evidence the 'case histories' provided by 'Ammār in Cairo testifying to its successful performance. In other words, while formal discourses on medicine and surgery are not necessarily always reliable guides to what procedures were actually undertaken – and are certainly not to be taken as evidence of the incidence or success of such undertakings – case histories and instruments must also be corroborated with other material.

Nor are pictures always a reliable source. Certain manuscript illustrations have frequently been interpreted as evidence that Caesarean sections were performed by medieval Islamic physicians. A miniature painting made in 1307 in a copy of a world history by the polymath al-Bīrūnī (d. c. 1051) illustrates the abdominal birth of Augustus, whom al-Bīrūnī erroneously considered the first of the Caesars (*wa-huwa awwal al-qayāṣirah*). Over the painting there is written in Arabic the statement: 'The reason for this was that his mother died in labour while she was pregnant with him; so her abdomen was opened, and he was taken out'. This statement by al-Bīrūnī demonstrates the common confusion amongst medieval writers regarding the Roman rulers, for the first 'Caesarean section' and the subsequent derivation of the term is usually associated with Gaius Julius Caesar, the founder of the line of Caesars, whose mother did supposedly die while giving birth to him. This particular miniature has often been reproduced and has been used to suggest that medieval Islamic physicians employed post-mortem sections.[54]

There are also a considerable number of preserved miniatures illustrating the birth of the mythical hero Rustam in copies of the *Shāhnāmah* (*The Book of Kings*) written in Persian at the end of the tenth century by Firdawsī. These have been used to support the statement that Caesarean sections on living women were performed in medieval Islam. In the course of the poem, it is said that the mother was given a drug to stupefy her and to dull any fear or anxiety in her mind, while incantations were recited. The operation, according to the poet, was performed successfully with her full recovery. These depictions of the abdominal birth of Rustam from a living woman are, however, merely illustrations of a legend attributing to its hero a miraculous birth, a common attribute in antiquity for great men. There is no mention in the surgical literature of such a procedure ever being attempted, even as a *post-mortem* effort to save the foetus after the mother had died. None of these illustrations should be taken as evidence that Caesarean sections, *post-mortem* or live, were performed in the medieval Islamic world. Only one medieval legal reference to the acceptability of *post-mortem* sections has so far been noted in the preserved literature, and no reference to a section birth on a living woman has been found.[55]

Regimen, circumcision, and personal hygiene

The first line of treatment for virtually all complaints was diet and regimen. Regimen could include not just regulation of rest and exercise, but calming activities such as music therapy. Listening to instrumentalists or singing poetry to the accompaniment of instruments was considered beneficial for melancholy and related complaints. The Brethren of Purity (*Ikhwān al-Ṣafā'*), a secret club of Neo-Platonic philosophers in tenth-century Baghdad, even referred to a particular musical mode being used in hospitals of Ancient Greece at dawn, and quoted poetry indicating that this means of therapy was used in their own day. In the twelfth- and thirteenth-century hospitals of Syria and Egypt there are records of expenditures for troupes of musicians to perform daily. If alterations of regimen and nutrition were not successful, then drug therapy was undertaken. Next, recourse was had to bloodletting and cauterisation, with surgery using the knife resorted to only when all else failed.[56]

Medical care also took forms other than those practised by learned physicians. The majority of the population, many of whom did not live in urban centres, had little or no access to learned medicine or to hospitals. They relied upon home remedies transmitted usually through the women in the family, traditional drug vendors, and itinerant practitioners of various sorts. Bone-setters and surgeons were available in many market-places, as is evident from their attempted regulation by market-inspectors in the twelfth century.

Barbers, phlebotomists, and cuppers could also be found in market-places, for they also are mentioned in manuals regulating the markets. They were also part of the staff (male and female) of every steam bath (*ḥammām*) – an institution of fundamental importance in the everyday life of the population. Barbers and hairdressers were important in maintaining cleanliness of the skin, controlling infestation of lice, and carrying out general cosmetic and beautifying procedures. The manufacture of hard soap, often perfumed, became an important industry, especially in Syria, though other places, such as Bālis on the River Euphrates, also became famous for exporting their soaps.

A miniature painting illustrating one such steam bath is shown in Figure

4.3. Public baths were numerous in every town (57, for example, in Damascus in the twelfth century, 85 in the next), and private baths were common in the precincts of palaces and wealthy estates. Certain days or times were delegated for use by women and other times for men. People regularly attended in order to relax, to engage in social exchanges, to cleanse themselves, and to fulfil certain ritual ablutions. Washing and scrubbing with soap was hygienic, and the warm baths soothing to joint complaints. Women were required to attend 40 days after giving birth; brides before weddings; and boys before circumcision. The age at which circumcision was performed was usually between ages five and seven, though it varied according to locale and could be as early as a week after birth or as late as age fifteen. All segments of society availed themselves of the steam bath and the care provided there by the barbers and bloodletters, many of whom also performed minor removal of growths and warts as well as circumcision.[57]

Baths were specifically prescribed by physicians for recuperating from illness. For example, the celebrated Egyptian Jewish physician Isḥāq ibn Sulaymān al-Isrā'īlī (d. 950) said that, when the fever has definitely subsided, the physician

> should have their patients take fresh-water steam baths in a moderately heated atmosphere that is kept at about the same gentle temperature as freshly drawn milk. The baths, however, should not be too far from their houses, and they should be carried there on cloth litters or sedans, so that they may avoid moving on their own and thereby suffering one or two afflictions, namely, increased dehydration of the body through evaporation brought on by movement or else overheating and debilitation of the body. [If either affliction should occur there would be] a reduction of the length of time during which patients will be capable of staying in the baths at a time when they stand in need of a long stay in the bath-tank ... The best kind of bath-tank for the purpose is one that is roomy and close to the door of the baths, so that patients who need to be spared the effort of walking in the atmosphere of the baths do not have to go too far, for the heat of the baths, if combined with walking and fatigue, will draw off the body's moisture in sweat and impart to it dryness and dehydration ... Now when the patient gets out of the tank, his body should be embrocated with oil of violets or of sweet pumpkin seeds dissolved in white wax so as to close the body's pores and prevent the moisture that has been taken in from the water from getting out.[58]

Medical texts often mentioned circumcision of boys, though it was most frequently performed by barbers or phlebotomists rather than physicians, and it was usually accompanied by many and varied rites. Circumcision of girls, on the other hand, was not discussed in the medical manuals. Although al-Zahrāwī repeats an earlier Greek account of surgically removing an excessively large clitoris, in general female circumcision was not an attempt to remedy an abnormal deviation of the genitalia, but rather was a *rite de passage*, though performed without much ceremony. Female circumcision (*khafḍ*) of various types, including the radical infibulation, was and is still today practised in

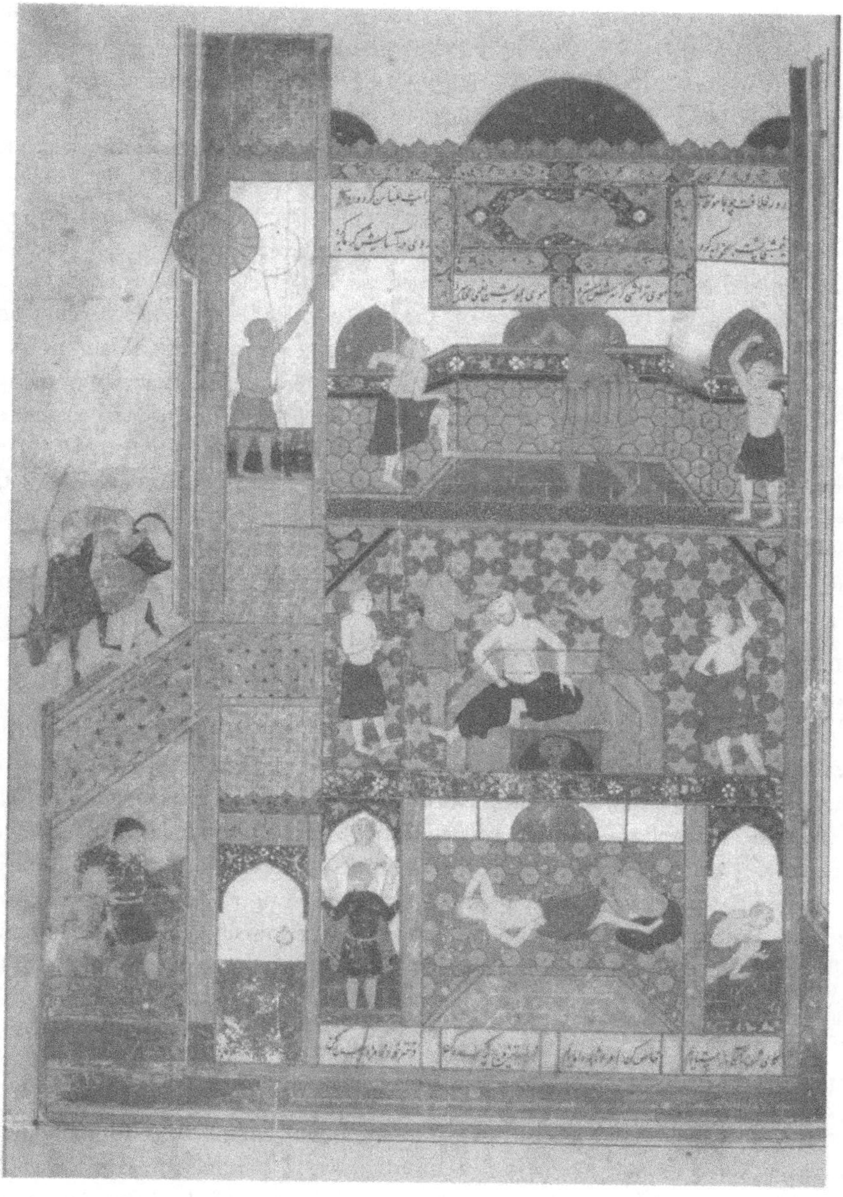

Figure 4.3 A scene in a steam bath (*ḥammām*), illustrating a copy made in 1529 of the *Khamsah* ('Quintette'), a classic of Persian literature by the poet Nizāmī (d. 1203). At the centre of the illustration, the ʿAbbāsid caliph Ma'mūn is having his head shaved by a barber. Three tiled rooms are depicted, each providing baths at a different temperature: cold, tepid, or hot. To the left, and outside the building, a well is being worked to supply the water.

certain Islamic countries, particularly Egypt and the Sudan, though it is now illegal in many areas. The Qur'ān does not mention the practice, although there are some *ḥadīths* (of questionable authenticity) suggesting that it was carried out in pre-Islamic Arabia. Most Muslim religious authorities did not consider female circumcision to be obligatory, but some said it was 'recommended', and its practice has been unevenly distributed across the Muslim world.[59]

Virtually all strata of the society regularly practised a form of dental hygiene in which they cleaned their teeth using a brush called *siwāk* (or *miswāk*), usually made from the bark, branches, or roots of the *arāk* tree, a variety of *Salvadora persica* L. Branches that had fallen off the tree and had remained for some time in the shade or been covered with soil (called *ṣurʿ*) were considered the most desirable source because they did not scratch the gums. The practice of using a *siwāk* was strongly recommended by jurists (though not considered absolutely obligatory) because of a saying attributed to the Prophet: 'Were it not for my desire not to burden my community, I would have ordered them to clean the teeth before every act of worship.' Relevant to the general health of the population, a recent study has shown that the wood of the *arāk* tree prevents plaque and inflammation of the gums, owing to fluoride, tannins, and a resinous substance in the wood.[60]

* * *

A person's general health, as well as available medical care, depended upon their wealth and rank and whether they lived in an urban or a rural setting – not unlike today in virtually every society. In the medieval Islamic world the everyday care of the educated and the illiterate, the affluent and the poor, encompassed a wide spectrum of practices not necessarily reflected in the formal medical literature preserved today. All attempts to maintain well-being or restore health are to be seen as part of medical care, including the recourse to magical therapies, folkloric traditions, and devout religious invocations that are the subject of the next chapter.

Suggested reading

For the effectiveness of drug therapy in medieval Islam, see Chipman, 'How Effective Were Cough Remedies', Chipman, *Minhāj al-dukkān*, Tibi, *Medicinal Use of Opium*, and (used with caution) Elgood, *Safavid Medical Practice*.

For general discussions of case histories and clinical accounts in antiquity and the Islamic world, see Álvarez-Millán, 'Practice versus Theory'; Álvarez-Millán, 'Graeco-Roman Case Histories'; Meyerhof, 'Thirty-Three Clinical Observations'; Savage-Smith, 'The Practice of Surgery', Savage-Smith, 'The Exchange of Medical and Surgical Ideas'; and Ullmann, *Rufus von Ephesos*. See also the index under authors al-Rāzī; al-Ḥāshimī; Abū al-'Alā' Zuhr; Abū al-'Alā' Zuhr; Muḥammad al-Shafrah. For surgery and the treatment of wounds in the crusader states, see Mitchell, *Medicine in the Crusades*, and for surgical and drug therapy in Spain in the Crown of Aragon (1285–1345), see McVaugh, *Medicine Before the Plague*.

For ophthalmic therapy, see Meyerhof, 'The History of Trachoma Treatment'; Sezgin, *Augenheilkunde im Islam* (four volumes of reprinted studies), and the treatises by authors Ḥunayn ibn Isḥāq; 'Alī ibn 'Īsá al-Kaḥḥāl; 'Ammār ibn 'Alī al-Mawṣilī; and Khalīfah ibn Abī al-Maḥāsin al-Ḥalabī. For partial translations of some relevant texts, see Blodi et. al., *Arabian Ophthalmologists*. For contemporaneous cataract surgery in Europe, see McVaugh, 'Cataracts and Hernias'.

Notes

1 Attributed to al-Rāzī by the historian Ibn Khallikān, *Deaths of Illustrious People*, v. 158, 17–18; a shorter version of the saying is given by Ibn Abī Uṣaybi'ah, *Sources of Information*, i. 315, 8–9.
2 A Persian proverb recorded by al-Karkhī, *Hope of the Hopeful*, 39; it was falsely attributed to al-Jāḥiẓ.
3 Ḥajjī Khalīfah, *Discovery of Opinions*, ii. 589, no. 4001.
4 Remains found in a cave cemetery near the town of Safed in present-day Israel have been analysed, but these were apparently Franks killed by Muslims at the time of the Crusades (see Mitchell, 'The Palaeopathology of Skulls'); there has also been one palaeopathological study of a Muslim woman from a Spanish grave site that revealed a calcified myoma (see Jiménez Brobeil, 'A Contribution to Medieval Pathological Gynaecology'). The scarcity of artefacts such as instruments contrasts markedly with classical antiquity and medieval Europe where the burial customs often included placement of important possessions, including surgical instruments. For instruments said to have been found at Fusṭāṭ (Old Cairo), see Hamarneh and Awad 'Medical Instruments' and for some now in the museum Dār al-Āthār al-Islamīyah (House of Islamic Antiquities) in Kuwait, see Institut du Monde Arabe, *L'Âge d'or des sciences arabes*, 174–5; most of these items could have had multiple uses, many of them non-medical. For so-called 'cupping glasses', of which there are a considerable number, see Maddison and Savage-Smith, *Science, Tools and Magic*, i. 42–7 and 48–57 and ii. 290–319 for other Islamic medical artifacts.
5 al-Rāzī, *Comprehensive Book*, (1st edn) xv. 122, 3. For a translation of the full passage, see Savage-Smith, 'Medicine', 917.
6 al-Rāzī, *Comprehensive Book*, iv. 67, 1–4 (2nd edn).
7 al-Rāzī, *Comprehensive Book*, xi. 227, 16–228, 2 (1st edn).
8 al-Rāzī, *Comprehensive Book*, xix. 416, 8–12 (1st edn). Case histories and clinical accounts are to be found not only in some of the Hippocratic writings but in other Greek sources as well, such as Rufus of Ephesus (*fl.* c. 100); See Ullmann, *Rufus von Ephesos*, and Álvarez-Millán, 'Graeco-Roman Case Histories'.
9 al-Rāzī, *Comprehensive Book*, xvi. 202, 14–203, 3 (2nd edn); translation is that of

the present authors. See also Meyerhof, 'Thirty-Three Clinical Observations', 344–5 (Case xxvii) and Arabic 10–11.

10 Istanbul, Topkapı Saray, Ahmed III, MS 1975, fols 47a–47b; translation is that of Álvarez-Millán, 'Practice versus Theory', 295.

11 Istanbul, Topkapı Saray, Ahmed III, MS 1975, fol. 10a; Álvarez-Millán, 'Graeco-Roman Case Histories', 34.

12 Pormann, 'Islamic Hospitals'. The cases described by al-Zahrāwī will be discussed below in this chapter.

13 Gohlman, *The Life of Ibn Sīnā*, 72–5. Al-Juzjānī gives two examples of medical cases (*tajārib*) that were contained on these lost pages: Ibn Sīnā curing himself of a headache by using an ice-pack, and a consumptive woman cured by doses of rose-honey. For literary anecdotes regarding Ibn Sīnā and his patients, see Browne, *Revised Translation of the Chahār maqála*, 88–93.

14 al-Hāshimī, *Book on Medical Sessions*, 21–2 (5th *majlis*). We wish to thank Cristina Álvarez-Millán for drawing this material to our attention.

15 The term 'cephalic' is derived (through a Latin rendering of the Arabic) from a Greek term *kephalikē* (*phleps*, 'head vein'), used by Paul of Aegina (*fl.* c. 640s), and possibly others; Arabic authors transliterated the Greek as *'irq al-qīfāl*, which al-Zahrāwī notes was popularly called *'irq al-ra's*, 'the head vein' (Spink and Lewis, *Albucasis*, 624–5). See Temkin, 'The Byzantine Origin of the Names for the Basilic and Cephalic Veins', and Goyanes, 'Todavia unas palabras sobre las venas cefalica y basilica'.

16 Álvarez-Millán, C., *Abū al-'Alā' Zuhr, Kitāb al-Muŷarrabāt*, entry no. 312; Spanish translation 193; Arabic 215.

17 Ibn Abī Uṣaybi'ah, *Sources of Information*, ii. 108, line 10; see also Hamarneh, 'Ibn al-'Ayn Zarbī and His Definitions of Diseases', 307–8.

18 Kahl, *Ya'qūb ibn Isḥāq*, 36 (Arabic), 55 (translation, slightly amended). The treatise by Ibn Zuhr has been edited and translated into Spanish by the late Rosa Kuhne Brabant and is being prepared for publication by Cristina Álvarez-Millán; we are grateful to her for giving us access to it before publication.

19 For the life of Muḥammad al-Shafrah, see Llavero Ruiz, 'La medicina granadina del siglo XIV' and McVaugh, *Medicine Before the Plague*, 53.

20 Álvarez-Millán, 'Practice versus Theory', 303.

21 See Milwright, 'The Balsam of Maṭariyya', for a discussion of the quotation from the historian Ibn Faḍl Allāh al-'Umarī, as well as a highly useful survey of the history and use of balsam. For wormwood (Arabic, *afsintīn*, Greek *apsinthion*), see Levey, *Medical Formulary*, 233, no. 17, and Tibi, *Medicinal Use of Opium*, 152, 178.

22 For a discussion of the chemical equipment and the production of distillates, see Hill, *Islamic Science and Engineering*, 83–91; and al-Hassan and Hill, *Islamic Technology*, 133–51.

23 See Chipman, *Minhāj al-dukkān*, and Tibi, *The Medicinal Use of Opium*. For an analysis of the effectiveness of medicaments in the treatise by Dioscorides, see Riddle, *Dioscorides*.

24 Spink and Lewis, *Albucasis*, 176–7, where the term for cupper is incorrectly translated as 'barber-surgeon'. For medical practitioners in the manuals of market inspection, see Chapter 3 above.

25 Budge, *Laughable Stories*, 86, no. 356.

26 Ibn Zuhr, *Easy Guide to Therapy and Dietetics*, 319, 2–3. For al-Kaskarī and the surgeon Sulaymān, see Pormann, 'Islamic Hospitals'.

27 For the account of al-Qurṭubī, see Ibn al-Qifṭī, *History of Learned Men*, 243; the account is repeated by Ibn Abī Uṣaybi'ah, who gives the name of the physician as 'Umar ibn 'Abd al-Raḥmān ibn Aḥmad ibn 'Alī al-Kirmānī (*Sources of Information*, ii. 40, last line).

28 Ibn Qayyim al-Jawzīyah, *Prophetic Medicine*, 105; tr. Johnstone, *Medicine of the Prophet*, 107. The translation given here is by the present authors. Al-Sulamī devotes a separate chapter to each category of specialist – oculist, surgeon, and bone-setter – and what questions are appropriate for each; see Leiser and al-Khaledy, *Questions and Answers*, 89–110.

29 Spink and Lewis, *Albucasis*, 376–9 and 536–51.

30 Ibid., 578–81.

31 al-Kaskarī, *Compendium*, fasc. fol. 142a1–4.

32 Ibn al-'Ibrī, *Abridged History of Nations*, 258–9; for Ibn Wāṣil's account see Richards, 'More on the Death'.

33 Spink and Lewis, *Albucasis*, 578–81.

34 For the diagnosis and therapy of cataracts, see Wood, *Memorandum Book*, 176–87; Meyerhof, *The Book of the Ten Treatises on the Eye*, 68–71 and 121–3; Spink and Lewis, *Albucasis*, 252–7; and Blodi et al., *Arabian Ophthalmologists*, 146–64 and 275–302. For fish-eating and cataracts, see Wood, *Memorandum Book*, 181; 'Ammār particularly mentions the fish-eating populations of Tinnīs and Damietta in the Nile delta as well as those on the Syrian coast (Meyerhof, *The Cataract Operations of 'Ammār ibn 'Alī al-Mawsilī*).

35 Spink and Lewis, *Albucasis*, 256–7.

36 McVaugh, 'Cataracts and Hernias', 326.

37 Iskandar, *Catalogue*, 43; the translation is that of Iskandar, slightly amended.

38 Ibn Juljul, *Classes of Physicians*, 81–2, no. 30; see also Álvarez-Millán, 'Medical Anecdotes'.

39 Elliot, *The Indian Operation of Couching* (22 per cent if one counted vision of 1/10 and upward, plus 17 per cent if one included finger-counting at two feet or less); for further details, see Feigenbaum, 'Early History of Cataract'. Couching continued to be practised in Europe until the technique of removal (extraction through an incision of the lower cornea) was developed by Jacques Daviel in the eighteenth century. In fact, couching continued for some time after that, for there were European oculists who maintained that couching was a better approach than the newly developed extraction methods. Before Daviel perfected his method of extraction, he performed many couchings, initially using a single-needle technique (that is, without the prior incision of a lancet), and with this method he found that five or six out of ten might be considered successful. He then switched to using a lancet followed by a needle (the method used by most medieval Islamic oculists) and found that the success rate increased to 61 out of 75.

40 al-Bīrūnī, *Epistle Cataloguing al-Rāzī's Books*, 5–6; translation by Savage-Smith, 'The Practice of Surgery', 320; for a fuller account see Savage-Smith, 'Medicine', 948.

41 See Tibi, *The Medicinal Use of Opium*.

42 For the sources for the quotations, and for a fuller account of varying versions of 'Urwah's amputation, see Savage-Smith, 'Medicine', 909.

43 Spink and Lewis, *Albucasis*, 578–80 and 480 for cases al-Zahrāwī did not perform himself, and 304, 330, 558–9, 374 for his own.

44 Llavero Ruiz, *Un tratado de cirugía hispanoárabe*, i. 157–8 (tr.) and ii. 60–1 (Arabic); for the case of the woman with boils, see ii. 23.

45 al-Rāzī, *Comprehensive Book*, ii. 138, 6–9 and ii. 174, 5–8 (1st edn). For the cases recorded by ʿAmmār, see Meyerhof, *The Cataract Operations of ʿAmmār ibn ʿAlī al-Mawsilī*, and for those of Khalīfah, see Blodi, et al., *Arabian Ophthalmologists*, 275–302.

46 Ibn al-ʿAdīm, *The Desire to Study Aleppo's History*, iii. 1291; see also Morray, *An Ayyubid Notable*, 51.

47 Khan, *Arabic Legal and Administrative Documents*, 274–5, no. 60.

48 al-Ṣafadī, *Illustrious People of the Age*, iii. 308–9. Al-Ṣafadī (ibid., i. 134–5) also provides an interesting account of the treatment of Baybars I (r. 1260–77) for obstruction to breathing (*al-khawānīq*) by Ibn Abī Ḥulayqah (d. 1308), who was Chief of Physicians in Egypt and Syria.

49 Meyerhof, *The Cataract Operations of ʿAmmār*, 47; a variant reading in one copy gives Baghdad rather than Tiberias.

50 Spink and Lewis, *Albucasis*, 256–7; for al-Rāzī's description, see al-Rāzī, *Comprehensive Book*, ii. 181–4 and 200–2 (1st edn)/ ii. 343–5 and 315–19 (2nd edn).

51 Meyerhof and Prüfer, 'Die angebliche Augenheilkunde des Ṯābit ibn Qurra', 4–8, 38–41.

52 Bethesda, Maryland, NLM MS A 29.1, fols 118a–120b (old pp. 235–9); unpublished. A full edition and translation of the entire chapter by al-Shādhilī will form part of the study under preparation by E. Savage-Smith, in collaboration with B. Inksetter, with the title 'Could Medieval Islamic Oculists Remove Cataracts?: The views of a fourteenth-century sceptic'.

53 See Feugère, et al., 'Les aiguilles à cataracte de Montbellet', and also Baker, 'Roman Medical Instruments', 16–18.

54 Edinburgh, University of Edinburgh Library, MS Or. 16, fol. 6b copied in 1307 (707 H); reproduced in M. Ullmann, *Islamic Medicine*, Plate 3. See Soucek, 'An Illustrated Manuscript', 109–11.

55 In the single instance so far noted, the Shīʿite jurist Muḥammad ibn Muslim al-Thaqafī (d. 767) is said to have told a woman who came to him in the middle of the night concerned about her daughter who had died in labour that it was permitted for the womb of the dead woman to be torn open and the child taken out (there is no record of the operation actually being performed or its outcome); see Sachedina, *Just Ruler*, 50. Most manuscripts illustrating the birth of Rustam date from the sixteenth through eighteenth centuries, with the earliest probably being the so-called 'Stephens Inju *Shāhnāmah*', made in Shiraz in 1352; see Maddison and Savage-Smith, *Science, Tools and Magic*, i. 27–9.

56 For the role of music in medical therapy, see Horden, 'Religion as Medicine'; Shiloah, 'Jewish and Muslim Traditions of Music Therapy'; Burnett, 'Spirtual Medicine in Music and Healing in Islam'; and Dols, *Majnūn*, 171–3.

57 For the statistics regarding numbers of public baths in various towns, see J. Sourdel-Thomine and A. Louis, art. '*ḥammām*', *EI*² iii. 139b–46a; see also W. Floor, W. Kleiss, art. 'Bathhouses', *Enc. Ir.*, iii. 863a–9b, and Benkheira, 'La maison de Satan'. For the manufacturing of soap (Arabic *sābūn*, from the Greek *sapōn*), see A. Dietrich,

art. '*sābūn*', *EI*[2] viii. 693a–b; and al-Hassan and Hill, *Islamic Technology*, 150–1. For housing and sanitation in general (a much overlooked topic in modern scholarship for this period), see Scanlon, 'Housing and Sanitation'.

58 Latham and Isaacs, *Kitāb al-Ḥummayāt*, 38 and 42. The *Canon* of Ibn Sīnā also has a fairly full discussion of various types of medicinal baths (see Shah, *The General Principles of Avicenna's Canon*, 195–9 and 307–9.

59 For studies of female circumcision, or female genital mutilation (FGM) as it is generally known today, see Knight, 'Curing Cut or Ritual Mutilation?'; Karim, *Female Genital Mutilation*. For Islamic sources and attitudes towards female circumcision, see the art. E. van Donzel et al., art. '*khafḍ*', *EI*[2] iv. 913a–4b, and Aldeeb Abu-Sahlieh, *To Mutilate in the Name of Jehovah or Allah*. For circumcision in general in Islam, see A. J. Wensinck, art. '*khitān*', *EI*[2] v. 20–2. For al-Zahrāwī's procedure for removing an enlarged clitoris, derived from the gynaecological text by the second-century Greek writer Soranus, see Spink and Lewis, *Albucasis*, 456–7.

60 For the effectiveness of using a *siwāk*, see Gazi *et al.*, 'The Immediate- and Medium-term Effect of Meswak'. The saying attributed to the Prophet is quoted in many compilations of *ḥadīth*; for precise references see A. J. Wensinck, art. '*miswāk*', *EI*[2] vii. 187a–b. For Islamic dental hygiene with a brush in general, see Wensinck, ibid.; Bos, 'The *miswāk*'; and Rispler-Chaim, 'The Siwāk'.

5

Popular medicine

Whoever eats honey three times a month will not meet with any great disaster
– Shams al-Dīn al-Dhahabī (d. 1348)[1]

Whoever eats seven dates between dawn and dusk will have no harm come to him between dawn and dusk
– Shams al-Dīn al-Dhahabī (d. 1348)[2]

Amulets are of no avail against death
  neither manna nor senna are of any use;
Neither enema nor cupping may help,
  neither bloodletting nor drinking potions
– Abū al-Ḥakam ʿUbayd Allāh ibn al-Muẓaffar (d. 1155)[3]

Throughout the society, in varying degrees, there was room for popular cures and explanations of disease and afflictions alongside the more learned – some might say more rational – approaches represented by the humoral medical system inherited from Late Antiquity and amplified and expanded by Islamic physicians. Magical and folkloric practices, as well as astrological medicine, formed part of the medical pluralism and reflected ancient beliefs and customs that long predated the advent of Islam. The reliance at times on astrology and magic can be seen at all levels of the society. Magical and astrological techniques, moreover, were an integral part, to one degree or another, of all medical practice, whether learned or traditional.

Wise women, known for their healing skills, were consulted especially for problems of childbearing and their knowledgeable dispensing of herbs and amulets. They generally treated a variety of ailments, frequently using methods of sympathetic magic, some of which employed articles of clothing. Popular Ṣūfī spiritual leaders often had considerable local followings because of their skills in supernatural healing. A dervish or experienced elder would recite prayers and Qur'ānic verses, sometimes holding ritual ceremonies or interpreting dreams to determine treatment.[4]

Most magic in the early Islamic world was protective in nature, asking for God's general beneficence. Occasionally, His intervention was sought against other powers – the Evil Eye, assorted devils (*shayṭāns*) and demons, in particular the *jinn* ('shape-shifting' supernatural creatures whose existence was recognised in the Qur'ān). Islam inherited this underlying assumption of the existence of evil beings, including a pantheon of demons, from pre-Islamic societies, as well as the methods of counteracting them.[5]

Amulets and talismans

Belief in the Evil Eye has been widespread in the Middle East for many centuries. People thought that individuals, by glancing at others or catching their eyes, could exert evil forces (sometimes unwittingly) and bring misfortune on the object. This could result in any number of calamities including sudden death, but the most common was a gradual wasting illness. Consequently, numerous instructions for making items to ward off the consequences of the Evil Eye are to be found in medieval writings.[6]

One of the most popular manuals on Prophetic Medicine, that by Ibn Qayyim al-Jawzīyah (d. 1350), contains an emphatic statement that the Evil Eye actually existed:

> One group of people, of those who have but a small share of transmitted knowledge and intelligence, have denied this matter of the Eye, saying this is merely imagination, with no truth in it. These are amongst the most ignorant of people, in knowledge and intelligence, and have the thickest of veil over their eyes, the heaviest of natures, and are furthest of all from knowledge of spirits and souls and their qualities, deeds, and effects. The intelligent people of all nations – with their differences of community and belief – neither reject nor ignore the question of the Eye, even though they disagree concerning its cause and impact.[7]

Talismans and amulets (there being virtually no distinction between the two English terms) were used not only to ward off the Evil Eye and misfortune, but could also be employed to increase fertility or potency or attractiveness and avert disease and sudden death. They encompassed not only magical symbols but also invocations and prayers nearly always addressed to God or one of His intercessors. The use of the English term 'charm' for such material is generally best avoided, for it implies an evocation of a lesser god or demon through recitations and incantations. The difference between magical invocations in the Islamic world and those of Antiquity and medieval Europe is that in Islam the invocations are most often (though not exclusively) addressed to God rather than to demons. Thus, while the artefact may have some magical writing and magical symbols, they are dominantly supplications to God to aid and protect the bearer.[8]

As early as the ninth century, Arabic treatises by learned physicians and scholars discussed the efficacy of amuletic remedies hung round the neck or bound to some part of the body. A particularly interesting essay on the topic was written by the Christian physician Qusṭā ibn Lūqā (d. c. 912), who emigrated to Armenia after working, like his contemporary al-Rāzī, in Baghdad. In this treatise Qusṭā argues that the strengthening of the mind that results from belief in the power of an amulet has much to do with its effectiveness. He presented many examples of amuletic techniques, citing Greek authorities as well as some Indian sources. He allowed for a little scepticism, saying: 'As for me, I have not tried these things, but neither are they to be denied by me, because if we had not seen a magnet drawing iron to itself we would not confirm or believe it.' Nonetheless, he believed that the state of the soul affected that of the body, and that, since talismanic procedures appear to strengthen the mindset of the patient, amulets should be employed where necessary. Learned physicians of his day and later seem to have generally agreed with this conclusion.[9]

Opinions differed amongst religious scholars as to the acceptability of wearing amulets. Ibn Qayyim al-Jawzīyah cited the opinion of Aḥmad ibn Ḥanbal (d. 855), founder of the Ḥanbalī school of jurisprudence. When asked about wearing amulets after the onset of affliction, the latter said: 'I trust that there should be no harm therein'. The son of Aḥmad ibn Ḥanbal reported seeing his father write talismans for someone suffering from fear and for someone with a fever after the onset of affliction, as well as for a woman undergoing a difficult childbirth. The texts of such talismans consisted primarily of quotations from the Qur'ān and pious phrases.[10]

One of the most obvious uses of amulets and incantations was to protect against epidemics, whose occurrences were devastating, unpredictable, and little understood. In such dire times many people naturally would attempt to propitiate the evil forces at work in a hostile world, and gain the blessing and protection of God. This could be done through certain incantations or prayers to be said at specified times or with amulets and talismans having special inscriptions which would both protect and alleviate. Many plague tracts contained texts for supplicatory prayers and directions for amulets to prevent or alleviate plague. Ibn Ḥajar (d. 1449), for example, recommended reading the 'Throne Verse' from the Qur'ān (*Āyat al-Kursī*, 2:255) in a house for three consecutive nights to prevent the plague entering. Virtually all authors of plague tracts specified prayers or magic squares or magical symbols that were to be written on paper, then washed off with water, and the water then drunk in order to avoid, or be cured of, the plague. An array of designs were given to be engraved on rings, or stones set in rings, that could protect the potential plague victim. Al-Shaqūrī cites al-Rāzī as the authority for the procedure of wearing a ring made of fresh myrtle on the little finger in order to quiet plague boils.[11]

Magical techniques were also used on a daily basis for protections against every sort of disease and misfortune. In popular opinion, verses of the Qur'ān

The *budūḥ* magic square

د	ط	ب
ج	ه	ز
ح	ا	و

=

d	ṭ	b
j	h	z
ḥ	a	ū

=

4	9	2
3	5	7
8	1	6

Figure 5.1 The *budūḥ* magic square.

were especially beneficial against all affliction and danger. The design of amulets sometimes combined magical alphabets and other sigla, which might include magic squares. The latter became an important part of the vocabulary of talisman-makers and compilers of magical manuals, particularly after the twelfth century. The earliest magic square (*wafq* in Arabic) was a 3 × 3 square having nine cells in which the numerals from one through nine were arranged so that every row and every column as well as the two diagonals had the same sum: fifteen (see Figure 5.1). These numerals appeared as Arabic letters of the alphabet, each assigned a specific value. For this reason, this ancient magic square (possibly of Chinese origin) was given its own special name of *budūḥ*, derived from the four letter/numerals that are placed in the corner squares (the letters *b* = 2, *d* = 4, *w*/*ū* = 6, and *ḥ* = 8).

So potent were the magical properties of this square that the name itself, *budūḥ*, acquired its own occult potency. Thus, when one did not wish, or know how, to write the magic square, one could invoke the name against stomach pains, temporary impotency, or even to become invisible, by writing or saying *yā budūḥ* (O Budūḥ). The names of the four archangels were frequently associated with the square, and it was often placed within a larger talismanic design. Magic squares of higher order (4 × 4, 6 × 6 and so on) do not become part of the magical vocabulary of symbols until after the twelfth century, although they were well-known to Islamic mathematicians from the late tenth century.[12]

Manuals of magical methods

Beginning in the late twelfth century, a vast number of general magical manuals were composed that concerned incantations, prayers, and talismans for all manner of illnesses and misfortunes, especially for aiding childbirth. The acknowledged authority on such matters was an Egyptian writer named al-Būnī, who is said to have died in 1225. Many treatises are ascribed to him, the most influential being the *Great Sun of Knowledge*, which, though printed many times, has never been critically edited or translated.[13]

A separate genre soon developed on the topic of the magical employment of plants, animals, and minerals. This continued an established late antique practice of ascribing hidden properties to various substances. The Arabic genre is usually called *khawāṣṣ* literature from the plural of the word *khāṣṣah* meaning 'special property'. The basic premise was that everything in nature had hidden or occult properties that could be activated. Some properties were compatible with others, while some were incompatible or opposite in nature. By recognising and utilising these properties, disease might be cured or good fortune attained. The type of magic represented by the *khawāṣṣ* literature did not usually involve prayers or invocations, for the material itself, or the inscribed symbols, was regarded as sufficient.[14]

An early example is a magical-medical pharmacopoeia written in the tenth century by al-Tamīmī (d. 980), who was originally from Jerusalem but spent the last ten years of his life in Egypt. Many others wrote treatises of this genre, usually with the title of *Kitāb al-Khawāṣṣ* (Book of Occult Properties) or sometimes *Kitāb al-Mujarrabāt* (Book of Tested Remedies) because prescriptions routinely ended with the word *mujarrab* 'tested'.[15]

Typical of the recommendations in such treatises are the following from a treatise titled *Book of Satisfaction in Treatment with Occult Substances* by a tenth-century writer in Muslim Spain, Abū al-Muṭrib ʿAbd al-Raḥmān:

> If you hang the long bone from the edge of the left wing of a goose on the person suffering from quartan fever, this will cure it.[16]
>
> If the stone called emerald is hung on the neck, it strengthens the external and internal parts of the body and abolishes torpor.[17]
>
> If you take peeled beans, cook them thoroughly and thereafter mix them with pulverized cumin, and bandage this on the region affected by a bruise and fall, doing this two or three times, he will be healed, by the decree of God.[18]
>
> [For gout], the fat of a cat kept for a month underground will help when used as an ointment, but first the patient should bathe his feet in a fox decoction, whereupon he should be immediately anointed with this laudable ointment; he will be cured thoroughly and without doubt, and this is a hidden secret.[19]
>
> When the woman drinks of the milk of a pregnant donkey, she will not abort, and this is 'tested'.[20]
>
> [For prevention of pregnancy] If you make a ring from a hoof of a white female mule for her to wear, she will not conceive while it is on her.[21]
>
> [For loss of memory] If the head and tongue of a cuckoo are taken and hung on this person, the result will be a manifest improvement of memory.[22]

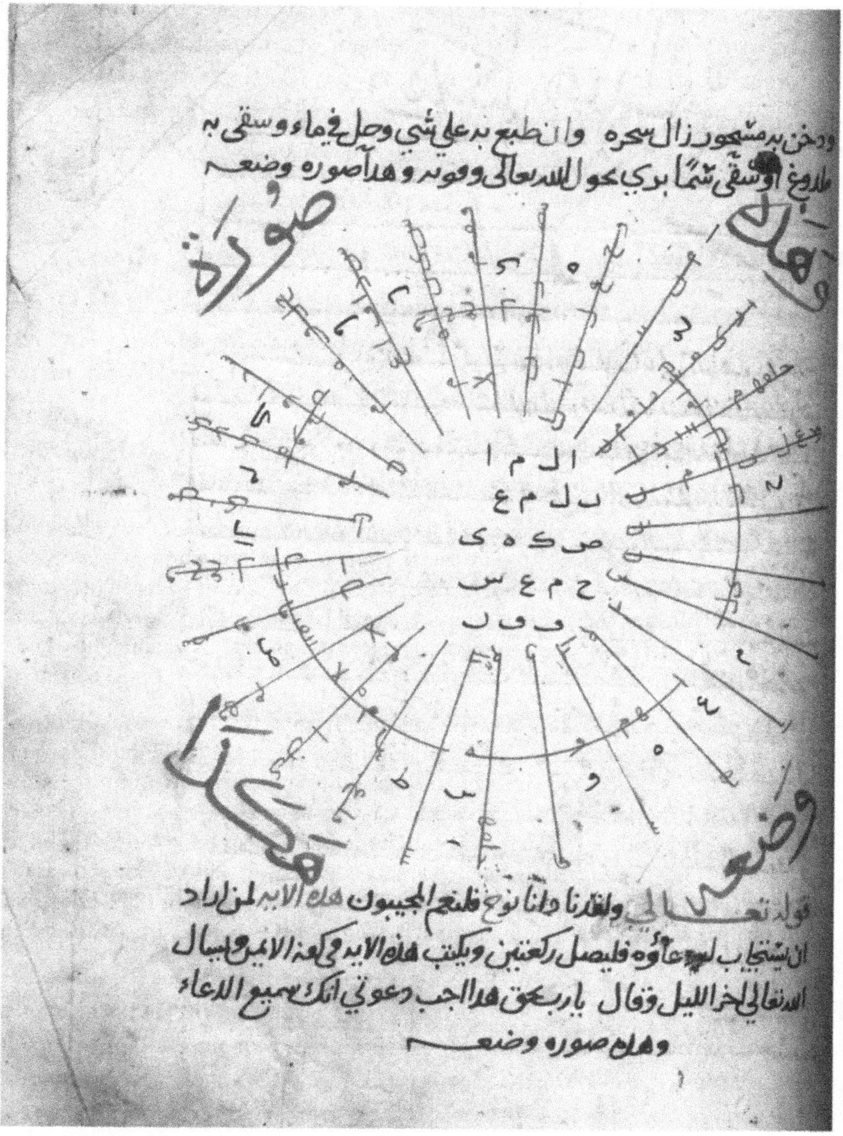

Figure 5.2 A design for a gemstone from a treatise on the magical uses of the names of God, *The Book of the Oblique* by al-Būnī, the Egyptian authority on magic said to have died in 1225. The enclosing text states that if it is inscribed with some additional magical words, on a ring, or on a gemstone set in a ring, and the ring is worn by a woman, then she will get married. If the ring is placed on the forehead of someone who has fainted, they will revive. If the ring is immersed in rain water, the water, when drunk, will relieve all pains. An impression of the inscription on the ring can be used to remove magic spells and cure poisonous bites.

A popular and distinct subset of *khawāṣṣ* literature were the 'stone-books', devoted to the magical virtues and uses of stones and minerals. Later treatises were often illustrated with designs to be engraved on gemstones and set into a ring – to help with capturing wild animals, releasing someone from a spell, gaining love, or a host of other uses. See Figure 5.2 for an example of such a design, in this instance one given by al-Būnī.[23]

Prophetic Medicine

Treatises on Prophetic Medicine also advocated in varying degrees folkloric and magical remedies in addition to numerous invocations for warding off afflictions and protecting from *jinn* and the Evil Eye. The early tract based on Shīʿite imams had, for example, the following prescriptions:

> He [the Prophet] said: 'Keep many domestic animals (*dawājin*) in your houses so that the demons are occupied with them instead of your children.'[24]

> [The imām Jaʿfar ibn Muḥammad] al-Ṣādiq said to him [one of his clients whose fever would not subside]: 'Undo the buttons of your shirt and put your head in it. Recite the call to prayer (*adhān*) and the introduction to prayer (*iqāmah*), and recite seven times the 'surah of praise' (*al-Ḥamd*, that is, the 'Opening', *al-Fātiḥah*, no. 1)'. The man said: 'I did that and recovered as quickly as a camel loosened from its cord.'[25]

> He [al-Ṣādiq] said to him [someone suffering from colic (or intestinal obstruction, *qawlanj*)]: 'Write for him the opening [surah] of the Qur'ān (*al-Fātiḥah*, no. 1), the surah 'Purity' (*al-Ilkhāṣ*, no. 112), and the two surahs for seeking protection (*al-maʿūdhatān*, the last two surahs of the Qur'ān, 'Dawn', *al-Falaq*, and 'People', *al-Nās*, nos. 113 and 114). Then write underneath: "I take refuge in the presence of God, the Great, and in His might, which is unceasing, and in His power, which nothing can resist, from the evil of this pain, and the evil within it." Then swallow it with rainwater on an empty stomach. You will be cured of it, God the Exalted permitting.'[26]

Ibn Qayyim al-Jawzīyah (d. 1350), in his popular treatise on Prophetic Medicine, defended the writing of talismans. He provided texts for some that he considered useful for fevers, for childbirth, for nosebleed, and toothache. For tertian fever, for example, he recommends writing on three thin sheets of paper: 'In the Name of God it has fled, in the Name of God it has passed, in the Name of God it has diminished'. Each day the physician is to place one sheet in the patient's mouth and have him swallow it with water.[27]

Ibn Qayyim's contemporary, Shams al-Dīn al-Dhahabī, cited authorities for the beneficial properties of stones:

> Aristotle said: 'Whoever wears a ring with cornelian set in it protects himself from fear of death. Whoever has a drink while wearing it, will stop bleeding.' A tradi-

> tional saying: 'If you wear a ring with a cornelian in it, then you will never experience poverty'.[28]

Al-Dhahabī, however, rejected the use of amulets and talismans, though he allowed that some words and phrases could have beneficial occult properties, through the will of God:

> The term amulet designates beads hanging around the neck – which some people think will ward off misfortunes. This is sheer ignorance! However, you should realize that there are some words that do indeed possess occult properties *(khawāṣṣ)* which do have an effect, by permission of God the Almighty.[29]

In general, al-Dhahabī remained sceptical of magical procedures. Of the uses of the hoopoe bird, for example, he said:

> It has been written in a volume called *Book of the Occult Properties* (*Kitāb al-Khawāṣṣ*) that the hoopoe possesses various occult properties. For instance, if it is tied to someone who is forgetful, then he will remember what he has forgotten. If a man carries one of these birds around with him, he will surely conquer his enemy. If someone – who has been enchanted or put under a binding spell – sniffs one, then he will be freed. Its flesh, when cooked, is good for people. However, I maintain that most of what has been attributed to it is not true.[30]

Broadly speaking, the medical-magical techniques in the Prophetic Medicine literature are more abundant than in any of the treatises written by formally trained physicians. Astrology, on the other hand, plays a much smaller role in Prophetic Medicine than it does in the scholarly medical literature.

Magic-medicinal bowls

It is evident that the twelfth century saw a marked increase of interest in magic. Present evidence suggests it was about this time that magic-medicinal bowls were first produced, that the magical use of higher-order magic squares occurred, and the production of magical texts began to increase dramatically. For us today, it is difficult to ascertain the exact reasons for this development, which may be linked to shifting patterns in medical literary activity and changing social attitudes.

The earliest Islamic magic bowl of which we know was made in 1167 for the Syrian ruler Nūr al-Dīn ibn Zangī – the same person who founded the famous Nūrī hospital in Damascus. Illustrated in Figure 5.3 is another bowl produced for the same Ibn Zangī just two years later. Thereafter magic-medicinal bowls were manufactured in considerable quantity. In origin they probably relate in some fashion to pre-Islamic Aramaic bowls, though in fact their design and function differed greatly. The latter are made of clay with spiral inscriptions invoking demons, while the Islamic ones are of metal and noticeably lacking in any reliance upon *jinn* and demons.[31]

Large numbers of Islamic magic-medicinal bowls survive today, the earlier ones originating in Syria and more recent ones in Iran and Turkey. In addition to Qur'ānic verses and magical writing, the early Islamic magic bowls were decorated with schematically, rather crudely-rendered, human and animal forms. Some scholars have designated a subgroup of Islamic magic-medicinal bowls as 'poison cups'. These so-called 'poison cups' always have representations of a scorpion, a snake (or serpent), an animal that is probably intended to be a dog (though some have called it a lion), and two intertwined dragons – imagery reminiscent of early tenth-century haematite amulets made in Persia. This combination of symbols perhaps represented sudden death. In addition to these images, every cup has an inscription on the outside specifying numerous uses, of which countering animal bites and poisons are only two among many.[32]

With all the Islamic magic bowls, the patients, or someone acting as their agent, were to drink from the bowl in order to be cured, sometimes following specific instructions, such as drinking hot water for colic, or saffron water if difficult labour was to be avoided. On the outside of the early (twelfth- to

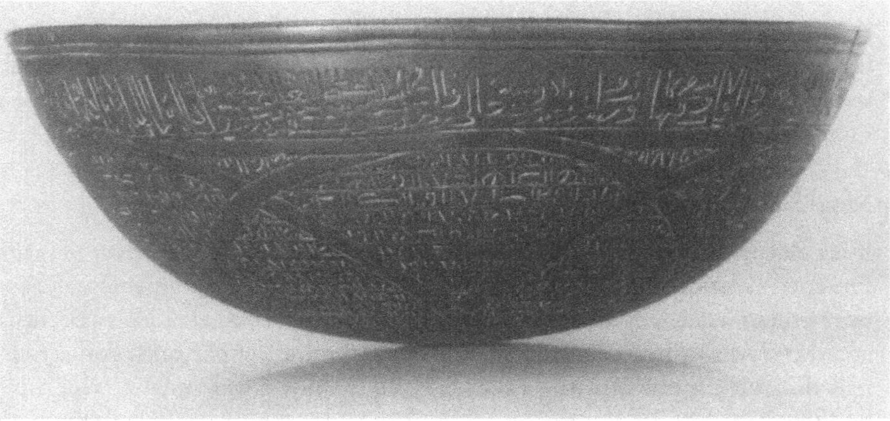

Figure 5.3 A magic-medicinal bowl made in 1169–70 (565 H) for Nūr al-Dīn Maḥmūd ibn Zangī, who ruled in Damascus from 1146 to 1174 and who founded the famous Nūrī hospital named after him. The inscription beneath the rim reads: 'This blessed cup is for every poison. In it have been gathered proven uses, and these are for the sting of serpent, scorpion and fever, for a woman in labour, the abdominal pain of a horse caused by eating earth, and the [bites of] a rabid dog, for abdominal pain and colic, for migraine and throbbing pain, for hepatic and splenic fever, for [increasing] strength, for [stopping] haemorrhage, for chest pain, for the eye and vision [or evil eye], for ophthalmia and catarrh, for *riyāḥ al-shawkah* [? an ulcerated skin disorder or stinging effects of sand-laden winds], for [driving out] spirits, for releasing the bewitched, and for all diseases and afflictions. [If] one drinks water or oil or milk from it, then they will be cured, by the help of God Almighty.'

fourteenth-century) magic-medicinal bowls, engraved statements give therapeutic uses. These inscriptions present an interesting view of the diseases and afflictions considered particularly prevalent, as well as responsive to magic – at least at the time the earliest bowls were designed. Fifty-nine bowls bearing therapeutic instructions have been either published or examined. From these it would appear that there was in the twelfth and thirteenth centuries an overriding concern with scorpion stings and the bites of snakes and mad dogs (mad-dog bites are mentioned 59 times, stings of scorpions 56 times, and bites of snakes 54), again perhaps indicating a fear of sudden death. The ailments that clearly dominate are various gastrointestinal complaints, with the next most frequent being labour pains accompanying a difficult birth. Headaches of one form or another figure prominently, as well as throbbing pain in general (toothache gets only one mention). Two-thirds of the bowls mention fevers, while their usefulness as an antidote to poisons (other than animal bites and stings) is suggested 35 out of 59 times. In later centuries, magic-medicinal bowls became increasingly Islamicised, leaving behind the pre-Islamic symbols and eventually evolving into bowls having nothing but Qur'ānic verses on them and no instructions for their use.

Learned physicians' attitudes

Even the writings of the highly learned physicians trained in Greek-based humoral theory are not entirely devoid of beliefs in sympathetic magic, occult powers, and astrology. For example, al-Rāzī records in his working notes that eating a scorpion or squashed earthworms breaks up bladder stones, or wearing an unwashed and sweaty garment which had been worn by a woman in labour cures a particular type of fever. Many a sympathetic remedy was recommended for easing the pains of childbirth – the use of a magnet being one example.[33]

Many extremely learned physicians, including al-Rāzī, composed entire treatises on occult medicinal properties of substances (*khawāṣṣ*). The progenitor of the famous family of physicians in Muslim Spain, Abū al-ʿAlāʾ Zuhr (d. 1131), himself the author of numerous medical works, composed a *Book of Occult Properties* (*Kitāb al-Khawāṣṣ*). In it, he presented substances in alphabetic order and employed abbreviations for earlier authorities who had recorded such uses. The resulting compilation includes advice, said to be from Ibn Sarābiyūn (*fl.* c. 870s), that a lock of hair from a dead person, when placed on a painful tooth, eases the pain, and if placed under the head of a sleeping person, will prolong their slumber. Abū al-ʿAlāʾ Zuhr provided magical-medical uses for 308 animal, vegetable, and mineral substances, including parts of lions, crocodiles, elephants, water buffalos, olives, saffron, artemisia, aloes, ambergris, amber, opium, pearls, lapis lazuli, coral, diamonds, and sal ammoniac.[34]

Astrology and divination

The services of fortune tellers and diviners offered an alternative for many to the diagnosis and prognosis of the established medical community. Thus itinerant astrologers, geomancers, and other prognosticators were consulted to determine the cause of an illness and what the outcome would be: whether recovery would occur soon or only after much suffering, or whether the illness might even bring death. Tracts preserved today on astrology and other forms of divination show that medical problems figured as one of the major reasons for consultation, as well as determining if a woman was pregnant, the sex of a child, and whether the delivery would be an easy one. An example of the diagnostic guidance commonly given in astrological manuals is that by Yuḥannā ibn al-Ṣalt (*fl.* 870–910), a personal acquaintance of Ḥunayn ibn Isḥāq in Baghdad, provided in his *Handbook of Astrological Medicine*:

> When you have ascertained the Ascendant [the planet that is closest to the eastern horizon at sunrise on a given day] of the patient, and Saturn is found to be at one of the four angles [that is, on the eastern or western horizon or at the upper or lower meridian] and in particular the Ascendant is in Aries, then it indicates a disease due to black bile, derangement of the intellect, decay of the brain, headache due to smoke, destructive thoughts, putridness, bad breath, toothache, cradle cap (*al-sa'fah*), earache, diminished hearing, deafness, and delusion (*waswās*).[35]

Today we tend to attribute such magical and astrological approaches to medicine to the less privileged. It is a fact, however, that prognosticators of various types worked in the entourage of every ruler. For example, when the Mamlūk sultan of Egypt al-Nāṣir Muḥammad, the son of the founder of the Manṣūrī hospital, became ill with diarrhoea in 1341, he consulted astrologers and geomancers as well as doctors.[36]

Many learned physicians were outspoken advocates of astrology, such as Ibn Riḍwān and al-Rāzī. To justify the physician's use of astrology, Islamic authors often alluded, in one form or another, to the dictum of Hippocrates in *Airs, Waters, and Places* that 'the science of the stars is no small part of the science of medicine'. The positions of the stars and planets could influence the crises of illnesses, determine the best time for bloodletting and other remedies, and serve as aids to diagnosis and prognosis of conditions. Horoscopic astrology, as well as simpler forms of zodiacal and lunar associations, were practised throughout Late Antiquity and continued in the Islamic period.[37]

The Alexandrian astronomer Ptolemy's defence of astrology in his *Tetrabiblos* (literally, 'The Four Books'), written in the second century and later translated into Arabic, was crucial in establishing astrology as the most important learned form of divination. Many other pre-Islamic customs, however, also influenced the development of the art in the early Muslim world. The Sabian inhabitants of Ḥarrān in northern Iraq, well-known as pagan star-worshippers, acquired particular fame for the practice of astrology, and had a considerable impact on the early Islamic period. Late antique Greek occult literature also provided a source of inspiration, particularly the writings usually referred to as 'Hermetic', after Hermes Trismegistus (meaning Hermes the 'Thrice Great' in Greek). In a divinatory text called *The Book of the Zodiac*, preserved in the Mandaic language of lower central Iraq, one sees the blending of Babylonian, Sasanian, and Hellenistic traditions in a popular form of astrological divination that also employed onomancy (divination based upon a person's name) and omens drawn from natural phenomena. A similar blending of divinatory techniques occurred in many of the Arabic astrological treatises preserved today.[38]

Most learned physicians employed some astrological techniques. For example, Bukhtīshū' ibn Jibrīl (d. 870), who served three caliphs in Baghdad as physician, reportedly 'used to prescribe an enema only when the moon reached its descending node, for then the colic (or intestinal obstruction, *qawlanj*) would immediately disappear. He ordered medications to be consumed only when the moon was in aspect [aligned] with Venus, for then the sufferer would immediately be restored.'[39]

Ibn Riḍwān (d. 1068), the cantankerous physician of Old Cairo, wrote an entire monograph on astrology, and he stated in his autobiography that he first earned his living as an astrologer. In the following century al-'Aynzarbī (d. 1153), a court physician in Egypt, devoted one third of his *What is Sufficient for the Medical Art* to the topic of astrological medicine as well as composing a separate essay on *What Every Physician Should Know about Astrology*.[40]

Others, such as Ibn Sīnā, wrote tracts refuting astrology, and anecdotal accounts abound recounting the failure of astrologers to treat patients properly. The following example concerns a physician by the name of Īsá ibn Ḥakam, also known as Masīḥ al-Dimashqī who was a contemporary of the caliph Hārūn al-Rashīd (d. 809). Two famous astrologers of the day also figure in the story: al-Abaḥḥ and 'Umar al-Ṭabarī (d. 815).

> 'Īsá ibn Ḥakam [Masīḥ al-Dimashqī] reported that Ghaḍīḍ, the mother of al-Rashīd's children, suffered from an attack of colic [or intestinal obstruction]. Therefore she called for him and for al-Abaḥḥ and al-Ṭabarī, the astrological calculators. I asked 'Īsá what was his opinion regarding her therapy, and 'Īsá said: 'I informed her that her colic has become inveterate and deep-rooted, and that unless she has an enema without delay, she would not escape the worst.'
>
> Thereupon she said to al-Abaḥḥ and al-Ṭabarī: 'Select a proper time for treating me.' But al-Abaḥḥ told her: 'Your illness is not one of those whose treatment may be postponed to a time that astrologers find favourable. I think you should be treated immediately before you undertake anything else.' That was also the opinion of 'Īsá ibn Ḥakam. Then she asked me, and I told her that al-Abaḥḥ had advised her correctly.

> But then she asked [the astrologer] al-Ṭabarī for his opinion, and he told her: 'Today the moon coincides with Saturn, tomorrow it will be with Jupiter. I think that it would be in your interest to postpone the treatment until the moon will be in conjunction with Jupiter' ... But Ghaḍīḍ died before the conjunction of the moon with Jupiter.[41]

Even those scholarly physicians who were not overt advocates of astrological and magical practices nearly all adhered in a fundamental way to what might be termed an astrological world view. According to it, events of the microcosm mirror – and hence relate to – those in the macrocosm. Such a view of the cosmos had permeated, to one degree or another, all learned thought well before the advent of Islam and continued to do so for centuries.

Between text and artefact

The artefacts present us with a different picture of magical practices than that which emerges from the written sources. Even if we allow that some of the more elaborate designs proposed in treatises might have been employed on very perishable materials, there is, nonetheless, a noticeable discrepancy between text and artefact as preserved today. A typical example of a talismanic design for a gemstone, as given by the acknowledged authority on magic the Egyptian writer al-Būnī, presents a large and intricate design involving circles, twenty-seven radiating lines, a couple hundred letters of the alphabet, magical symbols, and words written diagonally in the corners (see Figure 5.2). The design would take considerable space to reproduce and would require notable engraving or calligraphic skill on the part of the amulet maker. The enclosing text, nonetheless, states that if it is inscribed on a ring, with some additional magical words, or on a gemstone set in a ring, and the ring is worn by a woman, then she will get married. If the ring is placed on the forehead of someone who has fainted, they will revive. If the ring is immersed in rain water, the water, when drunk, will relieve all pains. An impression of the inscription on the ring can be used to remove magic spells and cure poisonous bites.

On the face of it, there is a problem trying to engrave these designs on a small gemstone. In the 'stone-books' devoted solely to the magical and therapeutic use of precious stones and minerals, even more elaborate designs are given, very often with figures of humans or angels. The reader is instructed to engrave the pictorial designs onto the surface of a gemstone set in a ring, with the gemstone usually specified as ruby or another precious stone. Such rings were said to have various powers, such as increasing the pleasure of sexual intercourse, easing childbirth, or warding off leprosy or the plague.

Moreover, and very importantly, these recommended designs are not reflected in *any* artefacts known to exist today – neither the abstract designs of al-Būnī nor the miniature figures from the stone books. Could we not here be encountering a literary tradition, possibly originating in Late Antiquity, that flourished separately from the actual production of amulets? How much actual *use* was made of such magical instruction books is very difficult to assess, though it is evident that there was much interest in compiling and copying them.

Various stones were of course used as amulets, some worn simply as pendants and others set in rings. There are hundreds, if not thousands, of small semi-precious or hardstone amulets and amuletic seals in collections around the world, and a considerable number have been studied and catalogued. Some have amuletic designs such as the common 3 × 3 magic *budūḥ* square, while most have Qur'ānic quotations and pious invocations. None, however, have human figures on them, nor even the intricate abstract designs given by al-Būnī.[42]

Amulets and magical equipment, on the other hand, sometimes have designs not to be found in any of the medieval written texts that have so far been examined. The most obvious example is that of the fish, which (judging from the artefacts) was a common and apparently early talismanic symbol, curiously lacking in the written texts. Another type of magical equipment with no counterpart in the literature are magic shirts, made of cloth and painted with magical symbols and verses from the Qur'ān. The only preserved examples are from the fifteenth century or later and were made in Ottoman Turkey, Safavid Persia, or Mughal India. There was, however, a tradition traceable to the ninth century of wearing a special shirt for curing fevers or aiding childbirth. It is likely that talismanic shirts were employed for avoiding or curing fevers, and other contagious conditions, and some have suggested, not unreasonably, that they were worn for protection in battle. Nothing written on them, however, details their intended use nor are they described or recommended in the magical manuals. A remarkable Judeo-Persian talismanic textile, though of recent date, nevertheless reflects an ancient magical tradition traceable to Mesopotamia and moderated through Jewish and Muslim communities.[43]

Magic-medicinal bowls are yet another example of artefacts not mentioned in written sources. Large numbers were made, at least since the twelfth century, and they continue, in variant forms, to be produced today (or at least until recently). Although this type of magical equipment was manufactured in large numbers over a wide geographical area during more than eight centuries, it appears to have been generally overlooked in the literature. Only two written references to the use of magic bowls have so far been found, and these occur outside the genre of formal medical or magical treatises: At the end of a thirteenth-century Arabic manuscript containing a summary (*jawāmi'*) of a treatise *On Urine* attributed to Galen, there is a magical formula against colic. It includes instructions to inscribe it on a red copper plate or bowl when Scorpio is in the Ascendant, or to carve it – at any time – on a bowl of walnut wood. If the sick person drinks from the vessel, the instructions say, the affliction is eliminated and the poison carried off immediately, or – if his agent drinks from it – after an interval of time. From the next century we have the recommendation given by al-Ṣanawbarī (d. 1412) in his treatise on Prophetic Medicine that protection against delusions (*waswās*) can be gained by drinking, before breakfast for three days, a liquid from a bowl on which Qur'ānic verses and the *budūḥ* magic square have been written.[44]

Virtually none of the artefacts preserved today were actually based on the detailed instructions presented in the popular medieval treatises. Some magical equipment preserved today is not mentioned in the magical or medical treatises, and, conversely, most of the intricate and complex designs presented in those treatises are not reflected in the preserved artefacts. Islamic magical artefacts deviate in yet another way from texts. Whilst the pre-Islamic belief in demons and spirits is evident in the magical literature, where invocations to *jinn* or even demons sometimes occur, the artefacts appear to direct the invocations only to God for protection and cure, with an occasional mention of angels. The latter are dominantly supplications to God to aid and protect the bearer.

The amulet and talisman makers (as opposed to the magical theorists) apparently maintained a simpler approach to magical inscriptions and designs, employing a more limited number of patterns, and producing a generic product useful for all calamities. At the same time they maintained a stricter adherence to the Muslim belief that it was only to God to whom one could turn for protection or cure.

It is evident, nonetheless, from both written sources and preserved artefacts of the material culture that, throughout the medieval Islamic world, people of all classes and all religious persuasions had frequent recourse to magical therapy, often turning to the preventive and curative power of talismans, amulets, and other magical equipment. It is also apparent that so-called 'rational' and 'irrational' medicine (to use modern and somewhat pejorative terms) co-existed in the thinking and practice of the learned physicians, as well as with their relatively uneducated competitors.

Suggested reading

For medieval Islamic magic and divination in general, see Savage-Smith, *Magic and Divination in Early Islam* and the bibliographic references therein. For studies of various aspects of medical magic, see Dols, *Majnūn*, 261–76; Morony, *Iraq after the Conquest*, 384–430; and Savage-Smith, 'Magic and Islam' in Maddison and Savage-Smith, *Science, Tools and Magic*, i. 59–148; and Ullmann, *Islamic Medicine*, 107–14. For contemporary magical practices, Kruk, 'Harry Potter in the Gulf'.

For astrological medicine, see Klein-Franke, *Iatromathematics in Islam*; Burnett, et al., *Abū Ma'shar. The Abbreviation of 'The Introduction to Astrology*;

and Wright, *al-Bīrūnī, The Book of Instruction*. For pre-Islamic influences of astrology in Islam, Ullmann's guide is particularly useful on this point (*Die Natur- und Geheimwissenschaften*, 271–358).

Notes

1 A *ḥadīth* given by al-Dhahabī, *Prophetic Medicine*, 169; translation that of Thomson, *As-Suyuti's Medicine of the Prophet*, 79.

2 A *ḥadīth* given by al-Dhahabī, *Prophetic Medicine*, 133; translation that of Thomson, *As-Suyuti's Medicine of the Prophet*, 45.

3 A poem by Abū al-Ḥakam 'Ubayd Allāh ibn al-Muẓaffar (d. 1155), a physician who ran an apothecary shop (*dukkān*) in Damascus. The translation is that of Van Gelder, 'The Joking Doctor', 222, slightly amended.

4 For a modern anthropological study of Ṣūfī healing, see Crapanzano, *The Ḥamadsha*.

5 See Henninger 'Beliefs in Spirits among the Pre-Islamic Arabs'.

6 For the Evil Eye, see Seligmann, *Die Zauberkraft des Auges*; Doutté, *Magie et religion dans l'Afrique*, 317–27; and Ph. Marçais, art. "*ayn*', *EI*² i. 786a–b.

7 Ibn Qayyim al-Jawzīyah, *Prophetic Medicine*, 120; translation that of Johnstone, *Medicine of the Prophet*, 122.

8 The many and various terms for amulets and talismans are discussed by Tewfik Canaan, 'The Decipherment of Arabic Talismans', 69–78. Our term talisman comes from the Arabic *tilsam* which in turn is from the Greek *telesma*, a magical inscription. For amulets and talismans in the Islamic world, see also J. Ruska, B. Carra de Vaux, and C. E. Bosworth, art. 'Tilsam', *EI*² x. 500a–2a (an excellent article except for over-use of the word 'charm' and over-emphasis on the difference between talismans and amulets); Anawati, 'Trois talismans'; see also Maddison and Savage-Smith, *Science, Tools and Magic*, i. 132–47; Porter 'Islamic Seals'.

9 For Qusṭā ibn Lūqā's treatise, see the Latin edition, translation and study by Wilcox and Riddle 'Qusṭā ibn Lūqā's *Physical Ligatures*'; the quotation is found on 45. The treatise is usually thought to be preserved only in a Latin translation (*De phisicis ligaturis*), but it is possible that the Arabic is preserved in a manuscript now in Munich (Bayerische Staatsbibliothek, MS Arab. 805, fols 76–81), which is an Arabic treatise attributed to Quṣṭā titled *Treatise on the Participation of Natures* (*Maqālah fī ishtirāk al-ṭabā'i'*); for the manuscript see Sezgin, *Medizin-Pharmazie*, 272, no. 21. For this treatise within the context of Qusṭā ibn Lūqā's other numerous writings, see Wilcox, 'Qusṭā ibn Lūqā and the Eastward Diaspora'.

10 For the quotation see Ibn Qayyim al-Jawzīyah, *Prophetic Medicine*, 278; translation that of Johnstone, *Medicine of the Prophet*, 253.

11 For the statements of Ibn Ḥajar and al-Shaqūrī, see Dols, *Black Death*, 126 and 136. For plague tracts in general, as well as treatises on Prophetic Medicine, see Chapter 2 above, and the section below.

12 For the *budūḥ* magic square and its uses, see D. V. Macdonald, art. '*budūḥ*', *EI*² suppl. 153a–4a; and for magic squares in general see the numerous publications of Jacques Sesiano, including *Un traité médiéval sur les carrés magiques*.

13 Pielow in *Die Quellen der Weisheit* has published a study of the principal features of al-Būnī's major magical manual, while Lory, 'La magie des lettres' has examined its

letter-magic.

14 For the *khawāṣṣ* literature, see M. Ullmann, art. 'Khāṣṣa', *EI*[2] iv. 1097b–8a; Qur'ānic verses and phrases were also said to have occult properties (*khawāṣṣ*), for which see T. Fahd, art. 'Khawāṣṣ al-Ḳur'ān', *EI*[2] iv. 1133b–4a.

15 For the magical-medical pharmacopoeia by al-Tamīmī, see the edition and translation of the chapter concerned with the occult properties (*khawāṣṣ*) of stones by Schönfeld, *Über die Steine*. See below for treatises on the same subject written by the learned physicians al-Rāzī and Abū al-'Alā' Zuhr.

16 Leibowitz and Marcus, *Sefer Hanisyonot*, 289, based on the Hebrew version of the treatise. This particular recommendation is attributed in the text to Ibn Māsawayh (d. 857). The editors and translators of the Hebrew version of this text attribute the treatise to Abraham ibn Ezra (d. 1167), saying that it is a reworking by him of an earlier tract by Ibn al-Haytham al-Qurṭubī (d. *c.* 951). A recent study of a copy of the original Arabic treatise, discovered amongst the holdings of the Institute of Oriental Studies of Uzbekistan (MS 9777/IV), has revealed the author's name to be Abū al-Muṭrib 'Abd al-Raḥmān ibn Isḥāq ibn al-Khaytham; see Hasani, 'A Unique Manuscript'.

17 Leibowitz and Marcus, *Sefer Hanisyonot*, 269.

18 ibid., 273.

19 ibid., 265.

20 ibid., 231, translation slightly amended.

21 ibid., 229.

22 ibid., 165; compare Hasani, 'A Unique Manuscript', 24.

23 For an excellent example of an Islamic 'stone-book', see Beeston, 'An Arabic Hermetic Manuscript'; numerous such treatises are preserved, but very few published. For other talismanic designs some of which are intended for rings, see Maddison and Savage-Smith, *Science, Tools and Magic*, i. 65–71.

24 Banū Bisṭām ibn Sābūr, *Medicine of the Imams*, 540; translation is that of Ispahany and Newman, *Islamic Medical Wisdom*, 145.

25 ibid., 219 (text)/60–61 (tr.), translation amended.

26 ibid., 156 (text)/38 (tr.); translation amended.

27 Ibn Qayyim al-Jawzīyah, *Prophetic Medicine*, 279; translation that of Johnstone, *Medicine of the Prophet*, 255.

28 al-Dhahabī, *Prophetic Medicine*, 172; translation that of Thomson, *As-Suyuti's Medicine of the Prophet*, 81–2.

29 al-Dhahabī, *Prophetic Medicine*, 238; translation that of Thomson, *As-Suyuti's Medicine of the Prophet*, 133, amended.

30 al-Dhahabī, *Prophetic Medicine*, 211; translation that of Thomson, *As-Suyuti's Medicine of the Prophet*, 108, slightly amended.

31 For the pre-Islamic bowls, see the work of Naveh and Shaked, *Amulets and Magic Bowls*.

32 For Islamic magic bowls, see Canaan, 'Arabic Magic Bowls'; Maddison and Savage-Smith, *Science, Tools and Magic*, i. 72–105; and Savage-Smith, 'Safavid Magic Bowls'. For the tenth-century amulets made of haematite with similar talismanic figures, see Maddison and Savage-Smith, *Science, Tools and Magic*, i. 138–9. For modern magic-medicinal bowls in the Islamic world, see Kriss and Kriss-Heinrich, *Volksglaube im Bereich des Islam*.

33 For al-Rāzī's use of sympathetic medicine, see Ullmann, *Islamic Medicine*, 109.

34 For Abū al-ʻAlā' Zuhr's treatise on occult medicinal substances, see Álvarez-Millán, 'El *Kitāb al-Jawāṣṣ*', and for al-Rāzī's treatise on occult medicinal substances (*Kitāb al-Khawāṣṣ*), see Ullmann, *Medizin im Islam*, 133.

35 Klein-Franke, *Iatromathematics in Islam*, 84; translation is by the present authors.

36 See Ullmann, *Islamic Medicine*, 112, n. 16

37 The Hippocratic dictum is given in the form translated into Arabic (*anna ʻilma l-nujūmi laysa bi-juz'in ṣaghīrin min ʻilmi l-ṭibbi*); see Mattock and Lyons, *Kitāb Buqrāṭ*, 13, 16–17 (text) and 14 (tr.). The original Greek of this quotation could be translated as 'astronomy contributes not a small part to medicine (*ouk elachiston meros sumballetai astronomiē es iētrikēn*)'; see the recent edition by Jouanna, *Hippocrate. Airs, eaux, lieux*, 189 and notes.

38 For the late antique Greek occult literature, particularly the Hermetic literature and its influence on astrological thought, see Peters, 'Hermes and Harran'; and Burnett, 'Legend of the Three Hermes'. The Mandaic divinatory text has been translated by Drower, *The Book of the Zodiac*.

39 Ibn Abī Uṣaybiʻah, *Sources of Information*, i. 144, 7–9; translation that of Klein-Franke, *Iatromathematics in Islam*, 61, amended.

40 For Ibn Riḍwān's astrological writing, in part a commentary on Ptolemy's *Tetrabiblos*, see Sezgin, *Astrologie-Meteorologie*, 44. For the life of Ibn Riḍwān, see Dols, *Medieval Islamic Medicine*, 54–66. The treatise *What is Sufficient for the Medical Art* as well as the essay *What Every Physician Should Know about Astrology* by al-ʻAynzarbī are unpublished, but survive in manuscript; see Savage-Smith, *Islamic Medical Manuscripts*; and Ullmann, Medizin in Islam, 255.

41 Ibn Abī Uṣaybiʻah, *Sources of Information*, i. 120, 22–31, in the biography of ʻĪsá ibn Ḥakam al-Dimashqī. The translation given here is that of the present authors; an incomplete and confused translation is to be found in Klein-Franke, *Iatromathematics in Islam*, 57–8. ʻĪsá wrote an *Epistle to Hārūn* [*al-Rashīd*], recently edited and translated into French by Gigandet, *La* risāla. For the critical attitude of Ibn Sīnā and others towards astrology, see Michot, 'Ibn Taymiyya on Astrology'; and Saliba, 'The Role of the Astrologer'.

42 For some of the numerous collections of Islamic seal stones and amulets, see Kalus, *Catalogue of Islamic Seals*, and Kalus, *Catalogue des cachets*.

43 For magic shirts, see Maddison and Savage-Smith, *Science, Tools and Magic*, i. 106–121; and for the Judeo-Persian textile, see Shani, 'A Judeo-Persian Talismanic Textile'.

44 The manuscript with the annotation referring to a magic bowl is in Oxford, Bodleian Library, MS Marsh 663, copied in AD 1242 [640 H], with the annotation on 274; for the reference by al-Ṣanawbarī, see his *Book of Mercy*, 191.

6

Afterlife

With us ther was a Doctour of Phisyk
In al this world ne was ther noon hym lyk
To speke of phisik and surgerye, ...
Wel knew he the olde Esculapius,
And Deyscorides, and eek Rufus,
Old Ypocras, Haly, and Galyen,
Serapion, Razis, and Avycen
– Chaucer (d. 1400), *Canterbury Tales*[1]

So Geoffrey Chaucer wrote in his Prologue to the *Canterbury Tales*, naming the great physicians of the past that his fourteenth-century audience could be expected to recognise. In the list are five authorities from Greek antiquity: Esculapius, or Asclepios, the Greek god of healing, and four doctors whom we have frequently encountered in the earlier chapters, namely Hippocrates (written as Ypocras), Rufus; Dioscorides (Deyscorides); and Galen (Galyen). Chaucer also names four physicians from the Muslim world: Ibn Sarābiyūn (Serapion); al-Rāzī (Razis); ʿAlī ibn Riḍwān (Haly); and Ibn Sīnā (Avycen).

That Chaucer would so casually refer to medieval Islamic medical writers in a narrative poem that met with immediate popularity clearly illustrates the profound influence that the Islamic medical tradition had in Europe. Within Islamic lands, this medical tradition continues to have an enduring presence, evident in the respect which the *Canon of Medicine* by Ibn Sīnā still enjoys. It can be seen in particular on the Indian subcontinent, where a derivative form of this medicine is still practised, taught, and researched today.

In this short chapter on the afterlife we offer a panoramic view of how the medieval Islamic medical tradition spread to other regions of the world, north, south, east and west of the Arab heartland. We begin with Europe to the north-west, and then move south and east to look at the continuation of this tradition within other Islamic countries. Throughout the process of transmission, translations into a plethora of languages were required, and many subtle changes ensued. Islamic medicine also faced challenges from competing medical systems, most notably modern Western medicine, which ultimately led to its being pushed to the margins of medical care.

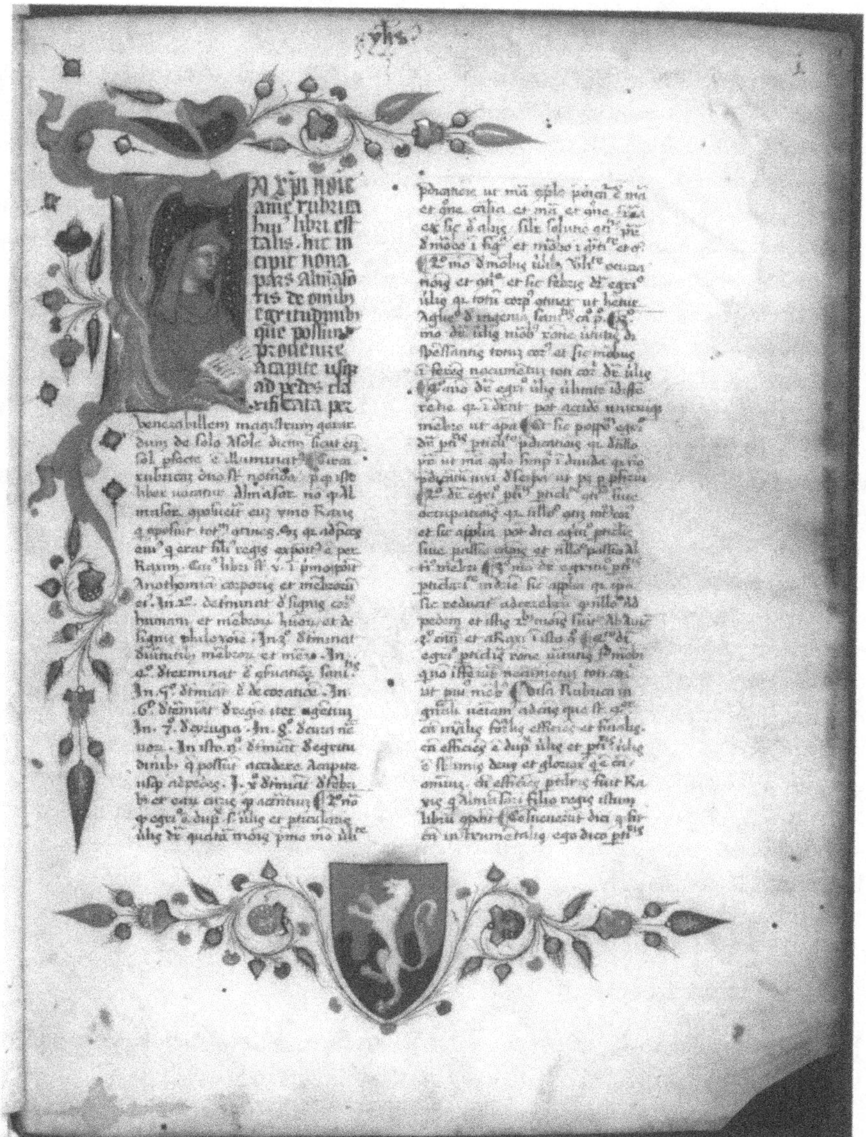

Figure 6.1 A copy made in 1443 of the ninth book, on therapeutics, of the Latin translation of *The Book for al-Manṣūr* by al-Rāzī, known to Europeans as Rhazes. The Latin translation, made in Toledo during the twelfth century by Gerard of Cremona, was one of the most widely read medieval medical manuals in Europe, and it continued to be used as a university textbook well into the sixteenth century, when even the most famous Renaissance anatomist, Andreas Vesalius (d. 1564), prepared a paraphrase of it. In this copy, an 'author portrait' of al-Rāzī – in Western garb – forms the initial decoration along with other European decorative elements unrelated to the text.

Medieval Latin and Byzantine Greek translations

An important vehicle for the transmission of knowledge from the Arabic-speaking world to medieval Europe and Byzantium was translation. As in Baghdad of the late eighth to the tenth century, so also in the Christian world, patrons sponsored, and scholars provided, translations of medical texts, from Arabic into Latin, Hebrew, or Byzantine Greek. Important centres for such activity were Salerno, linked through political ties to the monastery of Monte Cassino, both in southern Italy, and Toledo in southern Spain. Constantine the African (d. before 1099) arrived in Salerno in 1077 to study medicine and was the first to produce major translations from Arabic into Latin. Among his numerous renderings of Arabic medical texts there are, to name just the most significant ones, Ḥunayn's *Introduction to Medicine*, which circulated under the title *Isagoge of Iohannitius*, and al-Majūsī's *Complete Book of the Medical Art*, known as *Pantegni* ('The Whole Art') and attributed to al-Rāzī or Constantine himself. Roughly a century after Constantine, Gerard of Cremona (d. 1187) moved to Toledo in order to learn Arabic, and remained there for the rest of life. He translated many medical works from Arabic into Latin, his most momentous achievements in this area being his version of Ibn Sīnā's *Canon of Medicine*, and al-Rāzī's *Book for al-Manṣūr*. The ninth book of the latter became particularly famous and often circulated separately as *The Ninth Book for al-Manṣūr* (*Liber Nonus ad Almansorem*). Figure 6.1 shows a detail from a copy made in 1443 of the *Ninth Book*, in which the copyist or illustrator produced a 'portrait' of the author, al-Rāzī, in European dress. Over the next two centuries, a variety of Muslim, Christian, and Jewish scholars, working – and sometimes collaborating – in different parts of the Iberian Peninsula, continued to make available in Latin and Castilian the medical, philosophical and scientific heritage of the Muslim world.

Jews as transmitters

Jews, in particular, played their part in the transmission of medical knowledge. In Spain, Italy and southern France, many distinguished Jewish physicians translated medical treatises into Hebrew and Latin. For instance, the Tibbon family in twelfth- and thirteenth-century southern France rendered into Hebrew numerous works of religious, scientific, and philosophical content and thus put these texts at the disposal of Jews living throughout Europe. In the field of medicine, the most important member of the family was Moshe ibn Tibbon (*fl.* 1260), who translated, among other writings, Ibn al-Jazzār's *Provisions for the Traveller*, as well as Maimonides' treatise *On Poisons*. In Italy, there was the Meati family (thirteenth to fourteenth centuries), originally from Cento but later living in Rome. Its most prominent exponent was Nathan ha-Meati (*fl.* c.

1280), who prepared a Hebrew version of Hippocrates' *Airs, Waters, and Places*, of Ibn Sīnā's *Canon*, and of Maimonides' *Aphorisms*. His son Solomon (Shlōmō) translated Galen's commentary on the Hippocratic treatise *Air, Waters, and Places* from Arabic into Hebrew. We also know from an owner's note in a manuscript dated to September 1312 that Nathan's grandson Samuel (Shmū'el) possessed an Arabic copy of Ibn Sarābiyūn's *Small Compendium*. This copy, now kept in the Leiden University Library, also contains a number of Hebrew annotations in the margin, indicating that Jews not only translated Arabic medical texts, but used and perused them as well.[2]

Many of the Hebrew translations were then later rendered into Latin, such as the Galenic commentary by Solomon ha-Meati (just mentioned), translated into Latin by the Jewish doctor Moses Amram Alatino (d. 1605). But just as Arabic texts could reach a Latin reading public via intermediary Hebrew renderings, so people familiar with Hebrew could study Arabic works that had been translated first into Latin and then into Hebrew. An example for this path of transmission is Ibn Sarābiyūn's *Small Compendium*, translated from Syriac into Arabic, then into Latin, and finally into Hebrew by Moshe ben Maṣliaḥ.[3] Another work which travelled on both these tracks (Arabic-to-Hebrew and Arabic-to-Latin-to-Hebrew) is Ibn al-Jazzār's *Provisions for the Traveller*. It was translated, as we have seen, directly from Arabic into Hebrew, but was also rendered twice into Hebrew from the paraphrastic Latin version of Constantine the African.[4]

Ibn al-Jazzār's *Provisions for the Traveller* also exemplifies yet another route by which medical knowledge was conveyed from one culture to another, for there is a Byzantine Greek version of this text, attributed to 'Constantine the Protosecretary of Rhegion'. Other Byzantine texts related to medicine, such as the so-called *Oneirocriticon of Achmet*, an important book on dream interpretation written in the tenth century, drew on Arabic sources and therefore testify to the continuous cultural exchange between the different Eastern shores of the Mediterranean.[5]

University medicine

It is hard to overestimate the impact which these Latin translations had on the development of university medicine. They were at the very base of medical teaching in the first medical faculties set up in Montpellier (twelfth century, with a formal faculty of medicine founded in 1221), Paris (c. 1170), Bologna (c. 1200), and Padua (1222). Salerno, the first European 'medical school', had already arisen in the tenth century and illustrates the shift in theoretical outlook which occurred in the Latin West with the arrival of Arabic medical texts in translation. Prior to that time, the approach had been characterised by a certain eclecticism and plurality of concepts. For instance, methodist writings had circulated side by side with writings espousing the principles of humoral pathology.

The availability of Arabic texts in translation led, however, to a much more systematic and uniform treatment of the subject.

Consequently, by the late twelfth and early thirteenth century, Galenism in its Arabo-Latin guise – that is to say, the medical theory described in Chapter 2 above – dominated the curriculum and provided the medical theoretical framework. The basic textbook of the time was Ḥunain ibn Isḥāq's *Introduction to Medicine* (*Isagoge of Iohannitius*). It was subsequently incorporated into the *Articella* ('Small Art [of Medicine]'), a collection of introductory texts. Together with the medical encyclopedias written by al-Majūsī (*Complete Book of the Medical Art*) and Ibn Sīnā (*Canon*), the *Articella* came to form the core curriculum for medical students. The *Canon* proved so popular that it continued to be used for teaching purposes in some Italian universities until the eighteenth century.

This European university medicine, based largely on the medieval Islamic tradition, was characterised by a certain scholasticism. Theoretical structure and logical rigour were of paramount importance to university professors, which explains why Ibn Sīnā's *Canon*, an extremely well structured and logical work, found so much favour with both pupils and teachers. These scholastic tendencies are best illustrated by an example. Both Ibn Sīnā and Ibn Rushd (Averroes, d. 1198) explained the nature of fever. Yet, while the former defined it as an 'external heat (*ḥarārah gharībah, calor extraneus*)', not natural or innate to the body, the latter saw in it a combination of both natural heat (*ḥarārah ṭabī'īyah, calor naturalis*) and putrid heat (*ḥarārah 'ufūnīyah*). Things were further complicated through the Latin translation of the latter term, 'calor extraneus putredinalis (an *external* putrid heat)', which underscores the contradiction between Ibn Sīnā and Ibn Rushd. The definitions of these two authors, both great authorities in medical as well as philosophical matters could not easily be reconciled. The topic was, therefore, hotly debated not only in medieval commentaries but also in Renaissance treatises well into the seventeenth century.[6]

Learned university physicians often found themselves in competition and conflict with surgeons who, in many instances, were not integrated into the university structure. The former were fond of characterising the latter as little more than craftsmen with varying skills, lacking the theoretical underpinnings needed for sound practice. Yet even in the field of surgery, the influence of Arabic learned medicine was acutely felt. Gerard of Cremona translated into Latin the most important surgical text of the Islamic tradition, the thirtieth book of al-Zahrawī's medical encyclopedia. This book was a quite substantial treatise in its own right, and comprised some 200 pages in the 1531 Strasburg printing of the Latin translation. The most prominent surgeons of the Latin Middle Ages, such as William of Saliceto (d. 1277) and Guy de Chauliac (d. 1368), used it extensively. By drawing heavily on the surgical tradition of the

Arabs, they helped to put their discipline firmly on the map and paved the way for increased acceptance within learned medical circles. The services of surgeons were in considerable demand, especially during the great conflict of the Middle Ages – the Crusades.

The Crusades

From the twelfth century we have this Arab view of a Frankish surgeon in the Crusader States:

> The lord of al-Munayṭirah wrote to my uncle asking him to dispatch a physician to treat certain sick persons among his people. My uncle sent him a Christian [Arab] physician named Thābit. Thābit was absent but ten days when he returned. So we said to him, 'How quickly hast thou healed thy patients!' He said: 'They brought before me a knight in whose leg an abscess had grown; [...]. To the knight I applied a small poultice until the abscess opened and became well; [...]. Then a Frankish physician came to them and said, "This man knows nothing about treating them." He then said to the knight, "Which wouldst thou prefer, living with one leg or dying with both?" The latter replied, "Living with one leg." The physician said, "Bring me a strong knight and a sharp ax." A knight came with the ax, while I was standing by. Then the physician laid the leg of the patient on a block of wood and bade the knight strike his leg with the ax and chop it off at one blow. Accordingly he struck it – while I was looking on – one blow, but the leg was not severed. He dealt another blow, upon which the marrow of the leg flowed out and the patient died on the spot ...'
>
> I have, however, witnessed a case of their medicine which was quite different from that ...
>
> – Usāmah ibn Munqidh (d. 1188), *Book of Contemplation*[7]

The view of Crusader medicine as being far inferior to that of the Muslims is an interpretation often illustrated by this gory episode. The anecdote is taken from the memoirs of Usāmah ibn Munqidh, a Muslim warrior and courtier who lived during the heyday of the Latin Kingdom of Jerusalem. The story also includes a female patient dying at the hands of the Frankish physician, but is followed by a positive description of Frankish medical practice. It has been persuasively argued that this anecdote fulfilled primarily the literary function of juxtaposing contrasting events. In fact, a recent study has disclosed ample evidence for both emergency and elective surgery in the Crusader States, evidence that is at variance with the practice described in this episode. How much Frankish surgeons drew on Islamic practices which on occasion they must have witnessed, is still open to debate.[8]

It is clear, however, that there was a substantial exchange of medical ideas in general during the Crusades. The passage quoted above shows that a Christian lord during the Second Crusade could ask a Muslim, Usāmah's uncle, to provide him with a physician. There was, in fact, such a constant to-ing and fro-ing across the communities and boundaries that one scholar has talked of 'doctors without borders' when describing the medical activities in the Crusader States. In the city of Antioch, a Crusader stronghold, Stephen of Antioch produced a new and more literal Latin translation of al-Majūsī's *Complete Book of the Medical Art* than that by Constantine the African – another example of the cultural interchange and intellectual curiosity of the times. Moreover, some Latin physicians took such an interest in the Islamic medical tradition that they studied Arabic to read the texts in the original language. This can be seen from the fact that on occasion a Frankish medic in the Crusader States would annotate in Latin an Arabic medical text.[9]

A hotly debated topic is the question of whether the sophisticated Islamic hospitals influenced those set up by the Crusaders, and in particular, the large one run by the order of the Hospitallers in Jerusalem named after St John. A related question, equally eagerly discussed, is the extent to which hospitals in the Latin West took inspiration from their Islamic counterparts. Recent scholarship appears to be shifting towards the idea that Islamic medical institutions, and most notably the hospitals, had a clear impact on Western developments of similar structures. Some, however, continue to argue against this notion.[10]

As B. Z. Kedar, one of the most eminent scholars of the Crusades, has noted, a key passage for unraveling the question is a remark by Ibn Jubayr (d. 1217), commenting on the Christians living in Sicily in 1184:

> We observed along the way that the Christians had churches [*kanā'is*] fitted out [*mu'addah*] for Christians who are ill, and that in their cities they had something similar in form to Muslim hospitals [*mithla dhālika 'alá ṣifati māristānāti l-muslimīna*]. And we saw that they had similar [structures] in Acre and Tyre and were amazed at the extent of their [medical] care.[11]

Ibn Jubayr therefore clearly saw parallels between Muslim and Christian hospitals, although he is also aware of an important difference: that Christian hospitals were religious institutions ('churches', *kanā'is*) specifically designed for Christians. Kedar is therefore fully justified in pointing out the great difference between the St John's hospital in Jerusalem, and the great Islamic hospitals such as the Nūrī in Damascus. Although the former appears to have been able to cater for 900 patients on a regular basis, and double that in times of emergency, the medical care offered there was far inferior, as evidenced by the small number of physicians in attendance (only four).[12] Kedar concludes: 'In this respect, as in several others, twelfth-century Latins still played Third World *vis-à-vis* the First and Second Worlds of the realms of Islam and Byzantium.'[13]

The Renaissance

A popular view of the European Renaissance is that of a period of radical departure, when enlightened scholars and scientists freed themselves from the shackles of medieval tradition. On the other hand, the Middle Ages, at least in the Latin West, are portrayed as a time of scholasticism, idle speculation, and intellectual regression. In this view, the Islamic heritage is associated with all things medieval, whereas the 'return to the [Greek] sources' – the rallying cry of many Humanists – is interpreted as progress, not regress. This image is in large part due to the Renaissance writers themselves, who depicted their own time – like people living in most periods – as being the pinnacle of civilisation, looking back with contempt on previous ages and on those who still cherished 'the ways of old'. The idea of the Renaissance as the beginning of modernity and the great break with the 'dark' Middle Ages, however, has been challenged on numerous fronts.[14]

For our purposes, it is important to realise that during the Renaissance not only medical theory and learning, but also practice, continued to be informed and defined by a Galenism in Latino-Arabic garb. Ibn Sīnā's *Canon*, for instance, dominated the medical discourse and was printed in various forms at least sixty times between 1500 and 1674. Likewise, in the 1530s, five out of six lecture courses in Montpellier were concerned with Arabic authors in Latin translations. The Latin translation of al-Rāzī's *Book for al-Manṣūr* continued to be used as a university textbook well into the sixteenth century, when even the most famous Renaissance anatomist, Andreas Vesalius (d. 1564), prepared a paraphrase of it. But other voices made themselves heard over the course of the sixteenth century, demanding a return to the Greek sources, and vilifying the Arabic medical tradition. Prominent humanists such as Niccolò Leoniceno (d. 1524), Symphorien Champier (d. c. 1538), and Leonard Fuchs (d. 1566) endeavoured to remove all Arabic elements from their medical tradition. The latter, well known for his botanical studies and immortalised in the 'fuchsia', a plant named after him, was particularly violent in his attack of the 'Arabic' medical tradition, saying:

> ... It is best to sideline and simply reject the Arab authors, the barbarians of a bygone age, and learn – as if drawing water from the purest sources – from the writing of Greek physicians, who transmitted the art in the cleanest and most unpolluted way and through the soundest of methods, all that is necessary to exercise the art of medicine. Just as in the teachings of the Arabs all is dirty, barbarous, filthy, complicated, and riddled with the most horrendous errors, all things Greek, by contrast, are clean, clear, shining, brilliant, open, and uncontaminated by any error. ... The Arabs have nothing which they did not take from ... the Greeks, apart from the errors which are typical of them.[15]

Fuchs' opinion as expressed here, to be sure, was not universally shared, and other physicians attacked him for his anti-Arabic stance. It is, however, a viewpoint which gained widespread currency in later European historiography, even up to the twentieth century. In the field of philosophy, Alain de Libera has linked the rejection of the Arabic legacy to certain political and religious anti-Muslim trends of the time. In the area of medicine, similar tendencies were at work.[16]

In Europe, Arabic authors slowly disappeared from university curricula and the libraries of physicians during the eighteenth and nineteenth centuries. At the same time, many Greek authors such as Hippocrates, Galen, and Paul of Aegina continued to be taught and studied not only out of historical interest, but also to further medical practice. The theory of humoral pathology, which underlay both the Greek and the Islamic medical tradition, only fell out of favour with the advent of the germ theory of disease, and the discovery of bacteria and viruses in the late nineteenth century. It is fair to say that medicine has changed more in the last 150 years than it had in the previous 1500, and that, today, orthodox medicine is completely at odds with the humoral medical system which dominated for such a long time. But even in modern medical handbooks, one can find remnants of the Islamic legacy, although they are sometimes difficult to spot. For instance, the terminology used today occasionally had its origin in the Arabic of the Middle Ages. The term 'saphenous vein' or 'vena saphena' goes back to Constantine's Latin translation of al-Majūsī's *Complete Book*, where it translates *'irq … ṣāfin* ['clear vein']. Likewise, *dura mater* ('hard mother') and *pia mater* ('pious mother') are calques of Arabic expressions – *umm al-dimāgh al-jāfiyah* ('hard mother of the brain') and *umm al-dimāgh al-raqīqah* ('soft mother of the brain') – designating the meninges of the brain.[17]

Afterlife in the East – the later Ottoman empire

The nucleus of most Arabic, Turkish, and Persian medical compositions during the sixteenth, seventeenth, and eighteenth centuries continued the medieval Islamic tradition, despite some acquaintance with European medical ideas and the occasional contact with European doctors. For example, a Syrian physician named Dāwūd al-Anṭākī (d. 1599) composed a large and influential medical handbook called *Memorandum Book for Those Who Have Understanding and Collection of Wondrous Marvels*. It was for the most part based on medieval Islamic writers and earlier Greek sources (for which he learned Greek so as to study them directly). He did, however, incorporate into it a description of syphilis and the European treatment (not to be found in earlier Arabic or Persian treatises) of using China Root – *Chub-chīnī* in Persian, a rhizome of a species of smilax (*Smilax china* L.) native to eastern Asia, having steroidal sapogenins. In the fifteenth and sixteenth centuries, Europe had reacted with great enthusiasm to the introduction of China Root and considered it a panacea as well as a specific for treating syphilis, leprosy, dropsy, and melancholy.[18]

At the Ottoman court of the seventeenth century, the early-modern European concept of 'chemical medicine' was introduced through the writings of a court physician, a Syrian named Ṣāliḥ ibn Naṣr ibn Sallūm, who in 1655 translated into Arabic extracts of Latin treatises by Oswald Croll (d. 1609), professor of medicine at the University of Marburg, and Daniel Sennert (d. 1637), professor of medicine at Wittenberg. Both men were followers of Paracelsus (d. 1541), who had employed mineral acids, inorganic salts, and alchemical procedures in the production of remedies. Many of the medicaments required distillation processes as well as plants that were indigenous to the New World, such as guaiacum and sarsaparilla. Moreover, like Dāwūd al-Anṭākī a century earlier, Ibn Sallūm recommended China root for a variety of diseases. These new chemical procedures, the New World medicaments, and some new European items or items introduced via Europe such as China root, were combined with the rich heritage of medieval remedies. They formed a much expanded base for drug therapy in the Islamic world, firmly linked to the emerging field of chemistry.

Ibn Sallūm, however, drew his theoretical considerations of the causes and symptoms for the most part not from the Paracelsians. Rather, he relied on late medieval Islamic writers of the thirteenth to sixteenth centuries. His particular favourites were the *Book of the Blessed Gift*, an Arabic commentary on the *Canon* of Ibn Sīnā written in 1283 by Quṭb al-Dīn al-Shīrāzī, and the *Memorandum Book* by the Syrian physician Dāwūd al-Anṭākī (d. 1599). As a result, Ibn Sallūm's treatises were pastiches of late medieval Islamic medical thinking alongside seventeenth-century European medical chemistry. These versions of Paracelsian tracts were subsequently used in the eighteenth century by Turkish medical and chemical writers.

During the eighteenth century, complete translations of Ibn Sīnā's *Canon of Medicine* were made into both Turkish and Persian. Dietetics, drug remedies, and self-help manuals were the primary focus of medical writings, while in Arabic-speaking areas there seems to have been a renewed interest in didactic medical poetry concerned primarily with dietetics and drug lore. The vast majority of all medical writings in the Early Modern period were a mix of the old and the new, but with the 'new' only lightly sprinkled here and there into a dominantly traditional medical theory and practice.

European perspectives on the 'East'

European travellers of the eighteenth century frequently noted the failure of physicians to keep up with European developments in medicine or to maintain the best of the practices represented by the learned Arabic medieval medical compendia. A particularly interesting account of the medical care in Syria between 1742 and 1753 was given by Alexander Russell (d. 1768), who was physician to the English factory in Aleppo at that time. In his *The Natural History of Aleppo*, he commented on the streets of Aleppo being narrow but well paved and 'kept remarkably clean'. He also observed that 'the people here have no notion of the benefit of exercise, either for the preservation of health, or curing diseases.' In 1742, while describing an epidemic of smallpox, he noted that 'inoculation is only practised here among the Christians, and is not yet general even among them.' He went on to decry the poor state of medicine in Syria:

> Of the use of chemistry in medicine they are totally ignorant, but now and then one amongst them just acquires a smattering enough of alchemy to beggar his family by it. The books they have amongst them are some of the Arabian writers: Ebnsina [Ibn Sīnā] in particular, whose authority is indisputable with them. They have likewise some translations of Hippocrates, Galen, Dioscorides, and a few other ancient Greek writers. But their copies are in general miserably incorrect. Hence it may easily be seen, that the state of physic among the natives in the country, as well as every other science, is at a very low ebb, and that it is far from being in a way of improvement.[19]

Like Russell, Pierre-Charles Rouyer, a French army pharmacist who accompanied the Napoleonic expeditionary force to Egypt at the end of the century, expressed his criticism of indigenous medical practice, saying: 'The Egyptians, having become apathetic and indolent, have let a large number of their medications fall into disuse.' Of course, like most European travellers to the Middle East at that time, both Russell and Rouyer enthusiastically recorded the practices of an exotic culture while concluding that all comparisons with European ways only demonstrated the deficiencies of the foreign culture.[20]

In the larger commercial centres of the Middle East at this time, the practice of European physicians coexisted with traditional medicine. In North Africa, for example, the Turkish governors in Tunisia consulted European doctors while also employing local court physicians. In 1814, a North African physician by the name of Aḥmad ibn Muḥammad al-Salāwī composed an Arabic *Miscellany on the Art of Medicine*. In it he discussed the diseases most common in his day, incorporating much from medieval medical writings such as Ibn Sīnā. Yet he also warned against the use of some drugs approved by older authorities and occasionally advocated methods used by European doctors.[21]

Safavid Persia

Persia, ruled by the Safavids from the beginning of the sixteenth century until the demise of the regime in the early eighteenth century, had many European contacts through envoys from courts and religious missionaries. It was here that the earliest Islamic treatise on syphilis was composed in 1569. Its author, 'Imād al-Dīn Maḥmūd Shīrāzī, also wrote in Persian a treatise on the medical and addictive properties of opium. Moreover, he composed several Arabic medical treatises which reflect as much the medieval tradition as they do the then current European one.[22] The unsettled political conditions in Persia at the end of the seventeenth century and the beginning of the eighteenth prompted many physicians to move to the Mughal court, then in Delhi. In the nineteenth century, profound changes occurred in the teaching of medicine in most Islamic countries. Many European medical texts were translated into Arabic and Persian. In 1828, a medical school near Cairo was established at which French, Italian, and German professors taught European medicine. And in 1850, a military medical school, the Dār al-Funūn, was founded in Tehran where instruction was given in French by professors from Austria and Italy. As Western European ideas were introduced on a massive scale, the Islamic world was drawn more and more into the orbit of Europe.

The Indian subcontinent

> Modern medicine traces its origin to the Greeks. The Greek medicine was taken over by the Roman and then by the Arabs from whom, after its enrichment with Chinese and Indian medicine, it was taken over by modern Europe. The Muslim rulers introduced it into India and incorporated with it the native Ayurvedic medicine; this mixture is now known as Unani medicine or broadly speaking eastern medicine.
>
> No one feels more than we do that we must do research, for only 2–3 per cent plant wealth of, say, this [the Indian] subcontinent has been covered. But we still feel we must abide by our traditions and not follow the West in everything. Why should we resort to potent antibiotics when home remedies would do? Why burden the body with antibiotics and tranquillizers when milder drugs would achieve the same end?
> – Hakim Mohammed Said (1920–98), Founder and former President of the Hamdard National Foundation, whose mission is to 'preserve and promote the Eastern system of medicine'[23]

In India, the Islamic medical tradition was, for a long time, known by its Arabic name *ṭibb* 'medicine'. Only under the late Mughal rulers of India did the term 'Unani Tibb', or 'Unani medicine' come into fashion. The new name was a deliberate attempt to give greater prestige to the Islamic medical tradition on the subcontinent by linking it to Greek medicine, for *yūnānī* means 'Greek' in Arabic. As can be seen from the first quotation by Hakim Mohammed Said given above, advocates of Unani medicine present (rightly, one may add) Greek medicine as being at the origin of both the Western and their own medical traditions.

Unani medicine is practised today in India and Pakistan, alongside the classical Indian medicine called Ayurveda and modern Western European

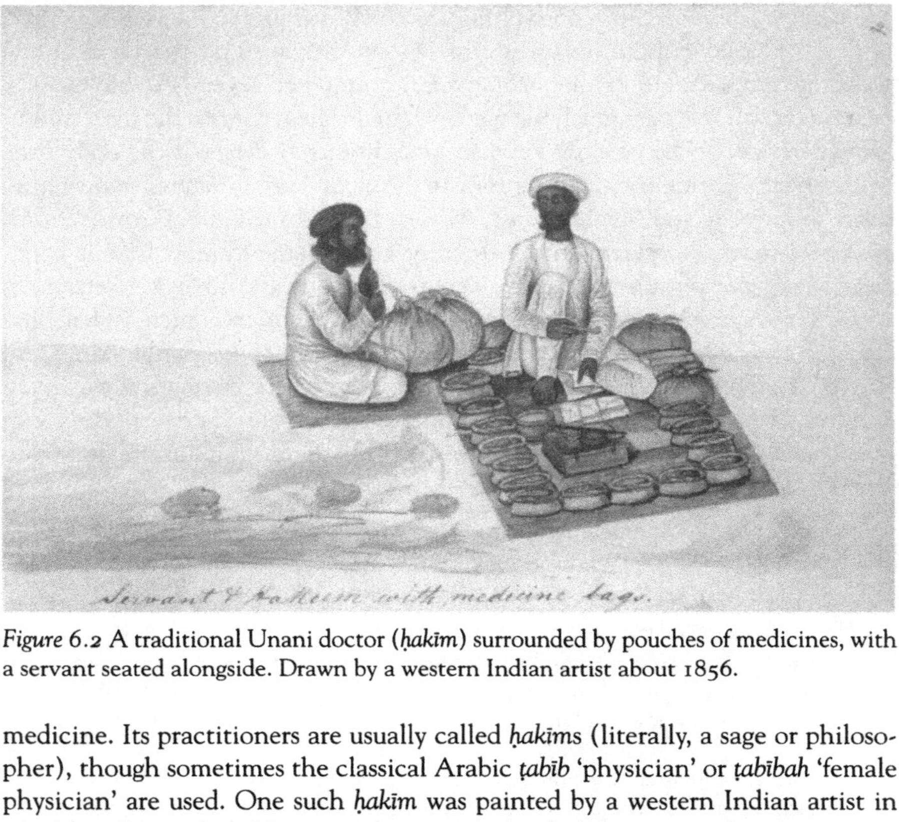

Figure 6.2 A traditional Unani doctor (*ḥakīm*) surrounded by pouches of medicines, with a servant seated alongside. Drawn by a western Indian artist about 1856.

medicine. Its practitioners are usually called *ḥakīms* (literally, a sage or philosopher), though sometimes the classical Arabic *ṭabīb* 'physician' or *ṭabībah* 'female physician' are used. One such *ḥakīm* was painted by a western Indian artist in 1856 (see Figure 6.2). Unani medicine stresses a holistic approach to patients as perceived in the medieval Arabic and Persian medical writings, and it accepts humoral pathology as the basis for the explanation and treatment of diseases. It advocates cure through the use of medicaments prepared in a traditional manner and rejects chemical synthesis of drugs. Hospitals play a prominent role in both medical teaching and medical provision. The view of practitioners is that they are continuing a more or less unadulterated form of medicine advocated by Ibn Sīnā. Yet subtle differences have evolved. For example, over time Unani medicine has taken into its arsenal of drugs some items from Ayurvedic medicine and has made extensive use of plants exclusively of Indian origin, while surgery plays a greatly diminished role in medical care.

Cordials, or drugs for chest pains and palpitations, are today a particularly important stock of Unani medicine. They often incorporate many ingredients and are prepared in a multitude of ways. They almost always include medicinal stones and precious metals such as pearl, yellow amber, coral, silver or gold filings, ruby, lapis lazuli and so forth, all very finely powdered like dust. These are combined with other ingredients – such as one or more of the three types of myrobalans (a genus of fruit-bearing trees indigenous to India; unknown to Greek physicians, it was introduced into Islamic medicine as early as the ninth century), rose petals, lettuce seed, cinnamon, cardamom, lavender – which have separately been pounded lightly and soaked in water for 12 to 20 hours. The combined ingredients are then boiled and filtered, with ambergris added during the boiling process and saffron and musk added after triturating in rose-water. Camphor is one of the final ingredients to be added, and the mixture is then kneaded with honey to form tablets.[24] Precious stones as well as gold and silver are thought to be particularly good for the heart – an idea traceable to Ibn Sīnā and other medieval physicians. In modern Pakistan and India very fine silver (or even gold) foil will occasionally be placed on top of a delicacy being offered to guests in order to preserve their health.

In the early twentieth century, the governments of India and Pakistan gave Unani medicine official recognition and set about regulating the practice through the Ministries of Health. Colleges and hospitals were established on the principles of Unani medicine, examples being the Nizamia Unani Hospital in Hyderabad and the Tibbiya College of Aligarh Muslim University. The curricula of most government-funded colleges of Unani medicine include 'integrated' courses in which texts such as the *Canon* of Ibn Sīnā are taught along with some components of modern European medicine and the employment of modern equipment. The Hamdard Foundation in Karachi, founded by Hakim Mohammed Said, who was quoted above, and the Institute of History of Medicine and Medical Research in New Delhi have been responsible for English translations and studies of several medieval Arabic texts, including *On Cardiac Drugs* by Ibn Sīnā which had earlier in 1956 been translated into Urdu and in 1966 into Uzbek.

Today

Unani *ṭibb* as practised in India and Pakistan is just one aspect of the continuous presence of the Islamic medical legacy today. Others include Prophetic Medicine: treatises on this subject are still in print in many countries throughout the Muslim world, with a growing market for English translations and updated compilations. In the bookstalls of Egypt one can buy numerous works on magical medicine by a twentieth-century astrologer named al-Ṭūkhī, and these same writings are being condensed and reworked in books printed in Malaysia and Indonesia. A popular booklet easily available in Egypt, Syria, and the Lebanon is a collection of magic squares and talismans for use in medicine, attributed to Ibn Sīnā and called *The Great Compilation*. Magical practices are, however, opposed by many orthodox Muslim clerics, particularly those of the Wahhabi persuasion.[25]

Moreover, traditional and folkloric practices still form part of the spectrum of medical care that can be obtained in any market or *sūq*. Figure 6.3 shows a

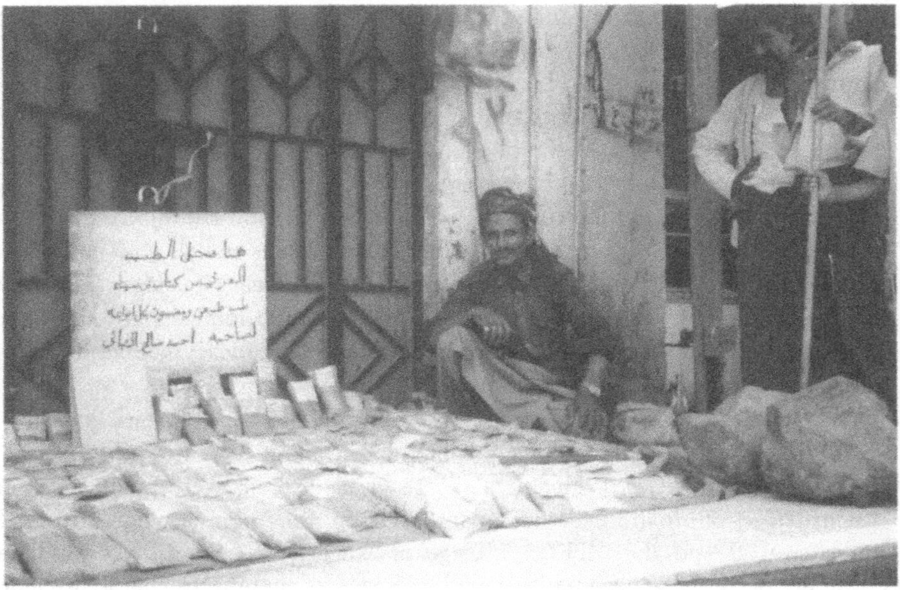

Figure 6.3 A vendor of traditional remedies in the city of Taʿiz (c. 150,000 inhabitants) in Southern Yemen. The Arabic placard above his packets of medicaments reads: 'Here is the place for Arabic medicine from the book of Ibn Sīnā. A natural and guaranteed medicine, the whole range. The proprietor: Aḥmad Ṣāliḥ al-Thabāʾī.'

Yemeni vendor of traditional remedies who advertises his medicinal herbs as being 'from the book of Ibn Sīnā, a natural medicine'. Throughout the Arab world, be it Casablanca or Cairo, Damascus or Doha, one can still purchase traditional drugs. The Yemeni vendor's methods are not that different from those of his colleague, shown in Figure 6.2 on p. 174, who, a century and a half before him, sold his herbs in India. Likewise, in many other countries throughout the Muslim world, practitioners can also still be seen, particularly in rural areas, making medicaments whose ingredients and methods of preparation – if not the very recipe – can be traced back to medieval Arabic or Persian manuals.

East and West

To date, only India and Pakistan have officially incorporated into their health care systems remnants of traditional Islamic medicine and drug therapy. But because of an increasing scepticism regarding orthodox Western medicine and its sometimes unpredictable side-effects, as well as the increasingly popular image of alternative practices, things might change in the West with regard to the Islamic medical tradition. At present, in 2005, there are only about 20 practitioners of Unani medicine active in the UK, and only one course granting diplomas in this area of alternative practice (a 'Diploma in Tibb' offered by the Mohsin Institute). Thus, in a variety of ways, strains of medieval Islamic medicine continue to coexist today with other ancient and modern approaches to health care.[26]

Suggested reading

For the transmission of medical knowledge from Arabic into Latin, see Jacquart, and Micheau, *La médecine arabe et l'occident médiéval*; more specifically on Constantine the African, M. H. Green, 'Constantine the African'; and on Toledo in the twelfth century, Burnett 'The Coherence of the Arabic-Latin Translation Programme'. For Arabic into Byzantine Greek, see Mavroudi, *Byzantine Book on Dream Interpretation*. For Jewish physicians, Shatzmiller, *Jews, Medicine, and Medieval Society*.

For university medicine and later developments, see Jacquart, 'Influence of Arabic Medicine', and Jacquart, *La médecine médiévale*; for medicine during the Crusades; Mitchell, *Medicine in the Crusades*. For the Renaissance, MacLean, *Logic, Signs and Nature*; for the strong presence of the Islamic tradition, Siraisi, *Avicenna in Renaissance Italy*; and Pormann, 'L'héritage oublié'.

For further discussion of the afterlife of medieval Islamic medicine within Islamic lands, see Savage-Smith, 'Islam'; Elgood, *Safavid Medical Practice*.

For Ibn Sallūm, see E. Savage-Smith, 'Drug Therapy of Eye Diseases'; Sari and Zülfikar, 'The Paracelsusian Influence on Ottoman'.

For eighteenth- and ninteenth-century European views of medicine in the Middle East, see Gunny, *Images of Islam*; Murphey, 'Ottoman Medicine and Transculturalism'.

For ninteenthth-century changes in medical education in Iran, see Ebrahimnejad, *Medicine, Public Health*; and for the situation in Tunisia, see Gallagher, *Medicine and Power in Tunisia*.

For Unani medicine, see Liebeskind, 'Unani medicine'; and Attewell, 'Medical Traditions in South Asia'.

An example of a recent compilation on Prophetic Medicine published in India, in English with Arabic text *ḥadīths*, is Sehban-ul-Hind, *Prophetic Medical Sciences*. For examples of al-Ṭūkhī's writings and the versions available in Malaysia, see Ṭūkhī, *Success in the Sciences of the Soul*, and Kabīr, *Crown of Kings*. For contemporary magical-medical practices, see Kruk, 'Harry Potter in the Gulf'.

Notes

1 General Prologue, vv. 411–32 (*Riverside Chaucer*, 30).

2 For Galen's commentary on the Hippocratic treatise *Air, Waters, and Places*, see Wasserstein, *Galen's Commentary*, 101–2. For Ibn Sarābiyūn, see Pormann, 'Further Studies', 242.

3 Pormann, 'Further Studies', 256.

4 P. E. Pormann, review of Bos, *Ibn al-Jazzār on Fevers* in: *Journal of the Royal Asiatic Society* 11 (2001), 65–9.

5 Mavroudi, *Byzantine Book on Dream Interpretation*, especially chapter 10, with medicine being discussed on 415–17.

6 Lonie, 'Fever Pathology', 21. We thank Karine van 't Land for kindly giving us access to unpublished material.

7 tr. Hitti, *An Arab-Syrian Gentleman*, 162; Arabic 132–3.

8 For an analysis of this episode see, Conrad, 'Usāma ibn Munqidh'. For surgery in the Crusader States, see Mitchell, *Medicine in the Crusades*.

9 For the notion of 'doctors without borders', see Pahlitzsch, *Ärzte ohne Grenzen*; for Latin annotations in Arabic medical manuscripts, see Savage-Smith, 'Between Reader and Text'. For Stephen of Antioch, Burnett, 'Stephen, the Disciple of Philosophy'.

10 For the view arguing for a clear impact, see Kedar, 'Twelfth-Century Description'; Mitchell, *Medicine in the Crusades*, ch. 2; Pormann, 'Islamic Hospitals'. For the contrary view, see Miller, 'Knights of Saint-John'; Conrad, 'Usāma ibn Munqidh', p. xl, n. 63.

11 Ibn Jubayr, *Travels*, 330, 1–3 (Arabic); tr. Broadhurst, *Travels of Ibn Jubayr*, 346 (the translation here is our own). See Kedar, 'Twelfth-Century Description', 11.

12 See also Edgington, 'The Hospital of St John in Jerusalem', xx–xxi, who remarks that 'in normal times the overwhelming concern of the hospital [sc. of St John in Jerusalem] was not *curing* but *caring*' (her emphasis).

13 Kedar, 'Twelfth-Century Description', 12.

14 Challenges include classics such as Yates, *Giordano Bruno*; and more specifically for medicine: MacLean, *Logic, Signs and Nature*.

15 Quotation from Fuchs, *Institutions of Medicine*, 807–8. For Ibn Sīnā in the Renaissance, see Siraisi, *Avicenna in Renaissance Italy*, 3; for lectures at Montpellier, Antonioli, *Rabelais et la médecine*, 43.

16 For the rejection of Arabic philosophy, see Libera, *Penser au Moyen-Âge*; for similar attitudes in medicine, see Pormann, 'L'Héritage oublié'.

17 Strohmaier, 'Constantine's Pseudo-Classical Terminology'.

18 For specifics, see Savage-Smith, 'Drug Therapy of Eye Diseases', 21–3.

19 Russell, *The Natural History of Aleppo*, 5, 194, and 99. See also Marcus, *The Middle East on the Eve of Modernity*, 252–68.

20 Estes and Kuhnke, 'French Observations'; quotation on p. 131.

21 The treatise by al-Salāwī is preserved in an autograph copy, but has not yet been published; see Savage-Smith, *Islamic Medical Manuscripts*. For medicine in Tunisia, see Gallagher, *Medicine and Power in Tunisia*

22 See E. Savage-Smith, art. "Emād-al-Dīn Maḥmūd Šīrāzī', *Enc. Ir.*, viii. 381a–2b; A. J. Newman, art. 'Ṣafawids' part IV.ii.1, *EI*² viii. 783a–5a; Elgood, *Safavid Medical Practice*.

23 Both quotations are by Hakim Mohammed Said; the first is from the preface to *Hamdard Pharmacopoeia of Eastern Medicine*; the second from the peroration of his lecture 'Al-Tibb al-Islami', a lecture presented on the occasion of the World of Islam Festival, London, April–June 1976, published in *Hamdard* 19 (1976), 1–117; quotation on 115–16. For more information about Said, see http://www.hakim-said.com.pk; for more information about Hamdard, http://www.hamdard.com.pk.

24 This example is given by the commentator to the English translation of Ibn Sīnā's book; Hameed, *Avicenna's Tract*, 61 n.

25 See Kruk, 'Harry Potter in the Gulf'.

26 According to the Home Office paper 'Unani Tibb Practitioners', March 2005, http://www.ind.homeoffice.gov.uk/documents/businessandcommericialoccsheet/occsheetunanitibb.pdf?view=Binary [accessed 4.8.06].

Conclusion

Medieval Islamic scholars made the rich intellectual traditions of older cultures around them – particularly that of ancient Greece – serve their own purposes, much as Renaissance thinkers were later to do when they encountered Greek culture first hand. Yet, were they innovative? Some scholars in the West from the Renaissance onwards have denied this, saying that Muslims only copied and transmitted what others had done before them. We have seen, however, that Islamic physicians, while maintaining great respect for the authority of ancient texts, at the same time often tested and challenged their precursors. Of those whom we can document, al-Rāzī is perhaps the most outstanding example of this analytical and questioning attitude. In our opinion, it is impossible to read the comments of this great clinician struggling to find a way of determining the true efficacy of a treatment recommended in antiquity as useful, or writing an essay on his doubts about Galen, or differentiating between measles and smallpox, and not to be impressed by the intelligence and originality at work. Lesser luminaries made their contributions as well during the millennium covered in this rapid survey. They described new medicinal substances, recognised new pathological conditions (even if they overlooked others that we feel with hindsight they ought to have spotted), illustrated the design of surgical instruments (obvious to us today, but entirely novel at the time), and vastly expanded the options available to a physician when treating patients.

Innovation was not, however, restricted to challenging authority and discovering new diseases and treatments. Undoubtedly one of the greatest success stories was the *Canon of Medicine* by Ibn Sīnā, as well as other medical compendia, which skilfully organised the medical precepts and principles. One might even say that they were too skilfully organised, for some physicians (both European and Islamic) were so impressed by the methodically construed system that they may have thought it required no further elaboration or development. The commentaries written on the *Canon*, however, could contain new insights, such as the discovery of the pulmonary transit by Ibn al-Nafīs, and commentaries in general provided a forum in which learned physicians could modify and debate issues.

The medieval Islamic community displayed its creativity, and applied the ethical principles of Islam, through another major avenue as well, namely what we would today label as 'public health care'. The extraordinary provision of public bath-houses, complex sanitary systems of drainage (more extensive even than the famous Roman infrastructures), fresh water supplies, and the large and sophisticated urban hospitals, all contributed to the general health of the population. In addition, it was an unprecedented initiative that the same physicians who treated the social and political elite also taught, practised, and observed the effects of various therapies in hospitals where the poor received medical care. Finally, although the evidence is sparse, it appears that at various times and places authorities set about to regulate, in one way or another, the performance and competency of those providing medical care or active in the medical market-place.

Medieval Islamic medicine, in all its diversity, emerged as a complex cluster of theories and practices. Two questions remain to be addressed: why did this multi-faceted tradition emerge when and where it did, and why do certain aspects of it still prove attractive to peoples in many parts of the world? With regard to the first question, openness to foreign cultures often engenders an atmosphere of creativity and growth, and medieval Islamic society tolerated other customs and confessions to a much larger degree than its medieval Christian counterparts. In particular, its medical tradition thrived through an infusion of outside influences. In the context of learned medicine, the underlying medical principles were secular and therefore permitted peoples of divergent backgrounds and beliefs to co-operate and to participate in a joint scientific discourse.

As for the second question, the basic medical system – inherited in its essence from Greece, but vastly expanded and developed in Islamic lands – was what we would today term 'holistic'. The overriding concern was for the improvement of the patient through manipulation of environmental factors, regimen, and diet. When those proved insufficient, medicaments were applied or taken internally. Intervention was kept to a minimum. This approach resonates with many current trends in medical care.

Throughout this book we have had to rely, regrettably, upon evidence that is often fragmentary and sometimes contradictory. Occasionally there is just a casual remark that provides only a brief or partial glimpse into what was occurring. It is left to us to speculate as to how to connect the dots between these disparate bits of evidence. Sometimes our generalities may have been too sweeping. In others we may have been too constrained. Our study has not been exhaustive, for there are a number of topics that could have been explored but have not been. In regard to many of the subjects we raised, much more evidence could have been presented and analysed than space permitted here. Our overall aim has been to draw not a comprehensive or detailed picture, nor just a skeletal outline of medieval Islamic medicine, but one that had some muscle and flesh on the basic structures, relying throughout on a fresh examination of the sources as well as the most recent scholarly studies. The end result, we hope, is a picture of a vibrant and varied society, one in which the medical care was not monolithic but rather configured with many shades and textures.

Bibliography

The bibliography contains works by modern scholars, as well as translations into modern European languages of the sources discussed here. The entries are arranged according to the names of the moderns authors, editors, and translators. References to the historical personalities and their works can be found in the Index of names and works beginning on p. 206.

Adams, F., *The Seven Books of Paulus Aegineta, translated from the Greek, with a commentary embracing a complete view of the knowledge possessed by the Greeks, Romans, and Arabians on all subjects connected with medicine and surgery*, 3 vols (London: 1844–7)

Adamson, P., *The Arabic Plotinus: A Philosophical Study of the* Theology of Aristotle (London: Duckworth, 2002)

Aguirre de Carcer, L. F., 'Sobre el ejercicio de la medicina en al-Andalus: una fetua de Ibn Sahl', *Anaquel de Estudios Arabes* 2 (1991), 147–62

Aldeeb Abu-Sahlieh, S. A., *To Mutilate in the Name of Jehovah or Allah: legitimisation of male and female circumcision* (Den Haag: Gegevenes Koninklijke Bibliothek, 1994)

Álvarez de Morales, C. and F. Girón Irueste, *Mujtaṣar fī l-ṭibb = compendio de medicina* (Madrid: Consejo Superior de Investigaciones Científicas, Instituto de Cooperación con el Mundo Arabe, 1992)

Álvarez-Millán, C. (ed. and tr.), *Abū al-'Alā' Zuhr, Kitāb al-Muŷarrabāt (Libro de las experiencias médicas)* [Fuentes Arábico-Hispanas, vol. 17] (Madrid: 1994)

Álvarez-Millán, C., 'El *Kitāb al-Jawāṣṣ* de Abū l-'Alā' Zuhr: materiales para su estudio', *Asclepio* 46 (1994), 151–73

Álvarez-Millán, C., 'Graeco-Roman Case Histories and their Influence on Medieval Islamic Clinical Accounts', *Social History of Medicine*, 12 (1999), 19–33

Álvarez-Millán, C., 'Practice versus Theory: Tenth-century Case Histories from the Islamic Middle East', in Horden and Savage-Smith, *The Year 1000* (2000), 293–306.

Álvarez-Millán, C., 'Medical Anecdotes in Ibn Juljul's Biographical Dictionary', *Suhayl* 4 (2004), 1–18

Amar, Z., et al. (eds), *Ha-Refu'ah bi-Yerushalayim le-doroteha* (Medicine in Jerusalem Throughout the Ages) (Tel-Aviv: ha-Mador le-toldot ha-refuah be-Erets-Yisrael, 1999)

Ambjörn, L. (ed. and tr.), *Qusṭā ibn Lūqā, On Numbness: A Book on Numbness, its Kinds, Causes and Treatment according to the Opinion of Galen and Hippocrates*, Studia Orientalia Lundensia n.s. 1 (Stockholm: Almqvist & Wiksell, 2000)

Anawati, G., 'Trois talismans musulmans en arabe provenant du Mali (Marché de Mopti)', *Annales islamologiques* 11 (1972), 287–339

Antonioli, R., *Rabelais et la médecine*, *Études rabelaisiennes*, vol. 12 (Geneva: Droz, 1976); repr. as id., 'La médecine dans la vie et dans l'œuvre de Fr. Rabelais', thèse Paris IV, 1974, Lille, Service de reproduction des thèses, Université de Lille III, 1977

Arberry, A. J., *The Spiritual Physick of Rhazes* (London: John Murray, 1950)

Attewell, G., 'Medical Traditions in South Asia', in W. and H. Bynum (eds), *Dictionary of Medical Biography* (Westport, CN: Greenwood, 2006) [forthcoming]

Baker, P., 'Roman Medical Instruments: Archaeological Interpretations of their Possible "Non-functional" Uses', *Social History of Medicine* 17 (2004), 3–21

Barhoum, N. A., 'Das Buch über die Geschlechtlichkeit (*Kitāb fī l-Bāh*) von Qusṭā ibn Lūqā', Doctoral Dissertation (Erlangen: Seminar für die Geschichte der Medizin, 1975)

Bar-Sela, A. and H. E. Hoff, 'Isaac Israeli's Fifty Admonitions to the Physicians', *Journal of the History of Medicine and Allied Sciences* 17 (1962), 245–57

Barthold, W., *An Historical Geography of Iran*, tr. Svat Soucek (Princeton, NJ: Princeton University Press, 1984)

Beeston, F., 'An Arabic Hermetic Manuscript', *The Bodleian Library Record* 7 (1962), 11–23

Beck, L. Y. (tr.), *De materia medica by Pedanius Dioscorides* (Hildesheim: Olms-Weidmann, 2005)

Benkheira, M. H., '"La maison de Satan": Le hammâm en débat dans l'islam mediéval', *Revue de l'histoire des religions* 220 (2003), 391–443

Bergsträsser, G. (ed. and tr.), *Ḥunain ibn Isḥāq über die syrischen und arabischen Galen-Übersetzungen*, Abhandlungen für die Kunde des Morgenlandes 17.2 (Leipzig: Brockhaus, 1925)

Berkey, J. P., *The Transmission of Knowledge in Medieval Cairo: a Social History of Islamic Education* (Princeton, NJ: Princeton University Press, 1992)

Bhayro, S., 'Syriac Medical Terminology: Sergius and Galen's Pharmacopia', *Aramaic Studies* 3 (2005), 147–65

Biesterfeldt, H. H., *Galens Traktat 'Dass die Kräfte der Seele den Mischungen des Körpers folgen'*, Abhandlungen zur Kunde des Morgenlandes 40.4 (Wiesbaden: Steiner, 1973)

Biesterfeldt, H. H., 'Some Opinions on the Physician's Remuneration in Medieval Islam', *Bulletin of the History of Medicine* 58 (1984), 16–27

Blodi, F. C., et al. (tr.), *The Arabian Ophthalmologists, Compiled from Original Texts by Hirschberg, J. Lippert and E. Mittwoch and Translated into English*, ed. M. Z. Wafai (Riyadh: King Abdulaziz City for Science and Technology, 1993)

Bos, G., 'The *miswāk*, an Aspect of Dental Care in Islam', *Medical History* 37 (1993), 68–79

Bos, G., *Ibn al-Jazzār on Sexual Diseases and their Treatment: A critical edition of Zād al-musāfir wa-qūt al-ḥāḍir*, The Sir Henry Wellcome Asian Series 3 (London: Kegan Paul, 1997)

Bos, G., *Ibn al-Jazzār on Fevers: A critical edition of Zād al-musāfir wa-qūt al-ḥāḍir*, The Sir Henry Wellcome Asian Series (London: Kegan Paul, 2000)

Bos, G., (ed. and tr.), *Maimonides, On Asthma* (Provo, UT: Brigham Young University Press, 2002)

Bos, G. (ed. and tr.), *Maimonides, Medical Aphorisms. Treatises 1–5* (Provo, UT: Brigham Young University Press, 2004) [further treatises in press and forthcoming]

Bray, J., 'The Physical World and the Writer's Eye: al-Tānūkhī and Medicine', in ead. (ed.), *Writing and Representation in Medieval Islam: Muslim Horizons* (London; New York: Routledge, Taylor & Francis Group, 2006), 215–49

Broadhurst, R. J. C. (tr.), *The Travels of Ibn Jubayr* (London: J. Cape, 1952)

Brock, S., 'Aspects of Translation Technique in Antiquity', *Greek, Roman and Byzantine Studies* 20 (1979), 69–87, repr. in id., *Syriac Perspective on Late Antiquity* (London: Variorum Reprints, 1984), item 3

Brosius, M., *The Persians* (London: Routledge, 2006)

Browne, E. G., *Arabian Medicine* (Cambridge: Cambridge University Press, 1921)

Browne, E. G., *Revised Translation of the Chahār maqála ('Four Discourses') of Nizámí-i-'Arúdí of Samarqand* (London: Luzac & Co., 1921; repr. 1978)

Buckley, R. P. (ed. and tr.), *The Book of the Islamic Market Inspector. Nihāyat al-Rutba fī Ṭalab al-Ḥisba (The Utmost Authority in the Pursuit of Ḥisba) by 'Abd al-Raḥmān b. Naṣr al-Shayzarī* (Oxford: Oxford University Press; University of Manchester, 1999)

Budge, E. A. W., *The Chronography of Gregory Abû'l Faraj ... known as Bar Hebraeus*, 2 vols (Oxford: Oxford University Press, 1932)

Budge, E. A. W., *The Laughable Stories Collected by Mâr Gregory John Bar-Hebræus* (London: Luzac & Co., 1897; repr. New York: AMS Press, 1976)

Budge, E. A. W., *The Syriac Book of Medicines: Syrian Anatomy, Pathology and Therapeutics*, 2 vols (London: Milford, 1913; repr. Amsterdam: Philo Press, 1976); the second volume, containing the translation, has recently been reprinted as Ernest Alfred Wallis Budge, *The Book of Medicines: Ancient Syrian Anatomy, Pathology and Therapeutics*, Kegan Paul Library of Arcana (London: Kegan Paul, 2002)

Bummel, J., 'Human Biological Reproduction in the Medicine of the Prophet: the Question of the Provenance and Formation of the Semen', in Greppin, et al. (eds), *Diffusion of Greco-Roman Medicine*, 169–84

Bürgel, J. C., 'Psychosomatic Methods of Cures in the Islamic Middle Ages', *Humaniora Islamica* 1 (1973), 157–72

Burnett, C., 'The Legend of the Three Hermes and Abū Ma'shar's Kitāb al-ulūf in the Latin Middle Ages', *Journal of the Warburg and Courtauld Institutes* 39 (1976), 231–4; repr. as item 5 in Burnett, *Magic and Divination*

Burnett, C., *The Introduction of Arabic Learning into England*, The Panizzi Lectures, 1996 (London: The British Library, 1997)

Burnett, C., *Magic and Divination in the Middle Ages: Texts and Techniques in the Islamic and Christian Worlds* (Aldershot: Ashgate, 1997)

Burnett, C., 'Spiritual Medicine in Music and Healing in Islam and Its Influence on Western Medicine' in P. Gouk (ed.), *Musical Healing in Cultural Contexts* (Aldershot: Ashgate, 2000) 81–91

Burnett, C., 'The Coherence of the Arabic-Latin Translation Programme in Toledo in the Twelfth Century', *Science in Context* 14 (2001), 249–88

Burnett, C., 'Stephen, the Disciple of Philosophy, and the Exchange of Medical Learning in Antioch', *Crusades* 5 (2006), 113–29

Burnett, C. and D. Jacquart (eds), *Constantine the African and 'Alī ibn al-'Abbās al-Maǧūsī: The Pantegni and Related Texts* (Leiden: Brill, 1994)

Burnett, C. et al., *Abū Ma'shar. The Abbreviation of 'The Introduction to Astrology': Together with the Medieval Latin Translation of Adlard of Bath*, Islamic Philosophy, Theology and Science: Texts and Studies 15 (Leiden: Brill, 1994)

Canaan, T., 'Arabic Magic Bowls', *Journal of the Palestine Oriental Society* 16 (1936), 79–127

Canaan, T., 'The Decipherment of Arabic Talismans', *Berytus* 4 (1937), 69–110 and 5 (1938), 141–51, reprinted in Savage-Smith, *Magic and Divination in Early Islam*, 126–77

Chamberlain, M., *Knowledge and Social Practice in Medieval Damascus, 1190–1350* (Cambridge: Cambridge University Press, 1994)

Chenery, T. and F. J. Steingass (tr.), *The Assemblies of al Harîri*, 2 vols (London: Williams and Norgate, 1867)

Chipman, L., 'How Effective Were Cough Remedies Known to Medieval Egyptians?', *Korot* 16 (2002), 135–57

Chipman, L., '*Minhāj al-dukkān* by Abū 'l-Munā al-Kūhīn al-'Aṭṭār: Aspects of Pharmacy and Pharmacists in Mamlūk Cairo', PhD thesis, Hebrew University of Jerusalem, 2006

Cholmeley, H. P. and M. McVaugh, 'The Galenic System' [*Kitāb al-Mudkhal*], translated from the Latin (*Isogoge*) in E. Grant (ed.), *A Source Book in Medieval Science* (Cambridge, MA: Harvard University Press, 1979), 705–15

Cohen, M. R., *Under Crescent and Cross: The Jews in the Middle Ages* (Princeton: Princeton University Press, 1994)

Cohen, M. R., *Poverty and Charity in the Jewish Community of Medieval Egypt* (Princeton, NJ: Princeton University Press, 2005)

Conrad, L. I., 'Arabic Plague Chronologies and Treatises: Social and Historical Factors in the Formation of a Literary Genre', *Studia Islamica* 54 (1981) 51–93

Conrad, L. I., '*Ṭā'ūn* and *wabā'*: Conceptions of Plague and Pestilence in Early Islam', *Journal of the Economic and Social History of the Orient* 25 (1982), 268–307

Conrad, L. I., 'Epidemic Diseases in Formal and Popular Thought in Early Islamic Society' in T. Ranger and P. Slack (eds), *Epidemics and Ideas: Essays on the Historical Perception of Pestilence* (Cambridge: Cambridge University Press, 1992), 77–99

Conrad, L. I., 'The Arab-Islamic Medical Tradition', in id., et al., *The Western Medical Tradition: 800 BC to AD 1800* (Cambridge: Cambridge University Press, 1994), 93–138

Conrad, L. I., 'Medicine: Traditional Practice', in J. L. Esposito (ed.), *The Oxford Encyclopedia of the Modern Islamic World*, 4 vols (New York: Oxford University Press, 1995), iii. 85–91

Conrad, L. I., 'Medicine and Martyrdom: Some Discussions of Suffering and Divine Justice in Early Islamic Society', in J. R. Hinnells and R. Porter (eds), *Religion, Health and Suffering* (London: Kegan Paul International, 1999), 212–36

Conrad, L. I., 'Usāma ibn Munqidh and Other Witnesses to Frankish and Islamic Medicine in the Era of the Crusades', in Amar, et al. (eds), *Ha-Refu'ah bi-Yerushalayim* (Medicine in Jerusalem) (1999), xxvii–lii

Conrad, L. I. and D. Wujastyk (eds), *Contagion: Perspectives from Pre-modern Societies* (Aldershot: Ashgate, 2000)

Crapanzano, V., *The Ḥamadsha: A Study in Moroccan Ethnopsychiatry* (Berkeley CA: University of California Press, 1973)

Crislip, A., *From Monastery to Hospital: Christian Monasticism and the Transformation of Health Care in Late Antiquity* (Ann Arbor, MI: University of Michigan Press, 2005) [see review in *Medical History* 51 (2007)]
Cruse, A., *Roman Medicine* (Stroud: Tempus, 2004)
Crussol des Epesse, B. T. de, *Discours sur l'œil d'Esmā'īl Gorgānī*, Bibliothèque iranienne 49 (Tehran: Presses universitaires d'Iran; Institut français de recherche en Iran, 1998)
Degen, R. and M. Ullmann, 'Zum Dispensatorium des Sābūr ibn Sahl', *Die Welt des Orients* 7 (1974), 241–58
Dietrich, A. (ed. and tr.), *Die Dioskurides-Erklärung des Ibn al-Baiṭār*, Abhandlungen der Akademie der Wissenschaften in Göttingen, phil.-hist. Kl., 3. Nr 191 (Göttingen: Vandenhoeck & Ruprecht, 1991)
Dodge, B., *The Fihrist of al-Nadim: a Tenth-Century Survey of Muslim Culture* (New York: Columbia University Press, 1970)
Dols, M. D., *The Black Death in the Middle East* (Princeton, NJ: Princeton University Press, 1977)
Dols, M. D., 'The Leper in Medieval Islamic Society', *Speculum* 58 (1983), 891–916
Dols, M. D., *Medieval Islamic Medicine: Ibn Riḍwān's Treatise 'On the Prevention of Bodily Ills in Egypt*, ed. Adil S. Gamal, tr. Michael Dols (Berkeley, CA: University of California Press, 1984)
Dols, M. D., 'The Origins of the Islamic Hospital: Myth and Reality', *Bulletin of the History of Medicine* 61 (1987), 367–90
Dols, M. D., *Majnūn: The Madman in Medieval Islamic Society* (Oxford: Clarendon Press, 1992)
Doutté, Ed., *Magie et religion dans l'Afrique du Nord* (Algiers: Typ. A. Jourdan, 1909; repr. Paris, 1984)
Drower, E. S., *The Book of the Zodiac*, Oriental Translation Fund 36 (London: Royal Asiatic Society, 1949)
Doufikar-Aerts, F., *Alexander Magnus Arabicus*, Diss. (Leiden: 2003)
Easterling, P., 'Menander, Loss and Survival', in A. Griffiths (ed.), *Stage Directions: Essays in Ancient Drama in Honour of E. W. Handley*, Bulletin of the Institute of Classical Studies. Supplement 66 (London: Institute of Classical Studies, 1995), 153–160
Ebrahimnejad, H., *Medicine, Public Health and the Qājār State*, Sir Henry Wellcome Asian Series 4 (Leiden: Brill, 2004)
*EI*² = *Encyclopaedia of Islam*, 2nd edn, ed. H. A. R. Gibbs, et al. (Leiden: Brill, 1960–2005), 11 vols
Eijk, Ph. van der, *Medicine and Philosophy in Classical Antiquity: Doctors and Philosophers on Nature, Soul, Health and Disease* (Cambridge: Cambridge University Press, 2005)
El-Abbadi, M., *The Life and Fate of the Ancient Library of Alexandria*, 2nd edn (Paris: Unesco/UNDP, 1992)
El Cheikh, N. M., 'Women's History: A Study of al-Tanūkhī', in M. Marín and R. Deguilhem (eds), *Writing the Feminine: Women in Arab Sources* (London; New York: I. B. Tauris, 2002), 129–48
El Cheikh, N. M., *Byzantium Viewed by the Arabs*, Harvard Middle Eastern Monographs 36 (Cambridge, MA; London: Harvard Unversity Press, 2004)
Edgington, S. B., 'The Hospital of St John in Jerusalem', in Amar, et al. (eds), *Ha-Refu'ah bi-Yerushalayim* (Medicine in Jerusalem), ix–xxv
Eldredge, L. M., *Benvenutus Grassus, The Wonderful Art of the Eye. A Critical Edition of the*

Middle English Translated of his De Probatissima Arte Oculorum (East Lansing, MI: Michigan State University Press, 1996)
Elgood, C., *A Medical History of Persia and the Eastern Caliphate* (Cambridge: Cambridge University Press, 1951)
Elgood, C., '*Ṭibb-ul-Nabbi* or Medicine of the Prophet' *Osiris* 14 (1962), 33–192
Elgood, C., *Safavid Medical Practice: The Practice of Medicine, Surgery and Gynaecology in Persia between 1500 AD and 1750 AD* (London: Luzac & Co., 1970)
Elkhadem, H., *Le 'Taqwīm al-ṣiḥḥa' (Tacuini sanitatis) d'Ibn Buṭlān: Un traité médical du XIe siècle. Histoire du texte, édition critique, traduction, commentaire*, Académie royale de Belgique, Classe des lettres, Fonds René Draguet 7 (Leuven: Peeters, 1990)
Elliot, R. H., *The Indian Operation of Couching for Cataract, Incorporating the Hunterian Lectures Delivered before the Royal College of Surgeons of England* (London: H. K. Lewis & Co., 1917)
Enc. Ir. = *Encyclopedia Iranica*, ed. E. Yarshater (London: Routledge and Costa Mesa, CA: Mazda Publications, 1985–)
Endress, G. and D. Gutas (eds), *A Greek-Arabic Lexicon* (Leiden: Brill, 1992–)
Estes, J. W. and L. Kuhnke, 'French Observations of Disease and Drug Use in Late Eighteenth-Century Cairo', *Journal of the History of Medicine and Allied Sciences* 39 (1984), 121–52
Fahd, T., 'Botany and Agriculture' in Rashed (ed.), *Encyclopedia*, iii. 813–52
Fähndrich, H. (ed.), *Treatise to Ṣalāh ad-Dīn on the Revival of the Art of Medicine by Ibn Jumay'*, Abhandlungen für die Kunde des Morgenlandes 46.3 (Wiesbaden: Kommissionsverlag F. Steiner, 1983)
Feigenbaum, A., 'Early History of Cataract and the Ancient Operation for Cataract', *American Journal of Ophthalmology* 49 (1960), 305–26
Feugère, M. et al., 'Les aiguilles à cataracte de Montbellet (Saône-et-Loire): Contribution à l'étude de l'ophtalmologie antique et islamique', *Jahrbuch des römisch-germanischen Zentralmuseums Mainz* 32 (1985), 436–508, and plates 53–67
Fierro, M., and J. Samsó (eds), *The Formation of al-Andalus, Part 2: Language, Religion, Culture and the Sciences*, The Formation of the Classical Islamic World 47 (Aldershot: Ashgate, 1995)
French, R., 'An Origin for the Bone Text of the "Five-Figure Series"', *Sudhoffs Archiv* 68 (1984), 143–58
Gallagher, N. E., *Medicine and Power in Tunisia, 1780–1900* (Cambridge: Cambridge University Press, 1983)
Garijo, I., 'Ibn Juljul's Treatise on Medicaments Not Mentioned by Dioscorides', in Fierro and Samsó, *Formation of al-Andalus, Part 2*, 419–30
Gazi, M. J., et al., 'The Immediate- and Medium-term Effect of Meswak on the Composition of Mixed Saliva', *Journal of Clinical Periodontology* 19 (1992), 113–17
Ghalioungui, P. (tr.), *Ḥunayn ibn Isḥāq, Questions on Medicine for Scholars* (Cairo: Al-Ahram Center for Scientific Translations, 1980)
Gigandet, S., *La* risāla al-Hārūniyya *de Masīḥ B. Ḥakam Al-Dimašqī, médecin* (Damascus: Institut français d'études arabes de Damas, 2001)
Gignoux, P., *Man and Cosmos in Ancient Iran* (Rome: Istituto Italiano per l'Africa e l'Oriente, 2001)
Gil'adi, A., *Children of Islam: Concepts of Childhood in Medieval Muslim Society* (Basingstoke: Macmillan in association with St Antony's College, Oxford, 1992)

Gil'adi, A., *Infants, Parents and Wet Nurses: Medieval Islamic Views on Breastfeeding and Their Social Implications* (Leiden: Brill, 1999)

Glick, T. F., et al. (eds), *Medieval Science, Technology and Medicine: An Encyclopedia* (New York; London: Routledge, 2005)

Gohlman, W., *The Life of Ibn Sina: a Critical Edition and Annotated Translation*, Studies in Islamic Philosophy and Science (Albany, NY: SUNY Press, 1974)

Goitein, S. D., 'The Medical Profession in the Light of the Cairo Geniza Documents', *Hebrew Union College Annual* 34 (1963), 177–94

Goitein, S. D., *A Mediterranean Society*, 5 vols (Berkeley, CA: University of California Press, 1967–88; repr. 1999)

Good, B. J., *Medicine, Rationality, and Experience: An Anthropological Perspective* (Cambridge: Cambridge University Press, 1994)

Goyanes, J. J. B., 'Todavia unas palabras sobre las venas cefalica y basilica', *Asclepio* 45 (1993), 61–70

Green, M. H., 'History of Science' in Suad Joseph (ed.), *Encyclopedia of Women and Islamic Cultures. Volume I: Methodologies, Paradigms and Sources* (Leiden: Brill, 2003), 358–61

Green, M. H., 'Constantine the African' in T. F. Glick, et al. (ed.), *Medieval Science, Technology and Medicine: An Encyclopedia* (New York; London: Routledge, 2005), 145–7

Greenhill, W. A., *A Treatise on the Small-Pox and Measles* (London: Sydenham Soc., 1848; repr. Birmingham, AL: Classics of Medicine Library, 1987)

Greppin, J. A. C. et al. (eds), *The Diffusion of Greco-Roman Medicine into the Middle East and the Caucasus* (Delmar, NY: Caravan Books, 1999)

Gruner, O. C., *A Treatise on the Canon of Medicine of Avicenna* (London: Luzac, 1930)

Gunny, A., *Images of Islam in Eighteenth-Century Writings* (London: Grey Seal, 1996)

Gutas, D., *Avicenna and the Aristotelian Tradition: Introduction to Reading Avicenna's Philosophical Works*, Islamic Philosophy and Theology 4 (Leiden: Brill, 1988)

Gutas, D., *Greek Thought, Arabic Culture: The Graeco-Arabic Translation Movement in Baghdad and Early 'Abbāsid Society (2nd–4th/8th–10th Centuries)* (London: Routledge, 1998)

Hamarneh, S. K., *The Physician, Therapist and Surgeon Ibn al-Quff* (Cairo: Atlas Press, 1974)

Hamarneh, S. K., 'Ibn al-'Ayn Zarbī and His Definitions of Diseases and Their Diagnoses' in A. Y. al-Hassan, et al. (eds), *Proceedings of the First International Symposium for the History of Arabic Science, April 5–12, 1976* (Aleppo: Institute for the History of Arabic Science, 1978), 305–23

Hamarneh, S. K., *Health Sciences in Early Islam*, ed. M. A. Anees, 2 vols (San Antonio, TX: Noor Health Foundation and Zahra Publications, 1983–4)

Hamarneh, S. K. and H. A. Awad, 'Medical Instruments' in *Fustat Finds: Coins, Medical Instruments, Textiles, and Other Artefacts from the Awad Collection* (Cairo: AUC Press, 2002), 176–83

Hameed, H. A., *Avicenna's Tract on Cardiac Drugs and Essays on Arab Cardiotherpy* (Karachi: Institute of Health and Tibbi Reserch; New Delhi: Institute of History of Medicine and Medical Research, 1983)

Hammami, S. M., *Kitāb al-Qūlang (Le livre de la colique) – al-Rāzī, édition critique et traduction* (Aleppo: Institute for the History of Arabic Science, 1983) [contains both the treatise by al-Rāzī and that by Ibn Sīnā]

Hampel, J., *Die Medizin der Zoroastrier im vorislamischen Iran* (Husum: Matthiesen Verlag, 1982)

Hasani, M., 'A Unique Manuscript of the Medieval Medical Treatise *al-Iktifā'* by Abū-l-Muṭrib 'Abd al-Raḥmān', *Manuscripta Orientalia* 5 (1999), 20–4

Haskell, H. D., 'Arabic Medical Literature', in M. J. L. Young, et al. (eds), *Religion, Learning, and Science in the 'Abbāsid Period* (Cambridge: Cambridge University Press, 1990)

al-Hassan, A. Y. and D. R. Hill, *Islamic Technology: An Illustrated History* (Cambridge: Cambridge University Press; Paris: Unesco, 1986)

Heinrichs, W., *Arabische Dichtung und griechische Poetik*, Beiruter Texte und Studien 8 (Beirut, Wiesbaden: F. Steiner, 1969)

Hirschberg, J., *Geschichte der Augenheilkunde*, Band I, Buch II, Teil 1, Graefe-Saemisch, *Handbuch der Gesamten Augenheilkunde* Bd. XIII (Leipzig 1908; repr. Hildesheim, 1977, and Sezgin (ed.), *Augenheilkunde*, iii. 1–250); tr. Fr. C. Blodi, *The History of Ophthalmology*, 11 vols (Bonn 1982–5)

Henninger, J., 'Beliefs in Spirits among the Pre-Islamic Arabs' in Savage-Smith (ed.), *Magic and Divination*, 1–53

Hill, D. R., *Islamic Science and Engineering*, Islamic Surveys (Edinburgh: Edinburgh University Press, 1993)

Hitti, P. K., *An Arab-Syrian Gentleman and Warrior in the Period of the Crusades* (New York: Columbia University Press, 1929; repr. 2000)

Horden, P., 'The Byzantine Welfare State: Image and Reality', *Bulletin: The Society for the Social History of Medicine* 37 (1985), 7–10

Horden, P., 'Religion as Medicine: Music in Medieval Hospitals' in P. Biller and J. Ziegler (eds), *Religion and Medicine in the Middle Ages*, York Studies in Medieval Theology 3 (Woodbridge: York Medieval Press in association with the Boydell Press, 2001), 135–53

Horden, P., 'The Earliest Hospitals in Byzantium, Western Europe, and Islam', *Journal of Interdisciplinary History* 35 (2005), 361–89

Horden, P., 'How Medicalized were Byzantine Hospitals?', *Medicina e Storia* 10 (2005), 45–74

Horden, P. and E. Savage-Smith, *The Year 1000: Medical Practice at the End of the First Millennium, Social History of Medicine* 13.2 (Oxford: Oxford University Press, 2000)

Horstmanshoff, H. F. J. and M. Stol (eds), *Magic and Rationality in Ancient Near Eastern and Graeco-Roman Medicine* (Leiden and Boston, MA: Brill, 2004)

Hoyland, R., *Arabia and the Arabs: From the Bronze Age to the Coming of Islam* (London: Routledge, 2001)

Hugonnard-Roche, H., 'Note sur Sergius de Reš 'Ainā, Traducteur du grec en syriaque et commentateur d'Aristote', in G. Endress and R. Kruk (eds), *The Ancient Tradition in Christian and Islamic Hellenism: Studies on the Transmission of Greek Philosophy and Sciences dedicated to H.J. Drossaart Lulofs on his Ninetieth Birthday* (Leiden: Research School CNWS, Leiden University: 1997), 121–43

Humphreys, R. S., *Islamic History: a Framework for Inquiry* (London: I. B. Tauris, 1991)

Institut du Monde Arabe, *L'Âge d'or des sciences arabes: exposition présentée à l'Institut du monde arabe, Paris, 25 octobre 2005–19 mars 2006* (Arles; Paris: Actes sud; Institut du monde arabe, 2005)

Isaacs, Haskell D. and C. F. Baker, *Medical and Para-Medical Manuscripts in the Cambridge Genizah Collections* (Cambridge: Cambridge University Press, 1994)

Iskandar, A. Z., *A Catalogue of Arabic Manuscripts on Medicine and Science in the Wellcome Historical Medical Library* (London: Wellcome Institute for the History of Medicine, 1967)

Iskandar, A. Z., 'An Attempted Reconstruction of the Late Alexandrian Medical Curriculum', *Medical History* 20 (1976), 235–58

Ispahany, B. (tr.) and A. Newman (rev.), *Islamic Medical Wisdom*: The Ṭibb al-a'imma (London: Muhammadi Trust, 1991)

Jacquart, D. and F. Micheau, *La médecine arabe et l'occident médiéval* (Paris: Maisonneuve et Larose, 1990)

Jacquart, D., 'The Influence of Arabic Medicine in the Medieval West', in Rashed (ed.), *Encyclopedia* (1996), iii. 963–84

Jacquart, D., *La médecine médiévale dans le cadre parisien (XIVe–XVe siècle)* (Paris: Fayard, 1998)

Jahier, H. and A. Noureddine, *Avicenne, Poème de la médecine* (Paris: Société d'Édition 'Les belles lettres', 1956)

Jiménez Brobeil, S. A., 'A Contribution to Medieval Pathological Gynaecology', *Journal of Paleopathology* 4 (1992), 155–61

Johnstone, P., *Ibn Qayyim al-Jawziyya, Medicine of the Prophet* (Cambridge: Islamic Texts Society, 1998)

Jouanna, J. (ed. and tr.), *Hippocrate. Airs, eaux, lieux* (Paris: Belles Lettres, 1996)

Kaadan, A. N., 'Albucasis and Extraction of Bladder Stone', *Journal of the International Society for the History of Islamic Medicine* 6 (2004), 28–33

Kahl, O., *Ya'qūb ibn Isḥāq al-Isrā'īlī's 'Treatise on the Errors of the Physicians in Damascus'. A Critical Edition of the Arabic Text Together with an Annotated English Translation*, Journal of Semitic Studies Suppl. 10 (Oxford: Oxford University Press on behalf of University of Manchester, 2000)

Kahl, O., *Sābūr ibn Sahl. The Small Dispensatory: Translated from the Arabic together with a Study and Glossaries* (Leiden: Brill, 2004)

Kalus, L., *Catalogue des cachets, bulles et talismans islamiques* (Paris: Bibliothèque nationale de France, 1981)

Kalus, L., *Catalogue of Islamic Seals and Talismans, Ashmolean Museum* (Oxford: Oxford University Press, 1986)

Karim, M., *Female Genital Mutilation (Circumcision): Historical, Social, Religious, Sexual, and Legal Aspects* (Cairo: National Population Council, 1998)

Kedar, B. Z., 'A Twelfth-Century Description of the Jerusalem Hospital' in H. Nicholson (ed.), *The Military Orders. Volume 2: Welfare and Warfare* (Aldershot: Ashgate, 1998), 3–26

Khan, G., *Arabic Legal and Administrative Documents in the Cambridge Genizah Collections*, Cambridge University Library Genizah Series 10 (Cambridge: Cambridge University Press, 1993)

Klein-Franke, F., *Iatromathematics in Islam: A Study on Yuḥanna Ibn aṣ-Ṣalt's Book on* Astrological Medicine, *Edited for the First Time*, Texte und Studien zur Orientalistik 3 (Hildesheim: Georg Olms Verlag, 1984)

Klein-Franke, F. and M. Zhu, 'Rashid ad-Din as a Transmitter of Chinese Medicine', *Le Muséon* 109 (1996), 396–404

Klein-Franke, F. and M. Zhu, 'Rashid ad-Din and the *Tansuqnamah*: The Earliest Translation of Chinese Medical Literature in the West', *Le Muséon* 111 (1998), 427–45

Klibansky, R., et al., *Saturn and Melancholy* (London: Nelson, 1964; repr. Nendeln: Kraus Reprint, 1979)

Knight, M., 'Curing Cut or Ritual Mutilation? Some Remarks on the Practice of Female and Male Circumcision in Graeco-Roman Egypt', *Isis* 92 (2001), 317–38

Koning, P. de, *Trois traités d'anatomie arabes* (Leiden: Brill, 1903; repr. Frankfurt, 1986)

Kraemer, J. L., 'Women Speak for Themselves', *The Cambridge Genizah Collections: Their Contents and Significance*, Cambridge University Library Genizah Series 1 (Cambridge: Cambridge University Press, 2002), 178–216

Kriss, R. and H. Kriss-Heinrich, *Volksglaube im Bereich des Islam. Band II. Amulette, Zauberformeln und Beschwörungen* (Wiesbaden: Otto Harrassowitz, 1962)

Kruk, R., '*De Goede arts*: Ideaalbeeld en werkelijkheid in de middeleuws-Arabisch wereld', *Hermeneus* 71.2 (April 1999), 140–8

Kruk, R., 'Harry Potter in the Gulf: Contemporary Islam and the Occult', *British Journal of Middle Eastern Studies* 32 (2005), 47–73

Kuhne, R., 'El Sirr ṣināʿat al-ṭibb de Abū Bakr Muḥammad b. Zakariyya' al-Rāzī', *Al-Qantara*, 3 (1982), 347–414; 5 (1984), 235–92; 6 (1985), 369–95

Kunitzsch, P., 'Über das Frühstadium der arabischen Aneignung antiken Gutes', *Saeculum* 26 (1975), 268–82

Kuriyama, S., *The Expressiveness of the Body and the Divergence of Greek and Chinese Medicine* (New York: Zone Books, 1999)

Lapidus, I. M., A *History of Islamic Societies*, 2nd edn (Cambridge: Cambridge University Press, 2002)

Latham, J. D. and H. D. Isaacs, *Kitāb al-Ḥummayāt li-Isḥāq Sulaymān al-Isrā'īlī (al-Maqāla al-Thālitha: fī al-sill) Isaac Judaeus: On Fevers (The Third Discourse: On Consumption)*, Arabic Technical and Scientific Texts 8 (Cambridge: Pembroke Arabic Texts, 1981)

Le Coz, R., *Les médecins nestoriens au Moyen Âge: Les maîtres des Arabes* (Paris: L'Harmattan, 2004)

Leibowitz, J. O. and S. Marcus, *Sefer Hanisyonot: Book of Medical Experiences Attributed to Abraham Ibn Ezra* (Jerusalem: Magnes Press, The Hebrew University, 1984)

Leiser, G., 'Medical Education in Islamic Lands from the Seventh to the Fourteenth Century', *Journal of the History of Medicine and Allied Sciences* 38 (1983), 48–75

Leiser, G., and N. al-Khaledy, *Questions and Answers for Physicians: A Medieval Arabic Study Manual by ʿAbd al-ʿAzīz al-Sulamī* (Leiden: Brill, 2004)

Levey, M., *The Medical Formulary or Aqrābādhīn of al-Kindī* (Madison, WI: University of Wisconsin Press, 1966)

Levey, M., *Medical Ethics of Medieval Islam, with Special Reference to al-Ruhāwī's 'Practical Ethics of the Physician'*, Transactions of the American Philosophical Society n.s. 57.3 (Philadelphia: American Philosophical Society, 1967)

Levey, M., *Substitute Drugs in Early Arabic Medicine: With Special Reference to the Texts of Masarjawaih, al-Rāzī, and Pythagoras*, Veröffentlichungen der Internationalen Gesellschaft für Geschichte der Pharmazie N. F. 37 (Stuttgart: Wissenschaftliche Verlagsgesellschaft, 1971)

Levey, M., *Early Arabic Pharmacology: An Introduction Based on Ancient and Medieval Sources* (Leiden: Brill, 1973)

Lewis, B., *Islam: From the Prophet Muhammad to the Capture of Constantinople*, 2 vols (Macmillan: London, 1974)

Lewis, B., *What Went Wrong* (London: Weidenfeld and Nicolson, 2002)

Libera, A., *Penser au Moyen-Âge* (Paris: Éditions du Seuil, 1991)

Liebeskind, C., 'Unani Medicine of the Subcontinent', in J. van Alphen and A. Aris (eds), *Oriental Medicine: An Illustrated Guide to the Asian Arts of Healing* (London: Serindia, 1995)

Littré, É., *Œuvres complètes d'Hippocrate*, 10 vols (Paris: Baillière, 1839–61, repr. Amsterdam: Hakkert, 1961–82)

Llavero Ruiz, E., 'Un tratado de cirugía hispanoárabe del siglo XIV: El *Kitāb al-Istiqṣā'* de Muḥammad al-Šafra. Edición crítica y traducción española con glosario de terminos técnicos y sustancias', Doctoral diss. (Granada, 1989), microfiche

Llavero Ruiz, E., 'La medicina granadina del siglo XIV y Muḥammad al-Šafra', *Revista del Centro de Estudios Históricos de Granada y su Reino* 6 (1992), 129–50

Lloyd, G. E. R. and N. Sivin, *The Way and the Word: Science and Medicine in Early China and Greece* (New Haven, CT; London: Yale University Press, 2002)

Lonie, I. M., 'Fever Pathology in the Sixteenth Century: Tradition and Innovation' in W. F. Bynum and V. Nutton (eds), *Theories of Fever from Antiquity to the Enlightenment, Medical History*, Supplement 1 (London: Wellcome Institute for the History of Medicine, 1981), 19–44

Lory, P., 'La magie des lettres dans le *Šams al-ma'ārif* d'al-Būnī', *Bulletin d'Études Orientales* 39–40 (1987–8), 97–111

Lyall, Ch. J. (ed.), *The Mufaḍḍalīyāt: An Anthology of Ancient Arabian Odes*, 3 vols (Oxford: Clarendon Press, 1918–24)

MacLean, I., *Logic, Signs and Nature in the Renaissance: The Case of Learned Medicine* (Cambridge: Cambridge University Press, 2002)

Mackie, G., 'Ending Footbinding and Infibulation: A Convention Account', *American Sociological Review* 61 (1996), 999–1017

Maddison, F. and E. Savage-Smith, *Science, Tools and Magic*, 2 vols (London; Oxford: Azimuth Editions; Oxford University Press, 1997)

Majeed, A., 'How Islam Changed Medicine', *British Medical Journal* 351 (24–31 Dec 2005) 1486–7

Makdisi, G., *The Rise of Colleges: Institutions of Learning in Islam and the West* (Edinburgh: Edinburgh University Press, 1981)

Makdisi, G., *The Rise of Humanism in Classical Islam and the Christian West with Special Reference to Scholasticism* (Edinburgh: Edinburgh University Press, 1990)

Marcus, A., *The Middle East on the Eve of Modernity* (New York: Columbia University Press, 1989)

Margoliouth, D. S., *The Table-talk of a Mesopotamian Judge* (London: Royal Asiatic Society, 1921–2)

Marmura, M. E., *Avicenna, The Metaphysics of The Healing* (Provo, UT: Brigham Young University Press, 2005)

Mattock, J. N. and M. C. Lyons, *Kitāb Buqrāṭ fī ṭabī'at al-insān: On the Nature of Man*, Arabic Technical and Scientific Texts 4 (Cambridge: Cambridge Middle East Centre, 1968)

Mattock, J. N. and M. C. Lyons, *Kitāb Buqrāṭ fī al-amrāḍ al-bilādiyya: On Endemic Diseases (Airs, Waters and Places)*, Arabic Technical and Scientific Texts 5 (Cambridge: Cambridge Middle East Centre, 1969)

Mavroudi, M., *A Byzantine Book on Dream Interpretation: The* Oneirocriticon of Achmet *and its Arabic Sources* (Leiden: Brill, 2002)

Menasce, J. P. de, *Le troisième livre du Dēnkart*, Travaux de l'Institut d'Études Iraniennes 5 (Paris: Librairie C. Klincksieck, 1973)

McVaugh, M. R., 'Cataracts and Hernias: Aspects of Surgical Practice in the Fourteenth Century', *Medical History* 45 (2001), 319–40

McVaugh, M. R., *Medicine Before the Plague: Practitioners and their Patients in the Crown of Aragon, 1285–1345* (Cambridge: Cambridge University Press, 1993)

Meyerhof, M., *The Book of the Ten Treatises on the Eye Ascribed to Ḥunain ibn Isḥāq (809–877 AD). The Earliest Existing Systematic Text-Book of Ophthalmology* (Cairo: Government Press, 1928); repr. in Sezgin (ed.), *Augenheilkunde* (1986), i. 1–517

Meyerhof, M., 'Ibn al-Nafīs und seine Theorie des Lungenkreislaufs', *Quellen und Studien zur Geschichte der Naturwissenschaften und der Medizin* 4 (1933), 37–88, abridged version in *Isis* 22 (1935), 100–20

Meyerhof, M., 'Thirty-Three Clinical Observations by Rhazes (circa 900 AD)', *Isis* 23 (1935), 321–56 and 14 pages of Arabic; reprinted in M. Meyerhof, *Studies in Medieval Arabic Medicine: Theory and Practice*, ed. P. Johnstone (London: Variorum Reprints, 1984), item 5

Meyerhof, M., 'The History of Trachoma Treatment in Antiquity and During the Arabic Middle Ages', *Bulletin of the Ophthalmological Society of Egypt* 29 (1936), 26–87; repr. in Sezgin (ed.), *Augenheilkunde* (1986), iii. 527–88

Meyerhof, M., *The Cataract Operations of 'Ammār ibn 'Alī al-Mawsilī, Oculist of Cairo* (Barcelona: Laboratorios del Norte de España, 1937); repr. in Sezgin (ed.), *Augenheilkunde* (1986), iii. 591–698

Meyerhof, M., *Šarḥ asmā' al-'uqqār (l'explication des noms de drogues): un glossaire de matière médicale, composé par Maïmonide*, Mémoires présentés à l'Institut d'Égypte 41 (Cairo: Institut français d'archéologie orientale du Caire, 1940)

Meyerhof M. and C. Prüfer, 'Die angebliche Augenheilkunde des Tābit ibn Qurra', *Zentralblatt für Praktische Augenheilkunde* 35 (1911), 4–8 and 38–41; repr. in Sezgin (ed.), *Augenheilkunde* (1986), iii. 360–8

Meyerhof, M. and C. Prüfer, 'Die Augenheilkunde des Juḥannā b. Māsawaih (777–857 n. Chr.)', *Der Islam* 6 (1915), 216–56; repr. in Sezgin (ed.), *Augenheilkunde* (1986), iii. 417–56

Meyerhof, M. and J. Schacht, *The Medico-Philosophical Controversy between Ibn Butlan of Baghdad and Ibn Ridwan of Cairo* (Cairo: Egyptian University, 1937)

Micheau, F., 'The Scientific Institutions of the Medieval Near East', in Rashed (ed.), *Encyclopedia*, iii. 985–1007

Michot, Y. J., 'Ibn Taymiyya on Astrology: Annotated Translation of Three Fatwas', *Journal of Islamic Studies* 11 (2000), 147–208, repr. in Savage-Smith (ed.), *Magic and Divination*, 277–340

Miller, T., 'The Knights of Saint-John and the Hospitals of the Latin West', *Speculum* 53 (1978), 709–33

Milwright, M., 'The Balsam of Maṭariyya: an Exploration of a Medieval Panacea', *Bulletin of SOAS* 66 (2003), 193–209

Mitchell, P. D., 'The Palaeopathology of Skulls Recovered from a Medieval Cave Cemetery near Safed, Israel (Thirteenth to Seventeenth Century)', *Levant* 36 (2004), 243–50

Mitchell, P. D., *Medicine in the Crusades: Warfare, Wounds and the Medieval Surgeon* (Cambridge: Cambridge University Press, 2004)

Montgomery, S. L., *Science in Translation* (Chicago, IL: Chicago University Press, 2000)

Morony, M. G., *Iraq after the Muslim Conquest* (Princeton, NJ: Princeton University Press, 1984)

Morray, D., *An Ayyubid Notable and his World: Ibn al-Adīm and Aleppo as Portrayed in his Biographical Dictionary of People Associated with the City* (Leiden: Brill, 1994)

Motzki, H., *Hadith: Origins and Developments*, Formation of the Classical Islamic World 28 (Aldershot: Ashgate Variorum, 2004)

Müller-Bütow, H. and Spies, O., *Anatomie und Chirurgie des Schädels, insbesondere der Hals-, Nasen- und Ohrenkrankheiten nach Ibn al-Quff*, Ars medica. III. Abteilung, Arabische Medizin vol. 1 (Berlin: Walter de Gruyter, 1971)

Murphey, R., 'Ottoman Medicine and Transculturalism from the Sixteenth through the Eighteenth Century', *Bulletin of the History of Medicine* 66 (1992), 376–403

Musallam, B. F., *Sex and Society in Islam: Birth Control Before the Nineteenth Century* (Cambridge; New York: Cambridge University Press, 1983)

Musallam, B. F., 'The Human Embryo in Arabic Scientific and Religious Thought', in G. R. Dunstan (ed.), *The Human Embryo: Aristotle and the Arabic and European Traditions* (Exeter: University of Exeter Press, 1990), 32–46

Naveh, J. and S. Shaked, *Amulets and Magic Bowls*, 1st edn (Jerusalem, 1985; 2nd edn, 1987)

Newman, A., '*Tašrīḥ-i Manṣūrī*: Human Anatomy between the Galenic and Prophetical Medical Traditions', in Ž. Vesel, et al. (eds) *La science dans le monde iranien à l'époque islamique* (Tehran: Institut français de recherche en Iran, 1998; 2nd edn, 2004), 253–71

Nutton, V., *Ancient Medicine* (London: Routledge, 2004)

O'Neill, Y. V., 'The Fünfbilderserie Reconsidered', *Bulletin of the History of Medicine* 43 (1969), 236–45

O'Neill, Y. V., 'The Fünfbilderserie: A Bridge to the Unknown', *Bulletin of the History of Medicine* 51 (1977), 538–49

Pahlitzsch, J., 'Ärzte ohne Grenzen. Melkitische, jüdische und samaritanische Ärzte in Ägypten und Syrien zur Zeit der Kreuzzüge', in K. Steger, K. P. Jankrift (eds), *Gesundheit–Krankheit: Kulturtransfer medizininschen Wissens von der Spätantike bis in die Frühe Neuzeit* (Cologne: Böhlau, 2004), 101–20

Perho, I., *The Prophet's Medicine: A Creation of the Muslim Traditionalist Scholars*, Studia Orientalia 74 (Helsinki: Finnish Oriental Society, 1995)

Peters, F. E., 'Hermes and Harran: The Roots of Arabic-Islamic Occultism', in M. Mazzaoui and V. B. Moreen (eds), *Intellectual Studies on Islam: Essays Written in Honor of Martin B. Dickson* (Salt Lake City, UT, 1990), 185–215; repr. in Savage-Smith, *Magic and Divination*, 54–85

Pielow, D. A. M., *Die Quellen der Weisheit: Die arabische Magie im Spiegel des* Uṣūl al-Ḥikma *von Aḥmad ʿAlī al-Būnī*, Arabistische Texte und Studien 8 (Hildesheim: Olms, 1995)

Plessner, M., 'The Natural Sciences and Medicine', in J. Schacht and C. E. Bosworth (eds), *The Legacy of Islam*, 2nd edn (Oxford: Clarendon Press, 1974), 425–60

Pormann, P. E., 'Theory and Practice in the Early Hospitals in Baghdad: al-Kaškarī On Rabies and Melancholy', *Zeitschrift für Geschichte der Arabisch-Islamischen Wissenschaften* 15 (2002–3), 197–248

Pormann, P. E., 'Jean le grammarien et le *De sectis* dans la littérature médicale d'Alexandrie', in I. Garofalo and A. Roselli (eds), *Galenismo e medicina tardoantica: fonti greche, latine e arabe* (Naples: Istituto universitario orientale, 2003), 233–63

Pormann, P. E., 'The *Parisinus Graecus* 2293 as a Document of Scientific Activity in Swabian Sicily', *Arabic Sciences and Philosophy* 13 (2003), 137–61

Pormann, P. E., 'The Alexandrian Summary (*Jawāmi'*) of Galen's *On the Sects for Beginners*: Commentary or Abridgment?', in P. Adamson, et al. (eds), *Philosophy, Science and Exegesis in Greek, Arabic and Latin Commentaries, Bulletin of the Institute of Classical Studies*, Supplement 83, 2 vols (London, 2004), ii. 11–33

Pormann, P. E., 'La querelle des médecins arabistes et hellénistes et l'héritage oublié', in V. Boudon-Millot et G. Cobolet (eds), *Lire les médecins grecs à la Renaissance: Aux origines de l'édition médicale, Actes du colloque international de Paris (19–20 septembre 2003)*, collection Médic@ (Paris: De Boccard Edition-Diffusion, 2004), 113–41

Pormann, P. E., *The Oriental Tradition of Paul of Aegina's 'Pragmateia'*, Studies in Ancient Medicine 29 (Leiden: Brill, 2004)

Pormann, P. E., 'Yūḥannā ibn Sarābiyūn: Further Studies into the Transmission of his Works', *Arabic Sciences and Philosophy* 14.2 (2004), 233–62

Pormann, P. E., 'The Physician and the Other: Images of the Charlatan in Medieval Islam', *Bulletin of the History of Medicine* 79 (2005), 189–227

Pormann, P. E., 'The Arab "Cultural Awakening (*Nahḍa*)", 1870–1950, and the Classical Tradition', *International Journal of the Classical Tradition* 13.1 (Summer 2006), 3–20

Pormann, P. E., 'Islamic Hospitals in the Time of al-Muqtadir', in *Abbasid Studies: Occasional Papers of the School of 'Abbasid Studies, Leuven, 27 June – 1 July 2004*, ed. J. Nawas, et al. (Leuven; Dudley, MA: Peeters, 2006) [forthcoming]

Porter, V., 'Islamic Seals: Magical or Practical?' in A. Jones (ed.), *University Lectures in Islamic Studies*, vol. 2 (London, 1998), 135–49; repr. in Savage-Smith, *Magic and Divination*, 178–200

Rāghib, Y., *Marchands d'étoffes du Fayyoum au IIIe/IXe siècle d'après leurs archives (actes et lettres)*, Supplément aux Annales islamologiques: cahier nos. 2, 5, 14, 16, 5 vols (Cairo: Institut français d'archéologie orientale, 1982–96)

Rahman, F., *Health and Medicine in the Islamic Tradition: Change and Identity* (New York: Crossroad, 1987) [see review in *History of Science* 26 (1988)]

Rapoport, Y., *Marriage, Money and Divorce in Medieval Islamic Society* (Cambridge: Cambridge University Press, 2005)

Rashed, R. (ed.), *Encyclopedia of the History of Arabic Science*, 3 vols (London: Routledge, 1996)

Richards, D. S., 'A Doctor's Petition for a Salaried Post in Saladin's Hospital', *Social History of Medicine* 5 (1992), 297–306

Richards, D. S., 'More on the Death of the Ayyubid Sultan al-Ṣāliḥ Najm al-Dīn Ayyūb', in Ç. Balım-Harding and C. Imber (eds), *The Balance of Truth: Essays in Honour of Professor Geoffrey Lewis* (Istanbul: Isis Press, 2000), 269–74

Richter-Bernburg, L., 'Abū Bakr Muḥammad Al Rāzī's (Rhazes) Medical Works', *Medicina nei Secoli* 6 (1994), 377–92

Riddle, J. M., *Dioscorides on Pharmacy and Medicine* (Austin, TX: University of Texas Press, 1985)

Rispler-Chaim, V., 'The Siwāk: A Medieval Islamic Contribution to Dental Care', *Journal of the Royal Asiatic Society*, ser. 3, 2 (1992) 13–20

Robinson, C., *Islamic Historiography* (Cambridge: Cambridge University Press, 2003)

Rosenthal, F., *The Muqaddimah: An Introduction to History* (London: Routledge and Kegan Paul, 1958)

Rosenthal, F., 'The Physician in Medieval Muslim Society', *Bulletin of the History of Medicine* 52 (1978), 475–91

Rosenthal, F., *The Classical Heritage in Islam* (London: Routledge, 1975; repr. 1992)

Rosner, F. and S. Munter (eds and tr.), *Maimonides' Treatise on Haemorrhoids: Medical Answers (responsa)*, The Medical Writings of Moses Maimonides 3 (Philadelphia, PA: Lippincott, 1969)

Rosner, F., *Maimonides' Medical Writings: Treatises on Poison, Hemorrhoids, Cohabitation* (Haifa: The Maimonides Research Institute, 1984)

Roueché, M., 'Did Medical Students Study Philosophy in Alexandria?', *Bulletin of the Institute of Classical Studies* 43 (1999), 153–69

Rubin, Z., '*Res Gestae Divi Saporis*: Greek and Middle Iranian in a Document of Sasanian Anti-Roman Propaganda', in J. N. Adams, et al. (eds), *Bilingualism in Ancient Society: Language Contact and the Written Text* (Oxford: Oxford University Press, 2002), 267–97

Russell, A., *The Natural History of Aleppo, and Parts Adjacent* (London: A. Millar, 1756)

Russell, G., 'The Anatomy of the Eye in 'Alī ibn al-'Abbās al-Magūsī: A Textbook Case', in Burnett and Jacquart (eds), *Constantine the African*, 247–65

Sabra, A., *Poverty and Charity in Medieval Islam. Mamluk Egypt, 1250–1517* (Cambridge: Cambridge University Press, 2000)

Sachedina, A. A., *The Just Ruler (al-sultān al-'ādil) in Shī'ite Islam: The Comprehensive Authority of the Jurist in Imamite Jurisprudence* (Oxford: Oxford University Press, 1988)

Sadek, M. M., *The Arabic Materia Medica of Dioscorides* (Quebec: Les Éditions du Sphinx, 1983)

Saeed, Ahmad (compiler), *Prophetic Medical Sciences*, tr. Badr Azimabadi (New Delhi: Saeed International, 1993)

Said, H. M., *Hamdard Pharmacopoeia of Eastern Medicine*, 2nd edn (Karachi: Hamdard Academy, 1970; repr. Delhi: Sri Satguru Publications, 1997)

Saliba, G., 'The Role of the Astrologer in Medieval Islamic Society', *Bulletin d'études orientales* 44 (1992), 45–67; repr. in Savage-Smith, *Magic and Divination*, 341–70

Sanagustin, F., 'La chirurgie dans le Canon de la medécine (*al-Qānūn fī-ṭ-ṭibb*) d'Avicenne (Ibn Sīnā)', *Arabica* 33 (1986), 84–122

Sanjana, Dastur Peshotan Bahramji, *The Ḍinkarḍ*, 19 vols (Bombay, 1869–1928)

Sari, N. and M. Bedizel Zülfikar, 'The Paracelsusian Influence on Ottoman Medicine in the Seventeenth and Eighteenth centuries', in E. İhsanoğlu (ed.), *Transfer of Modern Science and Technology to the Muslim World: Proceedings of the International Symposium on 'Modern Sciences and the Muslim World'* (Istanbul: Research Centre for Islamic History, Art and Culture, 1992), 157–79

Savage-Smith, E., 'Ibn al-Nafīs's *Perfected Book on Ophthalmology* and His Treatment of Trachoma and Its Sequelae', *Journal for the History of Arabic Science* 4 (1980), 147–204

Savage-Smith, E., 'Drug Therapy of Eye Diseases in Seventeenth-Century Islamic Medicine: The Influence of the "New Chemistry" of the Paracelsians', *Pharmacy in History* 29 (1987), 3–28

Savage-Smith, E., 'Attitudes toward Dissection in Medieval Islam', *Journal of the History of Medicine and Allied Sciences* 50 (1995), 67–110

Savage-Smith, E., 'Medicine', in Rashed (ed.), *Encyclopedia* (1996), iii. 903–62

Savage-Smith, E., 'Europe and Islam', in I. Loudon (ed.), *Western Medicine: An Illustrated History* (Oxford, Oxford University Press, 1997), 40–53

Savage-Smith, E., 'The Exchange of Medical and Surgical Ideas between Europe and Islam', in Greppin, et al. (eds), *Diffusion of Greco-Roman Medicine* (1999), 27–55

Savage-Smith, E., 'The Practice of Surgery in Islamic Lands: Myth and Reality', in Horden and Savage-Smith (eds), *The Year 1000* (2000), 307–21

Savage-Smith, E., 'Galen's Lost Ophthalmology and the *Summaria Alexandrinorum*', in V. Nutton (ed.), *The Unknown Galen*, Bulletin of the Institute of Classical Studies Supplement 77 (London: Institute of Classical Studies, 2002), 121–38

Savage-Smith, E., 'Islam', in R. Porter (ed.), *The Cambridge History of Science. Volume 4: Eighteenth-Century Science* (Cambridge: Cambridge University Press, 2003), 649–68

Savage-Smith, E., 'Safavid Magic Bowls', in J. Thompson and S. R. Canby (eds), *Hunt for Paradise: Court Arts of Safavid Iran, 1505–1576* (Milan: Skira, 2003), 240–7

Savage-Smith, E., *Magic and Divination in Early Islam*, The Formation of the Classical Islamic World 42 (London: Ashgate, 2004)

Savage-Smith, E., 'Between Reader and Text: Some Medieval Arabic Marginalia', in D. Jacquart and C. Burnett (eds), *Scientia in margine: Études sur les* marginalia *dans les manuscrits scientifiques du Moyen Âge à la Renaissance* (Geneva: Droz, 2005), 75–101

Savage-Smith, E., 'Anatomical Illustration in Arabic Manuscripts', in A. Contadini (ed.), *Arab Painting: Text and Image in Illustrated Arabic Manuscripts* (London: I. B. Tauris, 2007) [forthcoming]

Savage-Smith, E., *Islamic Medical Manuscripts at the National Library of Medicine* at www.nlm.nih.gov/hmd/arabic

Sbath, P., 'Le formulaire des hôpitaux d'Ibn abi Bayan, médecin du bimaristan annacery au Caire au xiiie siècle', *Bulletin de l'Institut d'Égypte* 15 (1932–3), 9–78

Sbath, P. and M. Meyerhof, *Le livre des questions sur l'œil de Ḥonain ibn Isḥāq*, Mémoires présentés à l'Institut d'Égypte 36 (Cairo: Imprimerie de l'Institut Français d'Archéologie Orientale, 1938); repr. in Sezgin (ed.), *Augenheilkunde*, ii. 745–897

Scanlon, G. T., 'Housing and Sanitation: Some Aspects of Medieval Islamic Public Service', in A. H. Hourani and S. M. Stern (eds), *The Islamic City* (Oxford; Philadelphia: Cassirer; University of Pennsylvania Press, 1970), 179–94

Scarborough, J. (ed.), *Symposium on Byzantine Medicine*, Dumbarton Oaks Papers 38 (Washington, DC: Dumbarton Oaks, 1985)

Schoeler, G., 'Der Verfasser der Augenheilkunde K. *Nūr al-'uyūn* und das Schema der 8 Präliminarien im 1. Kapitel des Werkes', *Der Islam* 64 (1987), 87–97

Schönfeld, J., *Über die Steine: Das 14. Kapitel aus dem 'Kitāb al-Muršid' des Muḥammad ibn Aḥmad at-Tamīmī, nach dem Pariser Manuskript herausgegeben, übersetzt und kommentiert*, Islamkundliche Untersuchungen 38 (Freiburg: K. Schwarz, 1976)

Seligmann, S., *Die Zauberkraft des Auges und das Berufen. Ein Kapitel aus der Geschichte des Aberglaubens* (Hamburg: Friederichsen, 1922)

Serjeant, R. B. (tr.), *The Book of Misers*, rev. Ezzeddin Ibrahim (Reading: Garnet, 1997)

Serra, G., *Da 'tragedia' e 'commedia' a 'lode' e 'biasimo'*, Beiträge zum antiken Drama und seiner Rezeption 19 (Stuttgar; Weimar: Metzler, 2002)

Sesiano, J., *Un traité médiéval sur les carrés magiques: De l'arrangement harmonieux des nombres* (Lausanne: Presses polytechniques et universitaires romandes, 1996)

Sezgin, F., *Medizin-Pharmazie-Zoologie-Tierheilkunde bis ca 430 H.*, Geschichte des arabischen Schrifttums 3 (Leiden: Brill, 1970)

Sezgin, F., *Astrologie-Meteorologie und Verwandtes bis ca 430 H.*, Geschichte des arabischen Schrifttums 7 (Leiden: Brill, 1979)

Sezgin, F. (ed.), *Augenheilkunde im Islam: Texte, Studien und Übersetzungen*, 4 vols (Frankfurt: Institut für Geschichte der Arabisch-Islamischen Wissenschaften, 1986)

Shahîd, I., *Byzantium and the Arabs in the Sixth Century* (Washington, DC: Dumbarton Oaks, pt 1, 1995; pt 2.1, 2002; pt 2.2, in preparation)

Shah, M. H., *The General Principles of Avicenna's Canon of Medicine* (Karachi: Naveed Clinic, 1966)

Shani, R., 'A Judeo-Persian Talismanic Textile', in S. Shaked and A. Netzer (eds), *Irano-Judaica IV* (Jerusalem: Ben-Zvi Institute for the Study of Jewish Communities in the East, 1999), 251–7

Shatzmiller, J., *Jews, Medicine, and Medieval Society* (Berkeley, CA; London: University of California Press, 1994)

Shiloah, A., 'Jewish and Muslim Traditions of Music Therapy', in P. Horden (ed.), *Music as Medicine: The History of Music Therapy since Antiquity*, (Aldershot: Ashgate, 2000), 69–83

Sigerist, H., *A History of Medicine*, 2 vols (New York: Oxford University Press, 1950–61)

Siggel, A., *Die indischen Bücher aus dem Paradies der Weisheit über die Medizin des Ali ibn Sahl Rabban at-Tabari*, Abhandlungen der Geistes- und Sozialwissenschaftlichen Klasse 1950, no. 14 (Mainz: Verlag der Akademie der Wissenschaften und der Literatur; F. Steiner: Wiesbaden, 1951)

Siggel, A., *Die propädeutischen Kapitel aus dem Paradies der Weisheit über die Medizin des ʿAlī b. Sahl Rabban aṭ-Ṭabarī*, Abhandlungen der Geistes- und Sozialwissenschaftlichen Klasse 1953, no. 8 (Mainz: Verlag der Akademie der Wissenschaften und der Literatur; F. Steiner: Wiesbaden, 1953)

Siraisi, N. G., *Avicenna in Renaissance Italy: The* Canon *and the Medical Teaching in Italian Universities after* 1500 (Princeton, NJ: Princeton University Press, 1987)

Soucek, P., 'An Illustrated Manuscript of al-Bīrūnī's *Chronology of Ancient Nations*', in P. J. Chelkowski (ed.), *The Scholar and the Saint: Studies in Commemoration of Abu'l-Rayhan al-Bīrūnī and Jalal al-Din al-Rūmī* (New York: New York University Press, 1975), 103–68

Spink, M. S. and G. L. Lewis (ed. and tr.), *Albucasis, On Surgery and Instruments* (Berkeley, CA: University of California Press, 1973)

Steinschneider, M., 'Wissenschaft und Charlatanerie unter den Arabern im neunten Jahrhundert', *Virchows Archiv* 36 (1866), 570–86; 37 (1866), 560–5; repr. in *Beiträge zur Geschichte der arabisch-islamischen Medizin*, 3 vols, (Frankfurt: Institut für Geschichte der arabisch-islamischen Wissenschaften, 1987), i. 39–61

Strohmaier, G., 'Ärztliche Ausbildung im islamischen Mittelalter', *Klio* 61 (1979) 519–24, repr. in id., *Von Demokrit bis Dante: Die Bewahrung antiken Erbes in der Arabischen Kultur*, Olms Studien 43 (Hildesheim: Olms, 1996), 391–6

Strohmaier, G., 'Constantine's Pseudo-Classical Terminology and its Survival', in Burnett and Jacquart (eds), *Constantine the African* (1994), 90–8

Strohmaier, G., 'Reception and Tradition: Medicine in the Byzantine and Arab World', in M. D. Grmek (ed.), *Western Medical Thought from Antiquity to the Middle Ages* (Cambridge, MA; London: Harvard University Press, 1998), 139–69

Tabbaa, Y., 'The Functional Aspects of Medieval Islamic Hospitals', in M. Bonner et al., *Poverty and Charity in Middle Eastern Contexts* (Albany, NY: State University of New York, 2003), 95–119

Taschkandi, S. E., *Übersetzung und Bearbeitung des* Kitāb at-Tašwīq aṭ-ṭibbī *des Ṣā'id ibn al-Ḥasan: Ein medizinisches Adabwerk aus dem 11. Jahrhundert* (Bonn: Selbstverlag des Orientalischen Seminars der Universität, 1968)

Temkin, O., 'The Byzantine Origin of the Names for the Basilic and Cephalic Veins', *XVIIe Congrès international d'histoire de la médecine, Athènes-Cos, 4–14 septembre 1960*, 2 vols (Athens: The Congress, 1960), i. 336–9

Temkin, O., *Galenism: Rise and Decline of a Medical Philosophy* (Ithaca, NY: Cornell University Press, 1973)

Thomson, Ahmad (tr.), *As-Suyuti's Medicine of the Prophet* (London: Ta-Ha Publishers Ltd, 1994)

Tibi, S., *The Medicinal Use of Opium in the Ninth-Century Baghdad*, Sir Henry Welcome Asian Series 5 (Leiden: Brill, 2006)

Ullmann, M., *Wörterbuch der klassischen Arabischen Sprache* (Wiesbaden: Harrasowitz, 1955–) [abbr. *WKAS*]

Ullmann, M., *Die arabische Überlieferung der sogenannten Menander-Sentenzen*, Abhandlungen für die Kunde des Morgenlandes 34.1 (Wiesbaden: F. Steiner, 1961)

Ullmann, M., *Die Medizin im Islam*, Handbuch der Orientalistik, I Abt., Erg. vi. 1 (Leiden: Brill, 1970)

Ullmann, M., *Die Natur- und Geheimwissenschaften im Islam*, Handbuch der Orientalistik, I Abt., Erg. vi. 2 (Leiden: Brill, 1972)

Ullmann, M., 'Hālid ibn al-Yazīd und die Alchemie: Eine Legende', *Der Islam* 55 (1978), 181–218

Ullmann, M., *Islamic Medicine*, Islamic Surveys 11 (Edinburgh: Edinburgh University Press, 1978)

Ullmann, M., *Rufus von Ephesos, Krankenjournale* (Wiesbaden: Harrassowitz, 1978)

Ullmann, M., 'Die Schrift des Badīgūras über die Ersatzdrogen', *Der Islam* 50 (1973), 230–48

Ullmann, M., *Wörterbuch zu den griechisch-arabischen Übersetzungen des neunten Jahrhunderts* (Wiesbaden: Harrasowitz, 2002) [abbr. *WGAÜ*]

Unschuld, P. U., *Chinese Medicine*, tr. Nigel Wiseman (Brookline MA: Paradigm Publications, 1998)

Van Ess, J., *Der Fehltritt des Gelehrten: die 'Pest von Emmaus' und ihre theologischen Nachspiele* (Heidelberg: Winter, 2001)

Van Gelder, G. J., 'The Joking Doctor: Abū al-Ḥakam 'Ubayd Allāh Ibn al-Muẓaffar (d. 549/1155)', in M. de la C. Vázquez de Benito and M. Á. M. Rodríguez (eds), *Actas XVI Congreso UEAI* (Salamanca: Agencia Española de Cooperación Internacional; Consejo Superior de Investigaciones Científicas; Union Européenne d'Arabisants et d'Islamisants, 1995), 217–28

Varisco, D. M., *Medieval Agriculture and Islamic Sciences: The Almanac of a Yemeni Sultan* (Seattle, WA: University of Washington Press, 1994)

Vázquez de Benito, M. de la C., *Libro de la introducción al arte de al medicina o «Isagoge» de Abū Bakr Muḥammad b. Zakarīyā al-Rāzī* (Salamanca: Ediciones Universidad de Salamanca, 1979)

Von Staden, H., *Herophilus: the Art of Medicine in Early Alexandria* (Cambridge: Cambridge

University Press, 1989)
Waines, D., 'Dietetics in Medieval Islamic Culture', *Medical History* 43 (1999), 228–40
Wasserstein, A., *Galen's Commentary on the Hippocratic Treatise* Airs, Waters, Places *in the Hebrew Translation of Solomon ha-Me'ati* (Jerusalem: Israel Academy of Sciences and Humanities, 1982)
Weisser, U., *Zeugung, Vererbung und pränatale Entwicklung in der Medizin des arabisch-islamischen Mittelalters* (Erlangen: Lüling, 1983)
Wellhausen, J., *Skizzen und Vorarbeiten* (Berlin: Druck und Verlag von Georg Reimer, 1884)
West, M., *The Eastern Face of Helicon: West Asiatic Elements in Early Poetry and Myth* (Oxford: Clarendon Press, 1997)
Wilcox, J., and J. M. Riddle, 'Qusṭā ibn Lūqā's *Physical Ligatures* and the Recognition of the Placebo Effect', *Medieval Encounters: Jewish, Christian and Muslim Culture in Confluence and Dialogue* 1 (1995), 1–48
Wilcox, J., 'Qusṭā ibn Lūqā and the Eastward Diaspora of Hellenic Medicine', in Greppin, et al. (eds), *Diffusion of Greco-Roman Medicine* (1999), 73–128
Wilson, L. G., 'The Problem of the Discovery of the Pulmonary Circulation', *Journal of the History of Medicine and Allied Sciences* 17 (1962), 229–44
Wood, C. A., *Memorandum Book of a Tenth-Century Oculist for the Use of Modern Ophthalmologists: A Translation of the* Tadhkirat *of Ali ibn Isa of Baghdad (cir. 940–1010 AD), The Most Complete, Practical and Original of all the Early Textbooks on the Eye and its Diseases* (Chicago, IL: Northwestern University, 1936; repr. Birmingham, AL: Classics of Medicine Library, 1985)
Wright, R. R., *al-Bīrūnī, The Book of Instruction in the Elements of the Art of Astrology* (London: Luzac, 1934)
Wujastyk, D., *The Roots of Ayurveda* (London: Penguin, 2003)
Yates, F. A., *Giordano Bruno and the Hermetic Tradition*, new edn (London: Routledge, 2002)

Chronology

The 'West'		***The 'East'***
Hippocrates active	c. 450 BC	
Plato dies	347 BC	
Alexander the Great dies	323 BC	
Aristotle dies	322 BC	
Augustus, founder of Roman Empire, dies	AD 14	
Dioscorides dies	c. 90	
Rufus of Ephesus active	c. 100	
Galen dies	c. 216	
	224	*Ardashir I founds the Sasanian Dynasty in Persia, lasting until 651*
Plotinus dies	270	
Porphyry dies	c. 304	
Oribasius of Pergamon dies	395	
Alexander of Tralles dies after	c. 500	
Aëtius of Amida active	c. 530	
	536	Sergius of Rēsh 'Aynā dies
Justinian I, Roman Emperor, dies	565	
John Philoponus dies	c. 570	
	600	Vāgbhaṭa active in India
	622	*Emigration (Hijrah) of Prophet Muḥammad from Mecca to Medina*
	642	*Alexandria captured by Arab forces*
	c. 650	Paul of Aegina active in Alexandria
	661	*Umayyad Caliphate established in Damascus*
	749	*'Abbāsid Caliphate established*
	768	Jurjīs ibn Jibrīl ibn Bukhtīshū' dies in Baghdad
Charlemagne crowned Emperor	800	
	857	Yūḥannā ibn Māsawayg dies in Baghdad

The 'West'		***The 'East'***
	c. 860	Qusṭā ibn Lūqā and al-Ruhāwī were active
	868	al-Jāḥiẓ dies in Basra; the next year Sābūr ibn Sahl dies in Iraq
	870	Bukhtīshū' ibn Jibrīl dies, al-Kindī dies shortly thereafter, and Ibn Sarābiyūn active c. 850–90
	873	Ḥunayn ibn Isḥāq dies 873 or 877
	c. 880	Yuḥannā ibn al-Ṣalt active 870–910
	901	Thābit ibn Qurrah dies in Baghdad
	925	al-Rāzī [Rhazes] dies in Rayy, in Persia
		al-Kaskarī active in early 10th century in Baghdad
	c. 932	Isḥāq ibn Sulaymān al-Isrā'īlī dies in Egypt
	942	Sinān ibn Thābit dies in Baghdad
	949	*'Aḍud al-Dawlah, founder of 'Aḍudī hospital, begins 40-year rule in Baghdad*
	980	Ibn al-Jazzār dies in Qayrawān
		'Alī ibn 'Īsá al-Kaḥḥāl active in 10th century in Baghdad
	c. 983	'Alī ibn al-'Abbās al-Majūsī active in Persia
Ibn Juljul dies in Spain	c. 994	
	996	*al-Ḥākim, Fāṭimid ruler of North Africa and Egypt, begins 25-year reign*
al-Zahrāwī [Abulcasis] active in Spain	c. 1000	
	c. 1010	'Ammār ibn 'Alī al-Mawṣilī active in Egypt
	1037	Ibn Sīnā [Avicenna] dies in Persia
al-Ḥāshimī active in Spain	1056	
	1058	'Ubayd Allāh ibn Bukhtīshū' dies after 1058 in Baghdad
	1066	Ibn Buṭlān dies in Syria; two years later Ibn Riḍwān dies in Egypt
Christians capture Toledo	1085	
Constantine the African dies before 1099	c. 1099	*First Crusade, 1096–9; Crusaders capture Jerusalem in 1099*
Abū al-'Alā' Zuhr dies in Córdoba	1131	Ismā'īl ibn Ḥusayn Jurjānī active in Persia
	1154	Ibn al-Tilmīdh dies in Baghdad 1154 or 1165
Abū Marwān ibn Zuhr [Avenzoar] dies in Seville	1162	
	1169	*Ṣalāḥ al-Dīn [Saladin], Ayyūbid ruler of Egypt, begins 25-year reign*

The 'West'		***The 'East'***
Ibn Rushd [Averroes] dies in Marrakesh	1198	Ibn Jumayʿ al-Isrāʾīlī dies in Egypt
	1204	Ibn Maymūn [Maimonides] dies in Old Cairo (Fusṭāṭ)
	1208	ʿAbd al-ʿAzīz al-Sulamī dies in Egypt
	1217	Ibn Jubayr dies in Alexandria
	1227	*Genghis Khan, Mongol conqueror, dies*
	1230	al-Dakhwār dies in Damascus
	1231	ʿAbd al-Laṭīf al-Baghdādī dies in Baghdad
Fall of Córdoba to Christians	1236	
	c. 1240	Ibn Abī al-Bayān al-Isrāʾīlī dies in Egypt
Fall of Seville to Christians	1248	Ibn al-Bayṭār dies in Damascus
	1250	*Mamluk rulers of Egypt and Syria begin rule lasting until 1517*
	1258	*Fall of Baghdad to the Mongols*
Moshe ibn Tibbon active c. 1240–1283 in southern France	c. 1260	Khalīfah ibn Abī al-Maḥāsin al-Ḥalabī active in Syria and al-Kūhīn al-ʿAṭṭār al-Isrāʾīlī in Egypt
Eighth Crusade; Louis IX of France, its instigator, dies in Tunis	1270	Ibn Abī Uṣaybiʿah dies in Syria
Nathan ha-Meati active in Italy	1280	*al-Malik al-Manṣūr Qalāwūn, founder of the Manṣūrī hospital, begins 10-year reign in Egypt*
	1281	*Ottoman dynasty established in Anatolia, lasting until 1924*
	1283	Quṭb al-Dīn al-Shīrāzī active in Persia
	1286	Ibn al-ʿIbrī [Bar Hebraeus] dies in Maragha (Azerbaijan) and Ibn al-Quff in Egypt
	1288	Ibn al-Nafīs dies in Cairo
	1291	*Crusaders lose Acre and abandon Crusader States*
	1350	Ibn Qayyim al-Jawzīyah dies in Egypt; Shams al-Dīn al-Dhahabī two years earlier
Muḥammad al-Shafrah dies in Fez	1360	
Guy de Chauliac dies	1368	al-Shādhilī active in Egypt
	1370	*Tīmūr [Tamerlane] begins 35-year rule in Samarqand*
Chaucer dies	1400	Manṣūr ibn Ilyās active in Persia
	1453	*Fall of Constantinople to Ottomans*

The 'West'		The 'East'
Christian conquest of Granada	1492	
	1501	*Safavid dynasty established in Persia, lasting until 1732*
	1505	Jalāl al-Dīn al-Suyūṭī dies in Cairo
	1516	*Ottoman conquest of Egypt*
	1526	*Mughal Emperors rule India until 1858*
Andreas Vesalius dies	1564	'Imād al-Dīn Maḥmūd Shīrāzī active in Persia
	1599	Dāwūd al-Anṭākī dies in Cairo
William Harvey dies in England	1657	Ḥajjī Khalīfah dies in Constantinople; Ibn Sallūm active in same city
Alexander Russell dies	1768	
	1814	Aḥmad ibn Muḥammad al-Salāwī active in North Africa

Index of names and works

This index contains the names of all historical personalities mentioned in this book, as well as the titles of their writings. It also lists translations of the sources, insofar as they exist. References to Arabic editions are provided in square brackets, and, where possible, in abbreviated form according to the standards laid down in Ullmann's *Wörterbuch der Klassischen Arabischen Sprache* – see his *Vorläufiges Literatur- und Abkürzungsverzeichnis zum zweiten Band* (Lām), 3rd edn (Wiesbaden, Harrassowitz: 1996). The Arabic article 'al-' is to be disregarded for the purpose of the alphabetical order in which the entries are arranged.

General index

CPSIA information can be obtained
at www.ICGtesting.com
Printed in the USA
JSHW040843151220
10269JS00001B/4

9 781589 011618